Monographs in Epidemiology and Biostatistics

Volume 21

Principles of Exposure Measurement in Epidemiology

BRUCE K. ARMSTRONG
Australian Institute of Health and Welfare, Canberra

EMILY WHITE
University of Washington
and
Fred Hutchinson Cancer Research Centre, Seattle

RODOLFO SARACCI
International Agency for Research on Cancer, Lyon
and
National Research Council, Pisa

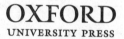
OXFORD
UNIVERSITY PRESS

OXFORD
UNIVERSITY PRESS

Great Clarendon Street, Oxford OX2 6DP

Oxford University Press is a department of the University of Oxford.
It furthers the University's objective of excellence in research, scholarship,
and education by publishing worldwide in

Oxford New York

Athens Auckland Bangkok Bogotá Buenos Aires Cape Town
Chennai Dar es Salaam Delhi Florence Hong Kong Istanbul Karachi
Kolkata Kuala Lumpur Madrid Melbourne Mexico City Mumbai Nairobi
Paris São Paulo Shanghai Singapore Taipei Tokyo Toronto Warsaw

with associated companies in Berlin Ibadan

Oxford is a registered trade mark of Oxford University Press
in the UK and in certain other countries

Published in the United States
by Oxford University Press Inc., New York

First published 1992
First published in paperback 1994
Reprinted 1995, 1999, 2000, 2001

A catalogue record for this book is available from the British Library

Library of Congress Cataloging in Publication Data
Armstrong, B. K.
Principles of exposure measurement in epidemiology / Bruce K.
Armstrong, Emily White, and Rodolfo Saracci.
(Monographs in epidemiology and biostatistics; v. 21) (Oxford medical publications)
Includes bibliographical references.
1. Epidemiology—Methodology. I. Armstrong, Bruce K. 1944–
II. White, Emily, 1946– . III. Saracci, Rodolfo, 1936–
IV. Title. V. Series. VI. Series: Oxford medical publications.
[DNLM: 1. Environmental Exposure. 2. Environmental Monitoring.
3. Epidemiologic Methods. W1 M0567LT v21 / WA 671 A735p]
RA652.4.A28 1992 92–8553
ISBN 0 19 262020 7 (pbk)

Printed in Great Britain
on acid-free paper by
Biddles Ltd., Guildford and King's Lynn

Principles of Exposure Measurement in Epidemiology

Monographs in Epidemiology and Biostatistics
edited by Jennifer L. Kelsey, Michael G. Marmot, Paul D. Stolley,
Martin P. Vessey

Preface

Valid measurements of exposure to known or suspected agents of disease are essential to epidemiological research. Exposure measurement, however, has been neglected for a long time as a topic of methodological research and teaching in epidemiology. While research on this subject has now increased substantially, there still exists no comprehensive review of it and, perhaps in consequence, it is rarely treated in any detail in graduate courses. The initial plan to try and fill this gap by writing an introductory book on the topic developed during exchanges of view between two of us (RS and BKA) in 1984. Following these discussions, one of us (BKA) taught a course entitled 'Exposure Measurement in Epidemiology' in the Department of Epidemiology, University of Washington, in the spring of 1986. Since then, the course has been taught by another of us (EW). This book has been developed from the notes prepared for that course and additional work that we have all done over the succeeding five years.

We have written this book primarily as a text for graduate courses in epidemiology, and as a reference book for use by graduate students and practising epidemiologists in the planning of their research. It only partially meets the need for a comprehensive review of exposure measurement. It deals only with principles—detailed reviews of methods of measurement of exposure to particular agents or classes of agents of disease are, for the most part, still required. Even the principles have been viewed from a limited perspective—the causation by external agents of non-infectious or 'chronic' disease. While many of them also apply to the measurement of genetic characteristics and exposure to infectious agents, specific treatments of these subjects require expertise that none of us professes.

Because of its main intended target, graduate students in epidemiology, who come from a range of backgrounds, the statistical treatment of the subject has been kept to a fairly basic level. Specifically, derivations of equations have not been given, although the assumptions and models used have generally been stated so that those with a strong statistical background could arrive at the derivations for themselves. Where possible, references to derivations have also been given.

Although this book is directed mainly towards epidemiologists, we believe that it will be useful to other scientists who, for whatever reason, need to obtain accurate measurements of exposure of humans to causes of disease. To facilitate their use of it, we have limited our use of epidemiological jargon as far as we could and, where we couldn't, have endeavoured to provide definitions of essential terms where they first appear. For jargon that we have used but not defined, non-epidemiologists may find Last's Dictionary of epidemiology (Last, J.M. (ed.) (1988). *A Dictionary of Epidemiology*, 2nd edn. Oxford University Press, Oxford) to be helpful.

We present this book with humility. There are many who could have done it better and will, we hope, do so in the future. But it needed to be done, and it seemed to us that by doing it now the gap would be at least temporarily filled and that others might be stimulated by our ideas and, perhaps, our errors to undertake the necessary empirical research and write on the subject too. If the book achieves only that, it will have been worthwhile.

Special thanks are due to Noel Weiss, Chairman of the Department of Epidemiology, University of Washington, who encouraged and provided support for the course on which much of this book is based, and read and commented on a final draft. We thank also our other colleagues who contributed ideas, encouragement, and criticism in the preparation of this book. In these respects, we especially acknowledge the assistance given by Shirley Beresford, Harvey Checkoway, Janet Daling, Dallas English, D'Arcy Holman, John Kaldor, Tom Koepsell, Alan Kristal, Margaret Pepe, Ross Prentice, Bruce Psaty, Judith Straton, Harri Vainio, and Jan Watt in reading and commenting on chapters at various stages in their production and, in some cases, the whole book. The students who have taken the course on which the book has been based have also, by their interest, questions, and observations, contributed much to its development; they have our thanks.

Without the special support given by the National Health and Medical Research Council of Australia and the Cancer Foundation of Western Australia to one of us (BKA), this book would never have been written.

While preparation of the book has been a team effort, each of us took major responsibility for different parts of it. Bruce Armstrong was mainly responsible for Chapters 1 (general aspects), 2, 6, 7, 8 (proxy respondents), 11, and 12; Emily White was mainly responsible for Chapters 3, 4, 5, and 8 (other methods); and Rodolfo Saracci was mainly responsible for Chapters 1 (dose and time), 9, and 10.

Lyon, Seattle, and Pisa   B.K.A.
September 1991   E.W.
                                                              R.S.

Contents

1

Exposure measurement

The first step facing an epidemiologist . . . is to specify the conceptual 'true' exposure. The answer will often be less than obvious since, in one sense, every measure is a surrogate for a more proximal cause of disease. . . . Even when a specific step in the causal sequence of events is selected as the 'true' exposure, the dimension of time will usually need to be considered since most epidemiologic exposures fluctuate and/or drift within persons. (Willett 1989)

INTRODUCTION

Epidemiology is a comparatively new science. Its methods were first developed when the study of diseases due to infectious organisms was its main focus. The measurement of exposure was then grounded in microbiology, and most epidemiologists had substantial training or experience in this discipline. Interest in non-microbiological determinants of disease was commonly confined to the more readily measurable host factors such as age, sex, race, etc. Measurement of the microbiological determinants was simplified by the possibility of isolation and culture of a specific organism from the presumed agent of disease, the short interval that commonly separated exposure from onset of clinical symptoms, and the possibility of serological documentation of exposure that had occurred in the distant past.

Exposure measurement has become substantially more complex with the growth of the study of non-infectious disease over the past 40 years. There are several reasons for this complexity:

- There may be no *necessary* cause for the disease under study, and any single component cause may make only a small contribution to aetiology

- The interval from onset, and perhaps cessation, of exposure to appearance of disease is more often measured in years than days, weeks, or months

- the agent of disease may leave no easily measurable indicator of past exposure

- the range of agents of interest has increased so much that it is no longer possible for one scientist to have an expert understanding of all those in which he or she may be interested.

Table 1.1 Distribution of the environmental exposure variables of main interest (one selected from each study) in 564 papers on the aetiology of non-infectious disease published in the *American Journal of Epidemiology* between January 1980 and December 1989

Variables	Distribution (%)
Demographic variables	
Socioeconomic status	2.3
Race	2.1
Religion	0.5
Maternal/paternal age	0.9
Medical history and use of medications	
Oral contraceptive use	3.4
Use of other medications	4.8
Other medical history	3.7
Reproductive and sexual history	8.5
Intake of alcohol and tobacco	
Active smoking	8.5
Passive smoking	1.8
Alcohol drinking	5.3
Diet and body size	
Diet	9.9
Coffee drinking	3.4
Body size	7.8
Physical activity and fitness	3.4
Psychosocial variables	
Mainly social variables	3.4
Other psychosocial variables	5.1
Occupation	
Specific occupations or exposures	9.6
Occupation in general	2.5
Radiation	
Ionizing radiation	3.0
Non-ionizing radiation	2.1
Other environmental variables	
Contaminants and pollutants of water	3.0
Pollutants of air	1.2
Other	3.7

To illustrate the range of agents now studied in the epidemiology of non-infectious disease, we reviewed all papers that were primarily concerned with causation by an environmental agent (i.e. an agent not endogenous to the human body) and published in the *American Journal of Epidemiology* between 1980 and 1989. Table 1.1 shows the distribution of the agents of main interest (one selected from each study) in the 564 papers reviewed.

It is no surprise that aspects of diet, use of tobacco and alcohol, occupation, and past medical history and use of medications were the most commonly studied exposures. Oral contraceptives were the most studied medications, and use of non-contraceptive oestrogens was the largest single category among 'other medications'.

Given the multiplicity and complexity of these exposures, it is remarkable that the subject of exposure measurement has, at least until fairly recently, received little attention in the epidemiological literature. Among the papers summarized in Table 1.1, only 83 (14.7 per cent) offered some data, or a reference to data, to support the reliability or validity of their measure of the main agent of interest. In addition, among a total of 756 papers considered *relevant to* the environmental aetiology of non-infectious disease published in the *American Journal of Epidemiology* from 1980 to 1989, 137 (18.1 per cent) dealt substantially with some aspect of exposure measurement. However, the proportion of papers of this type increased substantially during the

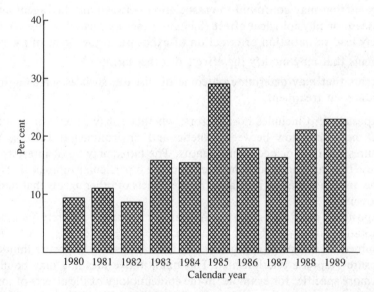

Figure 1.1 Proportion of all papers relevant to the environmental aetiology of non-infectious disease published in the *American Journal of Epidemiology* between 1980 and 1989 that dealt substantially with some aspect of exposure measurement.

second half of the 1980s (Figure 1.1), illustrating the increasing importance that is being attached to the measurement of exposure.

In this chapter we define some of the terms which are critical to an understanding of our subject, including exposure, measurement, and measurement instrument. We also address the subject of scales of measurement, both historically and in a modern context, and examine the objectives and scope of exposure measurement. We also discuss the representation of amount or 'dose' of exposure, and its relationship to time, because of the importance of these issues to the correct selection of variables for an epidemiological study.

Finally, we outline the contents of the rest of the book.

EXPOSURE

In epidemiology the term *exposure* denotes any of a subject's attributes or any agent with which he or she may come in contact that may be relevant to his or her health. This broad definition encompasses:

- agents that may cause physiological effects (e.g. food as determining body growth)
- agents that may cause or protect from disease
- agents that may confound the association between another agent and a disease or physiological effect (including factors related to disease that may lead to initiation or cessation of exposure to the agent of interest)
- agents that may modify the effects of other agents
- agents that may determine outcome of disease, such as screening procedures or treatment.

Exposure also includes host factors, whether solely genetic or resulting from the interaction between genetic and environmental factors, and measures such as socioeconomic status. The latter may be of interest, not because they are thought themselves to cause a particular biological effect, but because they may be indicators of the effects of other agents that remain unmeasured.

Exposure is often also given a quantitative rather than a merely qualitative connotation. It may designate the amount of an agent (or dose) with which the subject has come in contact — as in the expressions 'exposure limits' or 'exposure–response relationship'. This quantitative meaning may be made even more specific: for example, in the epidemiology of the effects of ionizing radiation it may be used to mean the production of ions in air external to the subject or actual irradiation of the human body (Kathren and Petersen 1989).

The word 'exposure' may also be employed by epidemiologists much as it is in everyday speech, i.e. as equivalent to 'contact'; as in the expressions 'exposure to an agent' or 'circumstances of exposure', for example.

MEASUREMENT

'In the broadest sense of the word, *measurement* might be regarded as a classification of objects and events in which a certain sign (numeral, letter, or word, etc.) is assigned to each defined class.' (Goude 1962). To this very general definition, two restrictions are commonly added: '. . . measurement is the assignment of *numerals* to objects and events according to *rules*.' (Stevens 1951; emphasis added). The near universality of numerical analysis in epidemiology means that the defining 'sign' is in most cases numerical, and the existence of a rule that determines the numerical classification of exposure (implied in any case by the process of classification) is essential to scientific rigour. Anderson and Mantel (1983) have drawn attention to the need for measurement 'rules' in epidemiology: 'One conspicuous cause of instability in survey data is the failure of field workers. . . . to follow operational methods of measurement. A method of measurement is considered operational if two requirements are satisfied. First, instructions for use of the method must [exist and] be understandable to other investigators who may wish to follow them. Second, there should be a demonstration (at least a pilot study) to show that measurements resulting from this method are reproducible.'

There have been objections to Stevens' (1951) definition of measurement on the grounds that it 'makes measurement an empirical, almost mechanistic process' (Zeller and Carmines 1980) and that many of the phenomena to be measured are, strictly speaking, neither 'objects' nor 'events' (Carmines and Zeller 1979). An alternative definition was proposed: 'We define measurement as the process of linking abstract concepts to empirical indicants.' (Zeller and Carmines 1980). This re-definition emphasizes the theoretical component of the measurement process and draws attention to the fact that what is measured may be not the variable of real interest but some indirect indicator of it. The variable of real interest, the *true exposure*, may not be directly measurable or it may be difficult or impossible to define.

Socioeconomic status is an example of such an abstract concept. Epidemiologists commonly measure it by means of 'empirical indicants' such as income, education, occupation, and place of residence to which, strictly speaking, it is only theoretically linked (Liberatos *et al.* 1988). In turn, socioeconomic status, when associated with disease (as it commonly is), is clearly not a cause of disease but an indicator of level or probability of exposure to some true cause which may be unmeasured or unknown. This example makes it clear that Zeller and Carmines (1980) have made a useful point, but it cannot be sustained as an objection to Stevens's (1951) definition of measurement. Rules can be made for measurement of the empirical indicants and numbers assigned to their measurement categories even if the variables of real interest are abstract or unknown.

SCALES OF MEASUREMENT

Four scales of numerical measurement have been defined, ordered according to the implied degree of sophistication of the measurement method (Stevens 1951).

Nominal scale

In a nominal scale the numerals are used only as labels and any other 'sign' (e.g., M or F, + or −) would do equally well. A nominal scale may have more than two categories, but the only empirical operation to which it lends itself is the determination of equality. That is, two subjects who share the same value are considered to be the same and two who have different values are considered to be different. The actual values taken by the latter tell us nothing about how different they are. Examples of nominal scales in common use in epidemiology include sex, occupation (if not ordered in some way to reflect socioeconomic status), race, and HLA type.

Ordinal scale

In an ordinal scale the numerals are used to indicate a rank ordering of classes of the variable, but differences between them cannot be taken to indicate the actual size of differences between the classes in the value of the underlying measurement. It is possible on an ordinal scale to go beyond simple statements of equality and inequality to statements about whether a particular subject has a value which is greater than or less than that of some other subject. Examples of ordinal scales in common use in epidemiology include socioeconomic status, some of the cruder measures of dietary intake and physical activity (e.g. the subject may score intake or activity by selecting one of a predetermined set of frequency ranges such as 'daily', '3–6 times a week', '1–3 times a week', '1–3 times a month', and so on) and any non-uniformly distributed, interval, or ratio scale variables (see below) that have been pre-coded into categories (e.g. 10–19 cigarettes smoked a day).

Interval scale

On an interval scale, the relative values of the numerals assigned to different classes or individuals reflect true differences in the values of the underlying measurements. However, the zero point for the scale may be arbitrary (as it is, for example, in the Fahrenheit and Celsius scales of temperature measurement). Examples of interval scale measurements in common use in epidemiology include year of birth and other variables measured in calendar time. These particular variables may be readily transformed to ratio scale measurements by, for example, conversion of year of birth to age at some fixed point.

Ratio scale

A ratio scale of measurement permits the valid comparison of measurements by calculation of a ratio; that is, one measurement may be said to be some multiple of another. This means that the zero point of the sclae is the 'true' zero.

Most exposure variables in epidemiological studies are, or can be, measured on a ratio scale. In a sample of 167 of the studies reviewed and summarized in Table 1.1, nearly a half (45.5 per cent) of the main variables were measured on a ratio scale, 3 per cent were measured on an interval scale, 21.6 per cent on an ordinal scale, and 29.3 per cent on a nominal scale. In one study the description of the exposure measurement was so inadequate that it was impossible to determine what the scale of measurement was!

These scales of measurement were originally defined as a way of identifying the types of statistical procedures that were permissible in the analysis of particular kinds of data (Stevens 1951). Nominal data were considered susceptible only to simple counts, identification of the mode, and contingency table procedures. Interval scale measurements were considered necessary before means and standard deviations could be calculated and linear regression techniques applied. While this approach has been criticized (see Stevens 1968) and statistical methods have advanced substantially since the scales were defined, it remains true that the options for analysis are greater when more sophisticated scales of measurement are used. For example, the now most commonly used statistical model in epidemiology, the *linear logistic model*, can readily be applied to nominal scale data, but statistical efficiency can be increased if variables are measured on interval or ratio scales and their effects modelled without conversion to categorical form (Dorfman *et al*. 1985). Of course, this is only acceptable if some continuous functional form for these effects (e.g. linear) can be justifiably assumed.

These observations have practical implications for the design and numerical coding of instruments of measurement. For example, in the collection of data on cigarette smoking it is better to record an estimate of the actual number of cigarettes smoked in a day than simply whether or not the subjects fall into a predetermined class. Even if the class intervals are of equal width, the expected value of observations in each class, and therefore the distance between classes, cannot be estimated accurately because the shape of the underlying distribution is not known. Thus, in this circumstance, only statistics that apply to ordinal scales of measurement can be *validly* used (although equality of 'distance' between intervals is often assumed to test for linear trend, or some other continuous underlying pattern of variation of effect with change in exposure).

The way scales of measurement are described in this book is more in line with current practice. The primary division in the classification is between *continuous variables* (those that in theory can take on an infinite number of values) and *categorical variables* (that take on a finite number of values). Categorical variables are further classified as *nominal categorical, ordered categorical*, or *dichotomous*. Nominal and ordered categorical variables are as described above for nominal and ordinal scale variables. Dichotomous (also called binary) variables are variables that take on only two values, so the distinction between nominal and ordinal is immaterial. Decisions about the appropriate statistical techniques are now usually based on the scales of measurement of the exposure and outcome variables, and on the distributions of values of the variables in the population of interest.

THE MEASUREMENT INSTRUMENT

In this book we use the term *measurement instrument*, or just instrument, to refer to a procedure or set of procedures designed to measure one or several of the variables of interest in an epidemiological study. The term is sometimes used interchangeably with the more general term, *measurement method*. Examples of measurement instruments include:

- self-administered questionnaires
- personal interviews
- biochemical analysis of blood or other biological specimens
- physical or chemical analysis of the environment.

We use the term measurement instrument in its broadest sense to include all aspects of the measurement process involving individual subjects, including:

- instructions for application of the main measurement method
- the method itself
- specification of procedures that follow application of the main method, up to the point of presentation of a 'clean' data file for analysis.

Thus, in the case of a personal interview, it will include:

- specifications for the training of interviewers and instructions given to them
- instructions or explanations given by interviewers to subjects

- the questionnaire used to elicit data from the subjects
- the subsequent editing of the interview schedule by the interviewer, or supervisor, and by use of a computer
- other quality control procedures (see Chapter 5).

In the case of the measurement of the concentration of some chemical in blood, it will include:

- procedures for the preparation of subjects
- procedures for the collection, transport, and storage of the specimen
- analytical procedures in the laboratory
- attendant quality control procedures (see Chapter 9).

A measurement instrument deserves to be so called, with the connotation of accuracy and reproducibility that the word 'instrument' implies, only when all of the procedures outlined above are written down in such detail that one set of investigators could, within the limits of biological or physical variability, reproduce the measurements obtained by another using only this written description.

OBJECTIVES OF EXPOSURE MEASUREMENT

For the investigation as a whole, the objective of exposure measurement is to obtain measurements that are the *minimum* necessary to meet the research objectives. In aetiological research, this will mean measurement of the variables defined by the study's hypotheses, measurement of any known or suspected confounding variables, and measurement of variables that may be thought to modify the effects of the main causal variables. Variables included in a study solely because they are possible confounders or effect modifiers should, like the main exposure variables, be the subject of specific hypotheses relating to their supposed confounding or modifying effects.

It need almost not be said, but is often forgotten, that it is impossible to select the appropriate measurements for a particular investigation unless a specific and detailed statement of research objectives has been made. Without such a statement the likelihood exists that key variables will not be measured, or will be measured in insufficient detail, or that too many variables will be measured so that the quality of measurement of the really important variable is compromised.

For each exposure variable, the objective of measurement is to obtain measurements that maximize validity; or, to put it another way, that minimize error. The subject of measurement error is dealt with in detail in Chapters 3 and 4.

SCOPE OF EXPOSURE MEASUREMENT

To characterize an exposure variable fully, it is necessary to record its nature, the amount (dose) of exposure to it, and the time relationships of that exposure.

Nature

As far as possible, the nature of exposure variables should be recorded in specific detail both to ensure observation of any associations that are there and to permit specific aetiological inferences.

Exposure variables should be *specific* in the sense that they permit isolation of the components of a broader class of exposure that are associated with a disease. Thus, for example, it is better to enquire about the different forms of tobacco smoking (cigarettes, pipes, cigars, etc.) separately, rather than simply to enquire about 'smoking'. The incidence of tobacco-induced disease is known to vary with the method of smoking. Use of the generic variable 'smoking' may lead to failure to observe true, but weak, associations with one of the specific types of smoking. Similarly, exposure variables should permit the distinction of the exposure of interest from possibly confounding exposures. In evaluations of the evidence for the carcinogenicity of chemicals in humans made by the International Agency for Research on Cancer, the commonest reason for applying a 'limited' or 'inadequate' evidence classification was that exposure to the agent of interest had not been distinguished from exposure to other potentially carcinogenic agents in the environment in which it had occurred (Armstrong 1985).

The exposure variables should also be *sensitive*, in the sense that they include all ways in which subjects may be exposed to the active agent of interest. For example, in testing the hypothesis that exposure to aluminium causes Alzheimer's disease, it is not sufficient to enquire only about use of aluminium-containing antacids. Aluminium is also ingested in some analgesics, applied topically in some anti-perspirants, and may be released into food from aluminium cookware. To select exposure to only one of these to test the hypothesis that aluminium causes Alzheimer's disease may so misclassify exposure to aluminium that an association that may exist is not observed (see Chapter 3).

Even when an hypothesis is not specific as to the important component of an exposure (e.g. that oral contraceptives rather than, say, the progestagenic potency of oral contraceptives, may cause breast cancer), the nature of the exposure should be recorded in as much detail as possible so that any role of specific components of it can be explored later. In the case of oral contraceptives, this would include the brand name and other details, such as dates of use, that would make it possible to find out the specific composition of the preparations used.

Other aspects of the nature of an exposure may also be important to specific and sensitive measurements of it, and to specific aetiological inferences. They include the route of exposure to the agent (e.g. oral but not nasal use of snuff may cause cancer of the mouth) and behaviours that may protect against exposure (e.g. in the study of the relationship of sun exposure to skin cancer, it is important to record the use of clothing and sun screens as well as the amount, pattern, and duration of outdoor exposure).

Dose

Dose may be measured either as the total accumulated dose (*cumulative exposure*), for example, the total number of packets of cigarettes smoked (usually expressed as 'pack-years'); or as the dose or exposure *rate*, for example, number of cigarettes smoked per day. The latter is a dose per unit time, the unit of time being chosen in practice in accordance with the time scale (hours, days, or years) on which the exposure varies. Cumulative exposure is calculated as the sum of the products of dose rates by durations of the periods of time for which they apply. When cumulative exposure is divided by the total duration of exposure, it provides an estimate of *average exposure* or average dose rate. The recording of dose rates and durations permits the most flexible and informative analysis of the data.

Dose should be described in accordance with its relationship to the exposed subject, whether as the available, administered, absorbed, or active dose, as summarized in Figure 1.2.

The *available dose* is measured in the subject's external environment. Examples of available dose include the concentration of asbestos fibres per ml of ambient air in a small time interval (an exposure rate), or average asbestos fibres per ml of ambient air multiplied by years of exposure (a cumulative exposure).

Although it is generally easy to measure, the available dose is not usually the same as the *administered dose* or intake, the actual amount of the agent coming into contact with the human body. How much of the available dose becomes administered dose depends on the subject's physiology and behaviour; for example, the respiratory volume at rest and during activity, and the quantities of food, drinks, and medications actually ingested. From a biological viewpoint, even the administered dose can only be regarded as a surrogate measurement of the *absorbed dose* or uptake, the dose which actually enters the body (unless the administered dose has direct effects at the surfaces with which it comes in contact).

The absorbed dose is, in turn, a surrogate for the dose that really matters, the *active or biologically effective dose* at the sites in the body (organs, tissues, cells, molecules) which are the specific targets of action of the agent. The relationship of the active dose to the absorbed dose is complex, depend-

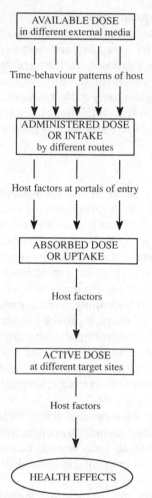

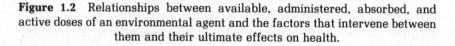

Figure 1.2 Relationships between available, administered, absorbed, and active doses of an environmental agent and the factors that intervene between them and their ultimate effects on health.

ing on the transport of the agent in the body, its distribution among different body compartments, its metabolism to both active and inactive forms, and its excretion from the body. Biological measurements are needed to measure absorbed or active doses, for example, concentration of alcohol in the blood (absorbed dose) or concentrations of adducts of DNA with benzo(*a*)pyrene in cells from the lung (active dose). These biological measurements are dealt with in more detail in Chapter 9.

When considering these various descriptions of dose it is also important to consider whether the agent being measured is in fact the actual cause or putative cause of disease of interest (e.g. one or several carcinogenic components of tobacco smoke) or some surrogate for it (e.g. cigarettes smoked). Usually, as one moves down the scale from available dose to active dose, the specification of the agent and the amount of exposure will move towards one which is more relevant to causation of disease.

The nearer that the dose specified (whether as dose rate and duration or as cumulative dose) can be to the active dose of the real agent of interest, the more likely it is that a study will demonstrate an association that may exist between an agent and a disease.

Measurement of dose (as opposed to simply the fact of exposure) does not just provide the opportunity for a more detailed and informative description of the relationship between an exposure and a disease. It is also important in inferring the presence, or absence, of a cause and effect relationship, because the presence or absence of a dose–response relationship (increasing incidence of disease with increasing or decreasing exposure to the agent) is part of the evidence considered when making inferences about aetiology (Weiss 1981). Without quantitative dose data, this evidence is not available. In addition, the power of a study to detect a particular association may be increased if a particular functional form of dose-response (e.g. linear) is expected and quantitative dose data are collected to permit expression of the results in that form.

Time

As far as possible, each exposure should be characterized as to when it first began, when it finally ended (if at all), and how it was distributed during the intervening period (was it periodic or continuous, and did the dose rate vary in any measurable way during the periods of exposure?). For discrete exposures (e.g. an episode of head injury), it may be sufficient to record only the year or age at which it occurred. For complex exposures (e.g. dietary intake of vitamin A) it may be impossible to describe lifetime exposure. For such exposures, one or more time periods in which exposure may be relevant to disease should be specified (see below), and the emphasis of exposure recording placed on those periods.

The time relationships of exposure are important for several reasons. First, duration of exposure is obviously a critical determinant of the total amount of exposure that has occurred. Next, for many (if not all) diseases there almost certainly exists a *critical time window* (also referred to as the aetiologically relevant exposure period) in which occurrence of a particular exposure may possibly be relevant to causation of the disease (Rothman 1981). Inclusion of exposure outside that time window in the exposure variable used in analysis of the data may lead to misclassification of exposure (see Chapter 3), and reduce the likelihood that an association that exists will be observed. On the positive side, a knowledge of the location of the critical time window in relation to the time of onset of the disease may assist in making inferences about the mechanism by which the agent produces disease (e.g. the point in the multistage process of carcinogenesis at which a carcinogen exerts its effect; Day 1984).

Often the time of the beginning and end of the critical time window is not known with any certainty, but collection of details of the timing of exposure will at least permit analyses that allow its extent to be examined. Such analyses may include examination of the effects of time since first exposure and time since last exposure on risk of disease, or more complex analyses of the variation in risk of disease with time period of exposure (Breslow and Day 1987; Checkoway *et al.* 1990).

The critical time window is usually defined in relation to disease diagnosis for cases and a similar time period for controls (e.g. the time period between 5 and 20 years before the diagnosis of the case). It may also be defined in physiological time (by an age interval, for example) or a period of physiological change, such as menarche or menopause. Examination of the effect of particular agents on disease in relation to these physiological events will present no difficulty provided that the time relationships of exposure have been measured.

A recent example of the consideration of time, as well as dose, in an epidemiological study can be found in the UK National Case-Control Study of Breast Cancer (UK National Case-Control Study Group 1989). In this study, duration of use of oral contraceptives could be used as a reasonable surrogate for cumulative dose because of the relative constancy of dose rate in individuals. Risk of disease was examined by duration of use of oral contraceptives, also taking into account age at start of use, whether use began before or after the first pregnancy, and use in various periods before diagnosis of cancer. To address the issue of individual differences in dose rate of the possibly active agents, analysis was also carried out separately for duration of use of combined pills containing $< 50 \, \mu g$ and $> 50 \, \mu g$ of oestrogen, and use of progestagen-only pills.

Examination of exposure within time periods defined by calendar year may be important when the nature of the exposure has changed over time. For example, the risk of lung cancer and cancer of the nasal sinuses in Welsh nickel refinery workers was dramatically less in those employed after 1925 than in those employed before this date (Peto *et al.* 1984). This change in risk is believed to have been due to changes in some of the processes used in the refinery.

Pattern of exposure during the exposure period may also be important. Exposure occurring in periodic intense bursts may have different effects from a similar total exposure which accumulates continuously but at low intensity. For example, to explain the apparently anomalous occurrence of a higher incidence of malignant melanoma of the skin in indoor workers than in outdoor workers, it has been postulated that a particular total dose of sunlight may be more effective in causing melanoma if it is received intermittently or irregularly rather than frequently or continuously (Holman *et al*. 1983). There is empirical evidence to suggest that this hypothesis is true (Armstrong 1988).

REPRESENTATION OF DOSE AND TIME OF EXPOSURE

Once time-specific measurements of exposure to a given agent have been assembled for each study subject, a decision has to be made on how best to represent dose in relation to time in analysing the relationship of exposure to disease. Three common representations are *peak exposure*, *cumulative exposure*, and *average exposure*. Cumulative exposure and average exposure are as defined on page 11. *Peak exposure* is the highest exposure level (exposure rate) ever experienced by a subject, or the highest level sustained over a given period (e.g. one year) or fraction of the total exposure time (say 10 per cent). Each of these three variables may be derived for the whole lifetime or for a particular part of it; for example, what is believed to be the critical time window.

Representation of the exposure presents no real difficulty in the investigation of the effects of brief exposures, because the short period of aetiologically relevant exposure does not have much room for complex patterns of exposure with time. In this situation, peak exposure, cumulative exposure and average exposure each have roughly constant quantitative relationships to the others across subjects and are essentially interchangeable. When the effects of long-term exposures are being studied, however, it is common to find complex patterns of exposure, including variable and intermittent exposure.

The importance of correct representation of dose has been underlined recently in a study of different approaches to representation of exposure to formaldehyde in a cohort study of formaldehyde workers in the United States (Blair and Stewart 1990). The representations used were:

- duration of employment
- duration of exposure
- level for job with the highest 8-hour time-weighted average exposure
- estimated highest peak exposure
- cumulative exposure
- average exposure.

Duration of employment and duration of exposure were highly correlated, as were highest 8-hour time weighted average exposure and average exposure. Average exposure showed little correlation with duration of employment, duration of exposure, or peak exposures. Other correlations between the variables studied were moderate. These correlations clearly show that different representations of dose will rank subjects differently according to their exposure and are, therefore, likely to give quite different results for the relationship between exposure and disease.

The effect of representation of exposure on results of analyses was illustrated by Lee-Feldstein (1989) who examined the effect of different representations on risk of lung cancer in several cohorts of men exposed to arsenic in copper smelting. In none of the cohorts was simple duration of employment a significant risk factor for lung cancer. In the cohort employed in the earliest time period (before 1925), job with maximum level of exposure to arsenic, cumulative exposure, and time-weighted average exposure, were significantly associated with risk of cancer. For a later cohort (first employed 1925–1947), neither cumulative exposure nor duration of employment was significantly associated with risk of cancer. These studies indicate that the choice of the representation of exposure can substantially influence the results obtained.

The choice of the optimum representation of exposure for analysis needs to be made in the light of the specific information that each representation carries. It depends first on the scale of the exposure measurements. For example, if it is known only that subjects were exposed or not exposed, this variable will be used as a surrogate for average exposure. If only duration of exposure is available, it can be used as a surrogate for cumulative exposure. However, this use assumes that there is little variation between subjects in the average exposure rate, and that variation in exposure rate across the period of exposure is not important to the effect of the exposure. The former assumption, at least, is likely to be wrong, especially when exposure over several years is considered. For example, as exposure to many pollutants in the workplace has fallen over the years, one year of exposure 30 years ago may well have entailed a cumulative exposure two or three times higher than a year of exposure in the same workplace 10 years ago. Under these circumstances, use of duration as a surrogate for cumulative exposure may lead to serious misclassification of exposure.

When exposure measurements have been made on an ordered rather than a nominal categorical scale, it may be tempting to use the product of the exposure rank and duration to represent cumulative exposure. However, because the 'distance' between successive units in an ordered categorical scale is not necessarily constant, and is usually not known, the resulting estimate of the cumulative exposure may be seriously in error. Only when measurements are made on a continuous scale can the true cumulative exposure be calculated.

The question also arises as to what is the biologically relevant representation of exposure. Cumulative exposure is commonly used to summarize the total exposure experience of a subject in a single figure. This implies that total accumulated exposure is the effective biological variable and, in particular, that once the pertinent measurement units have been fixed, exposure rate and length of exposure can be interchanged with equal weight over the whole period of exposure. In this very simple model, neither the average exposure nor the distribution of the exposure rate over time can modify the effect of a given cumulative exposure. This model is often only a crude approximation to the truth, and sometimes it may be entirely wrong (as suggested by the results of Lee-Feldstein 1989). Prolonged exposure to a chemical at low average rate can stimulate detoxification processes that would become saturated and ineffective at higher rates. In such a situation, the relationships of exposure rate and duration of exposure to outcome should be analysed separately. In several carcinogenic processes, average exposure rate and duration of exposure have been shown not to be equivalent, with duration carrying more weight than exposure rate. For example, lung cancer risk in lifelong smokers increases with about the second power of the number of cigarettes smoked a day, but with the fourth power of duration of smoking.

Where cumulative exposure does not correctly represent the biological relationship between exposure rate and duration in causing disease, other approaches to the representation of exposure rate and duration must be sought, including separate analysis of these two variables. For example, where the time distribution of exposure is important (e.g. where an intermittent high exposure may overwhelm protective mechanisms that would otherwise adjust to a continuous dose rate) some measure of periodicity of exposure – together, perhaps, with the relative size of peaks and troughs of exposure – may be useful. In examining the effect of intermittency of sun exposure on risk of malignant melanoma, a variable was created to indicate the proportion of outdoor exposure that was recreational. The assumption was that, for most people, recreational sun exposure is confined to weekends and holidays and is thus intermittent in character (Holman *et al*. 1986).

In some situations, length of the induction period of the disease (Rothman 1981) and retention time of the agent within the body will determine the aetiological weight of exposures occurring in different periods of time in relation to onset of disease. Some form of weighted cumulative exposure may be appropriate here, with different time windows carrying different weights. This approach has been used for silica crystals and asbestos, which have long retention times (see, for example, Dement *et al*. 1983).

In summary, the correct representation of exposure is essential to the valid use of exposure measurements. The information contained in valid measurements may be wasted by an inappropriate representation. The choice of representation is intrinsic to the construction of exposure–response relationships, either when seeking evidence for a causal link between exposure and disease or at the more exacting stage of attempting to establish a quantitative exposure–response relationship. Whenever the biological effects of a particular exposure and their linkage to the disease under study are not well understood, it is wise to examine the effects of several representations of exposure, within the limits of what is possible given the data that have been collected. This underlines the need for adequately specified and comprehensive measurements of exposure variables. A more comprehensive account of the representation and modelling of the relationships between exposure, time, and response can be found in Breslow and Day (1987), Thomas (1988), and Checkoway *et al.* (1990).

ABOUT THIS BOOK

In Chapter 2, we introduce the methods of exposure measurement and outline the considerations that go into deciding which method, or methods, to use in a particular study. Chapters 3, 4, and 5 deal extensively with measurement error and its effects, measurement and control, including the design, conduct, and analysis of validity and reliability studies. We then discuss the main methods of exposure measurement: first the design of questionnaires (Chapter 6), then the personal interview (Chapter 7), the use of diaries, proxy respondents, and records (Chapter 8), measurements in human subjects themselves (Chapter 9), and measurements in the environment (Chapter 10). In dealing with response rates and their maximization, Chapter 11 departs from the preceding theme of measurement of exposure *in individuals* to measurement of exposure in *whole populations*. It has been included because response rates vary with the method of measurement and influence the choice of a method. In addition, strategies to maximize response are an important aspect of the implementation of any measurement method. Finally, in Chapter 12, the ethical issues raised by the methods of exposure measurement are discussed and advice is given regarding ethical practice in epidemiology with particular reference to exposure measurement.

   We do not deal with the measurement of specific exposures in epidemiology except by way of illustration of general principles. Some recent reviews of the measurement of specific exposures include: for diet, Lee-Han *et al.* (1988), Willett (1990); for alcohol intake, Bernadt *et al.* (1982); for socioeconomic status and other psychosocial variables, Ostfeld and Eaker (1985), Liberatos *et al.* (1988); and for exercise, Blair *et al.* (1985), Washburn and Montoye (1986). Feinstein (1985) has prepared a bibliography of reliability and validity studies for methods of measurement of various exposures, and reference to which will assist in identifying the most valid methods for measuring particular exposures.

SUMMARY

In epidemiology, *exposure measurement* is the classification of attributes of subjects or environmental agents relevant to their health, with the assignment of numerals or other signs to these classes according to predetermined rules. Numerals are assigned according to four scales of measurement:

- *continuous*, where an infinite number of values is theoretically possible
- *ordered categorical*, in which the numerals assigned to classes indicate the rank ordering of the measurements but do not necessarily indicate the distance between them
- *nominal categorical*, in which the numerals are used only as labels and non-numerical signs would do equally well, that is, neither order of or distance between classes is known or is relevant
- *dichotomous*, where the categorical scale has only two classes.

A *measurement instrument* is a procedure or set of procedures designed to measure one or several of the variables of interest in an epidemiological study. It is essential to the reproducibility of exposure measurements that these procedures be documented fully in writing. Each measurement instrument should aim at obtaining measurements that maximize validity, and the totality of the measurements obtained in an epidemiological study should be the minimum necessary to meet the objectives of the study. The information obtained in the process of measurement should include details of the exact nature of the exposure, the amount or dose of the exposure, and the distribution of the exposure over time. Particular attention should be paid to:

- the accuracy of the measurement instruments in measuring the true exposure
- aspects of the mode of exposure that may influence the outcomes that may occur
- the proximity of the measurements actually made to the form of the agent that causes disease and the site in the body at which disease occurs
- the likely existence of a restricted period in time (*the critical time window*) in which the agent could have caused the disease in question.

When adequate data have been obtained on the nature, dose, and time relationships of the exposure, there remains the challenge of representing this information in the analysis in a way that reflects the underlying biological reality and maximizes the likelihood that a relationship that exists will be uncovered and described correctly. Our ability to do this depend most of all on collecting adequate data on the amount and timing of exposure in the first place.

REFERENCES

Anderson, D. W. and Mantel, N. (1983). On epidemiologic surveys. *American Journal of Epidemiology*, **118**, 613–9.

Armstrong, B. (1985). The use of epidemiological data to assess human cancer risk. In *Methods for estimating risk of chemical injury: humans and non-human biota and ecosystems*, SCOPE 26, SGOMSEC 2, (ed. V.B. Vouk, G.C. Butler, D.G. Hoel, and D.B. Peakall), pp. 289–301. John Wiley and Sons, Chichester.

Armstrong, B.K. (1988). Epidemiology of malignant melanoma: intermittent or total accumulated exposure to the sun. *Journal of Dermatological Surgery and Oncology*, **14**, 835–49.

Bernadt, M.W., Mumford, J., Taylor, C., Smith, B., and Murray, R.M. (1982). Comparison of questionnaire and laboratory tests in the detection of excessive drinking and alcoholism. *Lancet*, **i**, 325–8.

Blair, A., and Stewart, P.A. (1990). Correlation between different measures of occupational exposure to formaldehyde. *American Journal of Epidemiology*, **131**, 510–6.

Blair, S.N., Haskell W.L., Ho, P., Paffenbarger Jr., R.S., Vranizan, K.M., Farquhar, J.W., and Wood, P.D. (1985). Assessment of habitual physical activity by a seven day recall in a community survey and controlled experiments. *American Journal of Epidemiology*, **122**, 794–804.

Breslow, N.E. and Day, N.E. (1987). *Statistical methods in cancer research, Volume II – The design and analysis of cohort studies*, pp. 232–70. International Agency for Research on Cancer, Lyon.

Carmines, E.G. and Zeller, R.A. (1979). *Reliability and validity assessment*, p. 9. Sage, Beverly Hills, California.

Checkoway, H., Pearce, N., Hickey, J.L.S., and Dement, J.M. (1990). Latency analysis in occupational epidemiology. *Archives of Environmental Health*, **45**, 95–100.

Day, N.E. (1984). Epidemiological data and multistage carcinogenesis. In *Models, mechanisms and etiology of tumour promotion*, (ed. M. Borzsonyi, K. Lapis, N.E. Day and H. Yamasaki), pp. 339–57. International Agency for Research on Cancer, Lyon.

Dement, J.M., Harris, R.L., Symons, M.J., and Shy, C.M. (1983). Exposures and mortality among chrysotile asbestos workers. Part II: Mortality. *American Journal of Industrial Medicine*, **4**, 421–33.

Dorfman, A., Kimball, A.W., and Friedman, L.A. (1985). Regression modelling of consumption of exposure variables classified by type. *American Journal of Epidemiology*, **122**, 1096–107.

Feinstein, A.R. (1985). A bibliography of publications on observer variability. *Journal of Chronic Diseases*, **38**, 619–32.

Goude, G. (1962). *On fundamental measurements in psychology*. Almqvist and Wiksell, Stockholm.

Holman, C.D.J., Armstrong, B.K., and Heenan, P.J. (1983). A theory of the etiology and pathogenesis of human cutaneous malignant melanoma. *Journal of the National Cancer Institute*, **71**, 651–6.

Holman, C.D.J., Armstrong, B.K., and Heenan, P.J. (1986). Relationship of cutaneous malignant melanoma to sunlight exposure habits. *Journal of the National Cancer Institute*, **76**, 403–14.

Kathren, R.L. and Petersen, G.R. (1989). Units and terminology of radiation measurement: a primer for the epidemiologist. *American Journal of Epidemiology*, **130**, 1076–87.

Lee-Feldstein, A. (1989). A comparison of several measures of exposure to arsenic.

Matched case-control study of copper smelter employees. *American Journal of Epidemiology*, **129**, 112–24.

Lee-Han, H., McGuire, V., and Boyd, N.F. (1988). A review of methods used by studies of dietary measurement. *Journal of Clinical Epidemiology*, **42**, 269–79.

Liberatos, P., Link, B.G., and Kelsey, J.L. (1988). The measurement of social class in epidemiology. *Epidemiologic Reviews*, **10**, 87–121.

Ostfeld, A.M. and Eaker, E.D. (1985). *Measuring psychosocial variables in epidemiologic studies of cardiovascular disease. Proceedings of a workshop*. NIH Publication No. 85-2270. US Department of Health and Human Services, Washington, DC.

Peto, J., Cuckle, H., Doll, R., Hermon, C., and Morgan, L.G. (1984). Respiratory cancer mortality of Welsh nickel refinery workers. In *Nickel in the human environment*, (ed. F.W. Sunderman, A. Aitio, A. Berlin, C. Bishop, E. Buringh, W. Davis, *et al.*), pp. 37–46. International Agency for Research on Cancer, Lyon.

Rothman, K.J. (1981). Induction and latent periods. *American Journal of Epidemiology*, **114**, 253–9.

Stevens, S.S. (1951). Mathematics, measurement and psychophysics. In *Handbook of experimental psychology*, (ed. S.S. Stevens), pp. 1–49. Wiley, New York.

Stevens, S.S. (1968). Measurement, statistics and the schemapiric view. *Science*, **161**, 849–56.

Thomas, D.C. (1988). Models of exposure-time-response relationships with applications to cancer epidemiology. *Annual Review of Public Health*, **9**, 451–82.

UK National Case-Control Study Group (1989). Oral contraceptive use and breast cancer risk in young women. *Lancet*, **i**, 973–82.

Washburn, R.A. and Montoye, H.J. (1986). The assessment of physical activity by questionnaire. *American Journal of Epidemiology*, **123**, 563–76.

Weiss, N.S. (1981). Inferring causal relationships: Elaboration of the criterion of 'dose-response'. *American Journal of Epidemiology*, **113**, 487–90.

Willett, W. (1989). An overview of issues related to the correction of non-differential exposure measurement error in epidemiologic studies. *Statistics in Medicine*, **8**, 1031–40.

Willett, W. (1990). *Nutritional epidemiology*. Oxford University Press, New York.

Zeller, R.A. and Carmines, E.G. (1980). *Measurement in the social sciences: the link between theory and data*, p. 2. Cambridge University Press, New York.

2

Methods of exposure measurement

Accuracy and 'practicability' (of data collection methods) are often inversely correlated. A method providing more satisfactory information will often be a more elaborate, expensive or inconvenient one . . . Accuracy must be balanced against practical considerations, and that method chosen which will provide the maximal accuracy within the bounds of the investigator's resources and other practical limitations. (Abramson 1984)

INTRODUCTION

Methods used for the measurement of exposure in epidemiology range from objective methods of measurement of fixed human attributes (e.g. blood type) that are as precise and valid as any in biomedical science, to methods that depend totally on the imperfect capacity of human beings to recall information. Epidemiological practice is weighted heavily towards the second of these two extremes. Frequently, past exposure is important and there are usually no records that can provide the data required. Much of modern epidemiology deals with lifestyle. The subjects, recollections of their behaviour, or those of other people close to them, may be the only comprehensive evidence we have about exposure. Recent methodological work has emphasized the development of objective methods of exposure measurement (e.g. 'molecular epidemiology'; Perera and Weinstein 1982) and such methods are increasingly being used for validation purposes, if not for the measurement of exposure in all subjects (see Chapter 4)

In this chapter, we provide a classification and brief introduction to the methods of measurement of exposure that are used in epidemiology. The issues that must be considered in choosing a method for a particular study are outlined. The choice between face-to-face interview, telephone interview, and self-administered questionnaire is dealt with in detail because of the overwhelming importance of subjective self-report of information about exposure.

CLASSIFICATION OF EXPOSURES

Exposures can be classified in a number of ways that determine different approaches to their measurement.

Personal attribute or environmental agent?

The measurement of personal attributes implies access to data about individual subjects. On the other hand, it is possible to document *potential* exposure to environmental agents without any specific information about individual subjects except that they were resident in the environment measured and could have been exposed to the agent of interest. Measurements of environmental agents without knowledge of individual exposure to them is the hallmark of ecological studies of disease aetiology.

Subjective or objective data?

Whether recording an individual attribute or contact with an agent in the environment, we commonly depend on subjective statements about the attribute or contact. The person providing the subjective data may be either the subject of our study or a proxy respondent. Subjective responses are prone to manifold sources of error including, among others:

- lack of understanding of the task by the subject
- failure in recall of the required data
- the effects of the perceived threat of a topic of questioning on the subject's response to it (see also Table 3.1).

The alternatives to subjective data are reference to records of exposure, observation by the investigator (whose 'subjective' observations then replace or supplement those of the subject), or chemical or physical measurements on the subject or the environment. Subjectivity cannot be eliminated entirely from any of these alternatives, but responsibility for its control is moved away from the research subject towards the investigator and, to that extent, they are more 'objective' measurements.

Present or past exposure?

The documentation of past exposure is inevitably more difficult than the documentation of present exposure. It usually requires either records of the exposure or recourse to human memory. Data on present exposure are of limited usefulness in chronic disease epidemiology, first because present exposure may not correlate highly with aetiologically relevant exposure that occurred some time in the past (Rothman 1981) and, second, because of uncertainty, in some situations, over whether exposure preceded disease or disease preceded exposure. Present exposure is commonly recorded at a subject's entry to a cohort study. Unless this information is brought up to date periodically during the course of follow-up, and past exposure is also recorded, it may not be highly correlated with exposure in the aetiologically relevant period.

METHODS: AN INTRODUCTION

Table 2.1 lists the methods available for the measurement of exposure in epidemiology and classifies them according to the types of measurements that they can make in the terms that have been described above. The following paragraphs introduce these methods briefly; they are described in more detail in Chapters 6 to 10.

Personal interview

The personal interview, whether face to face or by telephone, is the most commonly used method of obtaining data about subjects themselves or their environments. It permits the collection of data on past as well as present exposure, although both are subject to errors in recall. There is a tendency for subjects to under-report most exposures, although socially desirable behaviours may be over-reported. Together with the under-reporting of socially undesirable behaviours, this is called *social desirability bias*. Over-reporting may also occur when recall is requested for a particular period in the past. Subjects tend to recall instances of exposure that occurred outside the exposure period, and report them as occurring within the exposure period; this is called *telescoping*.

The involvement of an interviewer in the data collection process has advantages in securing the subject's cooperation, reducing misunderstanding about the meaning of questions, and maximizing, by prompting, the collection of usable data. More data, and more detailed and complex data, can be collected in the course of an interview than, say, by means of a self-administered questionnaire. The specific disadvantages of personal interviews are their cost, and the potential for introduction of error by the interviewer.

Self-administered questionnaires

In principle, data that can be collected by interview can be collected by self-administered questionnaire. However, the amount of data that can be collected by this method is limited by the reduced response rate associated with very long questionnaires. In addition, detailed and complex data cannot be sought without risk of substantial error or non-response to individual complex items. The compensating advantages are a saving in costs and the elimination of interviewer error.

Some of these limitations may not apply if the questionnaire is presented by way of computer, rather than on paper. This is a not uncommon approach for the collection of data in multiphasic health screening facilities. Kiesler and Sproull (1986) observed that questionnaires presented by

Table 2.1 Methods of exposure measurement in epidemiology classified according to whether they collect mainly subjective or objective data, and can measure present or past exposure to personal attributes or environmental agents

Measurement method	Data		Time		Type of exposure	
	Subjective	Objective	Present	Past	Personal attribute	Environmental exposure
Personal interview	+	-	+	+	+	+
Self-administered questionnaire	+	-	+	+	+	+
Diary	+	-	+	-	+	+
Observation by investigator	-	+	+	-	+	+
Reference to records	-	+	+	+	+	+
Physical or chemical measurements on subject	-	+	+	-	+	+
Physical or chemical measurements on environment	-	+	+	+	-	+

computer can combine the advantages of interviews (e.g. the possibility of complex branching designs) with those of other self-administered questionnaires (e.g. standardization and anonymity). In a comparison of questionnaires presented by computer with those sent through the mail, they found that responses to the computer were less socially desirable, more extreme, and more disclosing (for open-ended questions) than those given on paper. This study, however, was undertaken in a computer-literate population of university students, and it may not be appropriate to generalize its results to the wider public.

Historically, mailed self-administered questionnaires have seen considered to have low response rates. Nevertheless, gradual trends towards lower response rates in surveys involving personal interview, and improvements in follow-up and other procedures for maximization of response to mail surveys, have combined to increase their attractiveness. An analysis of response rates in surveys, mainly in the USA and Canada (Goyder 1985), showed that after adjustment for number of contacts, salience of the topic, special incentives to response, sponsoring organization, and year of the survey, mail surveys experienced response about 7.5 percentage points lower than personal interview surveys. The present expected response rate for mail surveys in the USA is around 75 per cent, while for interview surveys it is 80–85 per cent.

Between the personal interview and the mailed self-administered questionnaire comes the 'drop and pick up' method of questionnaire delivery (Stover and Stone 1974) and the completion of self-administered questionnaires under supervision. In the 'drop and pickup' method, a questionnaire is delivered to the subject personally by a field worker who can solicit co-operation and explain the nature of the response tasks. The completed questionnaire may also be collected from the subject by the field worker, at which time missing or unclear responses can be dealt with. Completion of self-administered questionnaires under supervision is most common when data are being collected from groups of subjects (e.g. schoolchildren) or subjects must attend at a central location for some other measurement (e.g. the recording of blood pressures or the taking of blood). Again, it has the advantage over the mail approach that the nature of the task can be explained to the subject. Questions can be answered or problems dealt with during the course of the questionnaire or on completion.

Diaries

Diaries can only be used for the collection of *present* personal behaviour or experiences. For this purpose, however, they are more accurate than recall methods — at least if the amount of the behaviour recorded is any guide (Verbrugge 1980).

Diaries are better than interviews for recording experiences that are transient or of low impact. They minimize recall error, including lack of recall and telescoping. In addition, for the comparatively short periods of life that they cover, they present a more comprehensive picture of the pattern of exposure than is possible by recall methods. However, if they are to represent exposure over a fairly long period, there must be reasonably long recording periods distributed over the period of interest, especially if the behaviour recorded is highly variable. They may cost more than collecting the same data by personal interview, and they are generally more expensive to process and more difficult to analyse. Among other things, diary methods have been used in epidemiology to record current diet using dietary diaries extending from one to seven days.

Use of proxy respondents

The use of proxy or surrogate respondents — that is, people who provide information on exposure in place of the subjects themselves — is an important variation on the subjective methods of exposure measurement so far outlined. Proxy respondents are used in epidemiology when the subjects of study are for some reason (death, dementia, youth, lack of knowledge of their exposure) unable to provide the data required. They are used most commonly in case-control studies of fatal disease when the only alternative to proxies may be a small series of cases potentially biased by survival. The proxies may provide the data directly to the investigator, or use may be made of records in which the information about the subject was provided by a proxy (e.g. exposure data on birth and death records).

In 54 (9.6 per cent) of the 564 epidemiological studies referred to in Table 1.1, the exposure data were obtained wholly or for some subjects from proxy respondents. In most of these studies the data were obtained from the kin of a subject who was dead (usually) or very ill, and in a few from the parents for a child. The main exposure variables were occupation (15 studies), diet (9 studies), medical history (5), smoking (5), use of medications (4), and alcohol drinking (3).

Data on exposure provided by proxies are prone to all the errors of data provided by the subjects themselves, and some additional ones. The proxy may never have known the facts sought. In addition, when death is the reason for the subject's unavailablility for interview, the fact of his or her death may alter the proxy's recall of the relevant facts. In some circumstances, however, the proxy may be at least as likely to know of the exposure as the subject (as when a parent responds on behalf of a child in respect of exposures in early life). For some exposures (e.g. tobacco use) the proxy may give a more accurate account than the subject would have done.

Practical aspects of the use of proxy respondents and the validity of data obtained from them are dealt with in more detail in Chapter 8.

Observation of the subject by the investigator

Like diary methods, observation by the investigator can be applied only to the measurement of present exposure. Attributes such as sex and race are commonly measured by observation. Some other attributes, such as eye colour and hair colour, may be recorded entirely subjectively by a field worker or more objectively by comparison with a set of standards. In the latter situation, the distinction between what is observation by the investigator and what is a physical measurement on the subject becomes blurred.

The direct observation of variable attributes or behaviours of subjects requires that the observer 'participate' in the life of the subject during the period of observation. Such *participant observation* methods have been little used in epidemiology. One example is a dietitian or nutritionist observing mealtimes in the subject's household, and recording or even sometimes sampling (for analysis!) what the subject eats. Other examples include observation of infection control practices (Kelen *et al.* 1989) and measurement of physical activity (Patterson *et al.* 1988). Direct observation of behaviour has been used not so much as a primary method in epidemiology as for the validation of other methods of measurement (e.g. recall of diet, Karveti and Knuts 1985; self-reported seatbelt use at the population level, CDC 1988; and motion sensors as measures of physical activity, Klesges *et al.* 1985).

In the measurement of behaviour, direct observation of subjects has a number of strengths and weaknesses. On the positive side:

- it is more objective
- it can be used for low-impact behaviours
- it allows for a substantial amount of detail.

On the negative side:

- it can be applied to present behaviour only
- it is restricted generally to a comparatively short sampling period
- it can be applied only to quite frequent behaviours
- often it can only be implemented with a fairly highly selected group of subjects
- it requires extensive training of observers
- it is time consuming and expensive.

There are also some important sources of error, including inadequate sampling of time periods, biased sampling of time periods (for instance in dietary observation, only meals may be observed and food eaten between meals not recorded), too many events to record accurately, observer fatigue with 'drift' in recording, and an effect of the observation on the behaviour being observed.

Observation techniques will not be dealt with further in this book. More detailed treatments from the perspective of studies in psychology can be found in Cone and Foster (1982) and Nelson and Hayes (1986).

Reference to records

In this context 'records' means records that have not been collected specifically for the purpose of measurement of exposure. Medical, occupational and, sometimes, census records are those most commonly used in exposure measurement. Sometimes they are simply records of the subject's recall of the exposure, obtained nearer to the time that it occurred, or they may be records made by others who were associated with the exposure (e.g. dose of ionizing radiation given for treatment of disease, as recorded by the therapist) or records of measurements made on the subject or the subject's environment.

The use of records can be a valuable alternative to the collection of data directly from subjects. As with any other measurement of exposure, however, their validity for the research purpose must be carefully considered before they are used. Although they have achieved status as a means of evaluating the validity of subjective recall, records are themselves prone to error. A record may be incomplete or in error, or perhaps not even made. Records may be lost or altered, and (in medical records for example) there may have been systematic differences between multiple recorders in the items recorded and the way in which different items have been defined. Moreover, as in the case of records of prescriptions of medications, intended exposures may be recorded, but the subject may not have taken the stated dose.

Records of exposure have played a particularly important role in ecological studies of disease aetiology. Data in records, often collected for administrative purposes, that relate to whole populations or population subgroups rather than individual subjects, have been correlated with variation in disease incidence over time, between geographic areas, or among subgroups of the population defined in various ways (e.g. by sex, race, religion, birthplace, occupation, etc.). The collection of data on exposure for this purpose will not be dealt with further in this book. Some sources of data useful for ecological studies are listed in NCHS (1980, 1981), Stewart (1984), Jekel (1984, 1986, 1987, 1990), O'Brien and Wasserman (1986), and Gable (1990).

Physical or chemical measurements on the subject

The usefulness of physical or chemical measurements for epidemiology depends largely on whether they relate to fixed or variable attributes of the subject or the environment. How variable the attributes are is also important. At one extreme are measurements of genetic constitution (e.g. HLA type) which remain fixed throughout life and can be measured at any time. At the other extreme are measurements of carbon monoxide in expired air which, strictly speaking, relate only to intake of cigarette smoke (or another carbon monoxide source) within the preceding few hours. Only the present status of variable attributes can be measured by physical or chemical methods. This is true of stable attributes also, but their past status can to some extent be inferred from their present status. Anthropometric variables (e.g. height, weight, and skin-fold thicknesses), blood lipid levels, and the concentrations of trace elements in hair or nails, are examples of moderately stable attributes that can be measured physically or chemically. Occasionally past environmental contacts can be inferred from present measurements on the subject (e.g. presence of DNA adducts in cells as an indicator of past, as well as present, exposure to certain carcinogens).

A particular problem for physical and chemical measurements, and, to a lesser extent, all measurements made after the onset of disease, is the possibility that the presence of disease will interfere with the measurement process or alter the values obtained by measurement. This is a major weakness of cross-sectional studies, but it also arises in case-control studies when physical or chemical measurements are made. An example is the inverse relationship between plasma cholesterol concentration and incidence of colorectal cancer, which may be due to an effect of the cancer in lowering plasma cholesterol (McMichael *et al.* 1984).

Physical or chemical measurements on the environment

Physical or chemical measurements of the environment present similar problems, except that they are unlikely to be influenced by disease in the subject. Unless records exist, they can usually only relate to the current environment. It may sometimes be possible to make present measurements that reflect the past environment of subjects (e.g. lead in the water supplies of their former homes) but the use of such data to represent the existence or levels of exposure over periods in the distant past is very uncertain (see Chapter 10). They have been used most commonly in epidemiology in the analysis of retrospective cohort studies (also called historical or non-concurrent cohort studies) of occupation and disease, in order to add measurement of exposure to the agent of specific interest to data on the place, nature, and duration of employment.

Experience of use of different methods

Table 2.2 summarizes the methods used for measurement of exposure in the 564 epidemiological studies referred to in Table 1.1. Personal interview was the predominant method, and all but a handful of these interviews were face-to-face interviews with either the subject to whom the exposure had occurred

Table 2.2 Distribution of the main methods of exposure measurement (one selected from each study) in 564 studies of the aetiology of non-infectious disease published in the *American Journal of Epidemiology* between January 1980 and December 1989

Methods	Distribution (%)
Personal interview	49.1
Face to face	43.0
Telephone	4.1
Unclassifiable type	2.0
Self-administered questionnaire	14.0
By mail	6.4
Under supervision	7.6
Reference to records	22.3
Medical records	7.1
Other records	15.2
Physical or chemical measurements	13.3
On subject	10.8
On environment	2.5
Unclassifiable	1.2

or a proxy respondent. Records were the second most important source of exposure data, particularly non-medical records. Ecological studies were a major contributor to the use of records. Diaries or direct observation of subjects by the investigators were not the main method of exposure measurement in any of the studies. In 11 studies involving personal interview it was not stated whether the interview was carried out by telephone or face to face, and in seven studies the method of measurement of exposure was so inadequately described as to be defy classification under any of the specific headings of Table 2.2!

CHOICE OF METHOD

There is no simple way of choosing the best method of measurement of exposure in any situation. As often as not, the choice will depend on practical rather than theoretical considerations. The following factors all influence the choice of a method:

- type of study
- type, amount, and detail of data required by the study's objectives

- the impact of the exposure on the subjects' lives
- sensitivity of the subjects to questioning about the exposure
- the frequency of the exposure, and variability in the frequency and level of exposure over time
- the availability of records of exposure
- the availability of physical or chemical methods for measuring the exposure.

Inevitably, the costs of different possible methods relative to the funds available will also influence the choice.

Type of study

Prospective (also called *concurrent*) *cohort studies* or *randomized controlled trials* (for exposures other than the experimental exposure) usually require the recording of present exposure, or of both present and past exposure. Past exposure is particularly important in studies in adults, and when analysis is planned soon after the beginning of follow-up. In addition, if the exposure is highly variable over time it may be necessary to measure it again at intervals during the course of follow-up. For example, in the cohort study of male British doctors initiated in 1951 by Doll and Hill, doctors were re-surveyed regarding their smoking habits in 1957, 1966, and 1972 (Doll and Peto 1976). Over the period of this study the prevalence of current smoking in the cohort fell substantially. Essentially all methods of exposure measurement are applicable to prospective cohort studies. However, records of past exposure are rarely used in such studies, except in a prospective phase of an initially retrospective cohort study, probably because they are rarely available or are no more accurate than subjective recall on entry to the cohort.

Almost by definition, *retrospective cohort studies* depend on records for their measurements of exposure. They have been most commonly applied to the study of disease following exposure to workplace hazards. Thus the exposure records most commonly used have been records of employment, occasionally supplemented by measurements of the work environment.

The logic of *case-control studies* requires that the exposure measurements permit inferences about past exposure, at least in the period before onset of disease and often in periods long before that. Thus personal interviews, self-administered questionnaires, and reference to records about subjects or their environment have been the methods most commonly used in these studies. Diaries of a subject's present experiences, observation of subjects by the investigator, and physical or chemical measurements on subjects or their environment are sometimes used in case-control studies, but this assumes stability of the exposure over time. If this assumption is incorrect, misclassification of exposure in the aetiologically relevant time period is likely.

Cross-sectional studies are similar to case-control studies in that measurement of past exposure is usually required, although in some situations the study hypothesis may relate directly to the effects of *present* exposure on a rapidly responsive outcome variable such as blood pressure. Any of the methods applicable to past or present exposure may be chosen.

Amount and detail of data required

If large amounts of detailed data are required, and particularly if past exposure must be documented, the personal interview is almost the only method to use. It may be supplemented by records or physical or chemical measurements if they are available. A diary can provide very detailed data, for example the weights of foods eaten, but usually only about a few exposure variables and only in the present. Records are often neither sufficiently comprehensive nor sufficiently detailed for epidemiological purposes but they may provide more detail than the subjects themselves can recall (e.g. the pharmacy records of subjects in a closed medical care system). For small amounts of data and limited detail, the use of self-administered questionnaires may be worth considering. They are generally less expensive than personal interviews, and can achieve acceptably high response rates. Telephone interviews are also generally thought to be useful only for the collection of small to moderate amounts of data, although the detail sought can be the same as in a face-to-face interview.

Impact of the exposure on the subjects' lives

Recall of exposure is likely to be more accurate for exposures with a high impact on the subjects' lives (major surgery) than exposures with a low impact (eating a carrot). Diary methods are ideal for low-impact exposures but, if used for past exposures, require the assumption that the exposures are stable over time. Physical or chemical measurements are also suitable for low-impact exposures, subject to the availability of such measurements and, again, the assumption of stability over time. For example, the consumption of aflatoxin in food has esentially no 'impact' for impoverished residents of tropical countries. Measurement of its intake has thus depended on the sampling of foods eaten and measurement of aflatoxin concentration in the food; more recently, it has been possible to measure the concentration of aflatoxin or its reaction products in body fluids. For these measurements to be useful epidemiologically, however, it must be assumed that the sampling period chosen is representative of the generality of past (or future) exposure. Records are sometimes useful for the measurement of low-impact exposures. For example, in the occupational environment an exposure variable such as ionizing radiation may have been measured and recorded even though the subjects were unaware of their exposure to it.

Sensitivity

The sensitivity or threat of a particular exposure topic to the subject has been studied extensively by survey researchers, mainly in relation to the methods of questioning or response in personal interviews rather than the choice of the method of measurement. In general, it appears that response rates are not greatly influenced by coverage of a sensitive topic. But of course the exposure in question may be under-reported. There is a limited amount of evidence to suggest that distancing the investigator from the subject, as in the use of a self-administered questionnaire, may increase the reporting of sensitive behaviours. In theory we would prefer to have objective methods for the measurement of sensitive exposures, but these are rarely available.

The reporting of sensitive information can be increased by the combination of two methods of measurement in the so-called *bogus pipeline* approach (Jones and Sigall 1971). The term arose from social psychological research. The 'pipeline' is 'a direct pipeline to the soul'. It is 'bogus' because the pipeline is opened by convincing the subject that the investigator has some instrument (possibly fictional) that can measure the response that the subject is being asked to record. The bogus pipeline approach has been used to increase the quantity, and presumed validity, of self-reported consumption of tobacco, alcohol, and other drugs. For example, Evans *et al.* (1977) showed schoolchildren a film demonstrating how smoking could be detected by measurements on saliva; saliva samples were then obtained before the children completed a questionnaire on their smoking habits. This approach doubled the reported prevalence of weekly smoking. Similarly, Lowe *et al.* (1986) compared the responses of two groups of pregnant women to questions on their intake of alcohol, minor tranquillizers, and aspirin. The individuals in one group were randomly assigned to have blood and urine samples taken; they were told that laboratory tests on these samples would confirm their self-reported alcohol intakes. Of those so advised, 27 per cent admitted to consumption of alcohol since they had become pregnant; only 14 per cent of the other group did so.

Frequency and variability of the exposure

(a) Infrequent exposures of low impact on the subject are almost impossible to measure. The subject will be unable to recall them, it is unlikely that they will have been measured and recorded in the past, and any practical programme of sampling of the subject's present experience of them (by diary) or their concentration in the internal or external environment is unlikely to provide measurements that are sufficiently free of variability *within* individuals to be useful.

(b) Frequent exposures of moderate or high impact will be easily measurable by recall methods, may be the subject of records, and can be easily sampled by diary methods, observation by the investigator, or physical or chemical measurements where appropriate.

(c) Low-frequency exposures of high impact are best measured by subjective recall or by reference to records (if available).

(d) High-frequency exposures of low impact are best measured by diary or objective methods where applicable (observation by the investigator, or physical or chemical measurements on the subject or the environment).

All the methods of measurement of exposure listed in Table 2.1 can be used for the measurement of exposures that do not vary greatly over time. Objective methods are generally preferable to subjective methods. For exposures that vary with time, the method of measurement should be potentially valid for exposure in the period of time relevant to the objectives of the study. It may be necessary to make multiple measurements over time to minimize or eliminate seasonal effects, and to reduce the extent of within-person variability of the measure.

Availability of records and physical and chemical methods

The use of records or physical or chemical methods of exposure measurement is usually supplementary to data obtained by subjective report. In some situations, however, they may be the only practical or available measurements of the exposure, as in retrospective cohort studies and when the exposure of interest is defined in terms of a particular measurement (e.g. serum cholesterol concentration). Under those circumstances, the availability of these records or measurements will determine both the choice of exposure and the feasibility of the study.

Combinations of methods

It is common to combine a number of different methods of measurement of exposure within a single study. This may be done:

- for validation purposes only
- to combine results of two or more different approaches to measurement into a single, more accurate, measure of exposure (see page 115)
- because it may be better to use different approaches to collect different parts of the desired data.

For example, the investigator may carry out a personal interview and also collect some data by self-administered questionnaire. This might be done to save time or money, or because of the possible advantage of self-administered questionnaires over interviews in the collection of particularly sensitive data. In a case-control study of diet and colorectal cancer, Potter and McMichael (1986) first delivered to the subjects a self-administered food-frequency questionnaire and went through the instructions for completion of the 141 items. This questionnaire was then completed by the subjects themselves during the succeeding week, and checked and collected by the interviewer at the time of the main interview. The interview itself covered non-dietary variables of interest to the investigators. The major objective of this approach was to save time at interview. Combinations of methods will obviously be necessary when, for example, one measurement is of a physiological variable (e.g. plasma cholesterol concentration) and another requires subjective recall.

The Framingham study provides a good example of the multiplicity of types of exposure measurement that may be used in a single study. Initially, subjects were questioned about their medical history, family medical history, personal habits, history of weight change, and use of medications. Measurements were made of height, weight, other anthropometric variables, blood pressure, eye and hair colour, degree of freckling, distribution of hair and degree of baldness, and presence of arcus senilis or xanthelasma. A blood sample was taken for measurement of haemoglobin, cholesterol, other blood lipids, glucose, uric acid, and serology for syphilis and a routine urinalysis was performed (Dawber *et al.* 1951). Subsequent examinations were made every other year, mainly to detect the occurrence of new coronary heart disease, but exposure measurements were repeated and additional exposure measurements made (Dawber 1980). The latter included diet (by one-hour interview by a dietitian), physical exercise (24-hour recall), and a variety of psychosocial variables. The psychosocial measurements included some self-administered questionnaires (Haynes *et al.* 1978).

FACE-TO-FACE INTERVIEWS, TELEPHONE INTERVIEWS, OR SELF-ADMINISTERED QUESTIONNAIRES?

Subjective methods were the main methods of measurement of exposure in 64 per cent of the 564 epidemiological studies summarized in Table 2.2. So far the three main methods of collecting subjective data — face-to-face and telephone interviews and self-administered questionnaire — have been treated as more or less equivalent. In fact there are important differences between them. Table 2.3, derived from Dillman (1978), summarizes the performance characteristics of face-to-face and telephone interviews and mailed self-administered questionnaires. Of course, not all self-administered questionnaires are sent through the mail; less than half of the self-administered questionnaires used in the recent epidemiological studies summarized in Table 2.2 were mailed. Some of the disadvantages of self-administered questionnaires highlighted in Table 2.3 relate to distribution by mail, rather than self-administration as such.

Face-to-face interview

The face-to-face interview rates as high as or higher than the other two approaches on all the characteristics listed except with respect to the probability of social desirability bias, the possibility of interviewer effects on the accuracy of the data, and administrative requirements. The particular strengths of face-to-face interviews lie in the length and complexity of interview that is possible.

The administrative problem is that it may be difficult to obtain enough competent interviewers, especially if the sample is widely dispersed and the interviewer is required to visit areas that he or she would not normally enter. It is organizationally difficult to complete a large number of interviews quickly on a dispersed sample. The cost of data collection by face-to-face interview is almost invariably higher than it would be if the same data were collected by another method. For example, it has been estimated that for collection of data from a sample of subjects dispersed throughout the USA, the approximate *relative* costs would be (Dillman 1978):

- face-to-face interview, $100 each
- telephone interview, $20 each
- mailed questionnaire, $6 each

For a county-wide survey, the differences would be much smaller:

- face-to-face interview, $9–10 each
- telephone interview, $5–7 each
- mailed questionnaire, $4–6 each.

A study in a single large Australian city (Sydney) found that telephone interviews cost marginally more than home interviews ($74 vs. $71) while the cost of a mailed questionnaire was much less ($42) (O'Toole *et al.* 1986). Telephone interviewing may only have a cost advantage over face-to-face interviewing when the sample is widely dispesed.

From an epidemiological point of view, the administrative limitations probably have less force than they would in, say, an opinion survey. The cost savings in using the telephone or mail are important, however, as is the ability to enter almost any area. The use of random digit dialling instead of street sampling of households as a means of obtaining a sample of the population can add to the cost-efficiency of the telephone survey. Social desirability bias in face-to-face interviews is often a disadvantage when information is being sought on diet, alcohol and tobacco intake, exercise, or sexual behaviour.

Table 2.3 Comparison of face-to-face interviews, telephone interviews, and mailed questionnaires with respect to selected performance characteristics (adapted from Dillman, 1978; used with permission)

Performance Characteristics	Face-to-face interviews	Method Telephone interviews	Mail questionnaires
Obtaining a representative sample			
Opportunity for all members of population to be included in sample			
Completely listed populations	High	High	High
Populations not completely listed (e.g. household occupants)	High	Medium	Medium
Control over selection of respondents within sampling units	High	High	Medium
Likelihood that selected respondents will be located	Medium	High	High
Response rates			
Heterogeneous samples (e.g. general public)	High	High	Medium
Homogeneous specialized samples (e.g. doctors, nurses, students)	High	High	High
Likelihood that unknown bias from refusals will be avoided	High	High	Low
Questionnaire construction and question design			
Allowable length of questionnaire	High	Medium	Medium
Type of question Allowable complexity	High	Low	Medium
Success with open-ended questions	High	High	Low

Performance Characteristics	Method		
	Face-to-face interviews	Telephone interviews	Mail questionnaires
Success with screen questions	High	High	Medium
Success with controlling sequence in which questions are asked	High	High	Low
Success with tedious or boring questions	High	Medium	Low
Success in avoiding item non-response	High	High	Medium
Insensitivity to questionnaire construction procedures	High	Medium	Low
Obtaining accurate answers			
Likelihood that social desirability bias can be avoided	Low	Medium	High
Likelihood that interviewer distortion and subversion can be avoided	Low	Medium	High
Likelihood that contamination by others can be avoided	Medium	High	Medium
Likelihood that consultation will be obtained when needed	Medium	Low	Medium
Administrative requirements			
Likelihood that personnel requirements can be met	Low	High	High
Potential speed of implementation	Low	High	Low
Keeping costs low			
Overall potential for low cost interviews	Low	Medium	High
Insensitivity of costs to increasing geographical dispersion	Low	Medium	High

Telephone interview

In comparison with the face-to-face interview, the telephone interview has several specific advantages and disadvantages. In addition to the potential cost savings identified above, the telephone interview can be private in almost any surroundings because bystanders can hear only one side of the conversation. (One should not rely on this potential privacy in order to ask sensitive questions, however.) Studies using telephone interviews can also be completed very quickly.

On the negative side, telephone interview questionnaires usually have to be shorter and simpler than questionnaires administered face to face. It is difficult to present the subject with lists of possible alternative answers and other printed material (e.g. photographs of oral contraceptives) to support the telephone interview. If this difficulty has not been overcome by prior mail or other contact, the investigator may have to ask a long series of questions where in a face-to-face situation a single question and a list would suffice. On the other hand, computer-assisted telephone interviewing may permit the use of more complex branched questionnaire designs than are otherwise possible (see page 191).

While item non-response is no greater in telephone than face-to-face interviews, Groves (1978) noted that the number of items mentioned in response to an open-ended question ('What are the most important problems facing this country?') was less in telephone interviews. This may be explained by the observation that people need time to retrieve information (Bradburn *et al.* 1987), and because respondents are less confortable with pauses on the phone than in a face-to-face interview (or when completing a self-administered questionnaire), so their recall in telephone interviews may be less complete. There is also evidence that when a list of responses is read on the phone, subjects are more likely to choose the first or the last than when they can read the whole list for themselves (Jordan *et al.* 1980). This may be due to difficulties in recall in the telephone situation.

It is difficult to select a random sample of the population when telephone *interviewing* is linked with telephone *sampling*. Subjects without telephones are excluded from any strictly telephone-based sampling process, and sample bias is inevitable unless the proportion of households with telephones is very high. In the USA in 1981, only 6.8 per cent of households were without a telephone (Hartge *et al.* 1984). Other countries with over 90 per cent coverage of households by telephones include Sweden (99 per cent!), Canada, Finland, New Zealand, Denmark, France, Netherlands, Australia, and Hong Kong (Trewin and Lee 1988). In poorer countries, the coverage may be very low: 16 per cent in Hungary, Mexico, and Poland.

Even in countries with high telephone ownership, there is appreciable heterogeneity. Non-coverage is generally highest in the following categories (Trewin and Lee 1988):

- rural households
- single-person households or very large households
- low-income households
- households where the head of the household is very young, very old, single or divorced, unskilled, or unemployed
- rented and old accommodation
- ethnic minority households.

These differences can lead to appreciable bias in telephone sample results (Thornberry and Massey 1988).

Households with two telephones (1.5 per cent of residential connections in Australia; Cutler and Sharp 1985) and households with unlisted telephone numbers (19.3 per cent of households with telephones in the USA in 1970; Glasser and Metzger 1972) may also present problems. Both are likely to differ from other telephone-owning households (Cutler and Sharp 1985; Groves and Kahn 1979). Where two-telephone households can be identified, bias can be avoided by sampling in only half of them. The presence of an appreciable proportion of unlisted numbers substantially precludes the use of telephone directories for the selection of population samples, and has led to the use of random digit dialling methods for sample selection (Waksberg 1978; Hartge *et al.* 1984; Lepkowski 1988).

Sample bias may also be introduced in telephone sampling through the methods used to select a respondent in each household contacted. A request for a list of all household members may provoke refusal to participate further, so a variety of respondent selection rules have been introduced that do not require identification or enumeration of all members of the household. None of these is free from bias, however (Groves and Kahn 1979), and they do not allow ready selection of a sample stratified by age and sex, for example. Therefore, for epidemiological purposes, selection of the respondent from a full list of household members is probably the best. This approach has been shown to enumerate a sample of the population that is no more biased, in comparison with the census, than samples obtained through the best face-to-face surveys (Maklan and Waksberg 1988).

Where telephone ownership is low or concern about the possibility of sample bias is high, for whatever reason, the efficiencies of telephone interviewing may be obtained by mixed-mode interviewing (e.g. telephone, with face-to-face interviews or contact for those without telephones or for whom telephone numbers are unavailable). This approach assumes, however, that any population sample used will have been selected by means other than random digit dialling.

Self-administered questionnaires

Self-administered questionnaires have comparatively few advantages and a number of disadvantages in comparison with the other two methods. They may promote more truthful responses to sensitive questions, usually cost less to administer than either method of personal interview, and require fewer expert staff. Their particular disadvantages are the comparative brevity and simplicity of the questionnaires that can be used, and the lower expected response rate. Response rate should not be any lower, of course, if the questionnaire is completed under some form of supervision rather than just sent in the mail. Non-response to individual items is also more likely in a self-administered questionnaire. O'Toole *et al.* (1986) found 5.5 per cent of items in a mailed questionnaire had missing responses, compared with 0.4 per cent and 0.2 per cent in telephone and home interviews respectively. Rolnick *et al.* (1989) also found more item non-response in a mailed questionnaire than a personal interview, particularly in questions relating to sexual history, although the overall prevalence of missing data was low in both methods — 0.001–0.006 per cent of data items. It is often possible to complete missing items when the questionnaire is collected, or through a follow-up letter or phone call.

Sudman and Bradburn (1984) have presented a detailed discussion of the use of mailed questionnaires. They note that mail surveys work best with members of professional societies and other educated groups, less well in the general population, and especially poorly among the aged and the poorly educated. The latter two groups find self-administered questionnaires hard to read and understand and have generally had little experience with the completion of questionnaires. It has also been asserted that response rates to mailed questionnaires is higher in the USA than in most other countries (Goyder 1982). A recent study of identical approaches to getting responses to a mailed questionnaire in Japan and in the western USA, however, obtained nearly identical response rates, and acceptably high response rates have been reported from other countries with populations of mainly European origin (Jussaume and Yamada 1990). It seems probable that the use of mailed questionnaires is feasible in any population which is literate, can be sampled, and can be contacted through a dependable postal system.

As to the nature of the questionnaire itself, Sudman and Bradburn (1984) concluded that mailed questionnaires performed best when they were short, dealt with highly salient topics, did not contain open-ended questions, did not require complex branching, did not contain questions that required probes, and did not require that questions be answered in a strict order (because of the impossibility of controlling the order in which subjects answer questions in mailed questionnaires). On the positive side, if it is desirable that a subject consult records or other people when answering, this is more likely to happen with a mailed questionnaire. A mailed questionnaire also gives the subject more time to reflect on the questions and recall the relevant details. Of course, both of these advantages may become disadvantages when the questionnaire deals with opinions rather than facts or, in case-control studies perhaps, if they lead to greater efforts by cases than by controls to provide accurate data.

Comparative validity of data obtained face to face, by telephone, or through a self-administered questionnaire

Comparisons of the quality of data obtained by interviews and questionnaires have commonly relied on comparisons of the distributions of responses to particular questions in samples of subjects surveyed by different methods. These comparisons generally suggest that:

(a) Sensitive questions are more readily answered and socially undesirable behaviours more readily admitted in self-administered questionnaires.

(b) Responses to open-ended questions are less complete and acquiescence (a tendency to agree with propositions in the questionnaire), extremeness (choosing the first or last answer from a list of responses), and evasiveness (don't know and no answer) in response to attitude questions more evident in telephone interviews. (Groves 1978; Groves and Kahn 1979; Jordan *et al.* 1980; Siemiatycki *et al.* 1984).

These issues in the comparison of telephone and face-to-face interviews have been reviewed in detail in Groves *et al.* (1988).

A few studies have compared the approaches to collecting subjective data with respect to their validity against prior subjective observations or some external standard. For example, Hochstim (1967) found that a history of Pap smear, or pelvic examination without a Pap smear, could be confirmed in medical records in about 80 per cent of subjects. The confirmation rate was much the same whether the history was obtained by personal interview, telephone interview, or self-administered questionnaire. In the study of Battistutta *et al.* (1983), there was no difference in completeness of response among the three methods of study, and agreement between initial responses and those obtained at re-interview was similar among the methods. Weeks *et al.* (1983) found, on the other hand, that the confirmation rate in records was higher for histories of ambulatory care and hospital admission given by telephone than by personal interview, although this difference was not statistically significant. Siemiatycki *et al.* (1984) showed that confirmation rates of history of physician visits were at least as high or higher for self-administered questionnaires as for telephone interviews. O'Toole *et al.* (1986) found similar levels of agreement between an initial personal interview, telephone interview, and self-administered questionnaire and a subsequent personal interview with respect to histories of chemical exposure, harmful activities, smoking habits, and alcohol use. Herrman (1985), on the other hand, found less agreement between a self-administered questionnaire and a preceding or succeeding interview than between two interviews. Overall, there appears to be no consistent trend towards better or worse performance of any of the three methods.

SUMMARY

A variety of subjective and objective methods of exposure measurement directed towards present or past personal attributes or environmental contacts are used in epidemiology. They include personal interview, either face to face or by telephone, self-administered questionnaires, diaries of behaviour, reference to records, physical or chemical measurements on the subject, physical or chemical measurements in the environment and, infrequently, direct observation of the subject's behaviour by the investigator. When the subject is too young, too ill, or dead, it is also common to obtain data about him or her from a proxy respondent, usually a member of the subject's family.

The choice of a method is influenced by the type of study to be undertaken, the type, amount, and detail of data required by the study's objectives, the impact of the exposure on the subjects' lives, the sensitivity of the subjects to questioning about the exposure, the frequency of the exposure and variability in the frequency and level of exposure over time, the availability of records of exposure, the availability of physical or chemical methods for measuring the exposure, and the costs of the various possible methods. Combinations of methods are often necessary or desirable for validation purposes, to reduce error in measurement, or because different parts of the data require different approaches to collection.

Subjective recall of exposure, collected by way of face-to-face or telephone interview or self-administered questionnaire, is the predominant method of collection of exposure data in epidemiology. There appears to be little difference between these methods with respect to the validity of the data obtained. Self-administered questionnaires may perform better than the other approaches in the documentation of sensitive or socially undesirable behaviour, and telephone interviews may lead to less complete responses and a tendency to select the extremes from a distribution of responses. Face-to-face interviews are the dominant approach in epidemiology and are clearly best for the collection of large amounts of complex data. However, where subjects are widely dispersed and the questionnaire can be kept comparatively brief, telephone interviews may be favoured. Self-administered questionnaires, usually delivered and returned by mail, should be considered for low-budget studies for which the addresses of subjects are available and for which small amounts of reasonably simple data are required. Good response rates can be achieved with mailed self-administered questionnaires. There are usually substantial financial advantages in the use of telephone interviews or self-administered questionnaires.

REFERENCES

Abramson, J. H. (1984). *Survey methods in community medicine*, (3rd edn), p. 121. Churchill Livingstone, Edinburgh.

Battistutta, D., Byth, K., Norton, R., and Rose, G. (1983). Response rates: a comparison of mail, telephone and personal interview strategies for an Australian population. *Community Health Studies*, **7**, 309–13.

Bradburn, N. M., Rips, L. J., and Shevell, S. K. (1987). Answering autobiographical questions: the impact of memory and inference on surveys. *Science*, **236**, 157–61.

CDC (Centers for Disease Control) (1988). Comparison of observed and self-reported seat belt use rates—United States. *Morbidity and Mortality Weekly Reports*, **37**, 549–51.

Cone, J. D. and Foster, S. L. (1982). Direct observation in clinical psychology. In *Handbook of research methods in clinical psychology*, (ed. P. C. Kendall and J. N. Butcher), pp. 311–54. John Wiley and Sons, New York.

Cutler, T. A. and Sharp, K. F. (1985). Telephone interviewing in Australia: some aspects of using the telephone network. In *Survey interviewing, theory and techniques*, (ed. T. W. Beed and R. J. Stimson), pp. 128–35. George Allen and Unwin, Sydney.

Dawber, T. R. (1980). *The Framingham study: the epidemiology of atherosclerotic disease*. Harvard University Press, Cambridge, Massachussets.

Dawber, T. R., Meadows, G. F., and Moore, F. E. (1951). Epidemiological approaches to heart disease: the Framingham Study. *American Journal of Public Health*, **41**, 279–86.

Dillman, D. A. (1978). *Mail and telephone surveys: the total design method*. John Wiley and Sons, New York.

Doll, R. and Peto, R. (1976). Mortality in relation to smoking: 20 years' observations on male British doctors. *British Medical Journal*, **2**, 1525–36.

Evans, R. I., Hanse, W. B., and Mittelmark, M. B. (1977). Increasing the validity of self-reports of smoking behavior in children. *Journal of Applied Psychology*, **62**, 521–3.

Gable, C. B. (1990). A compendium of public health data sources. *American Journal of Epidemiology*, **131**, 381–94.

Glasser, G. J. and Metzger, G. D. (1972). Random digit dialing as a method of telephone sampling. *Journal of Marketing Research*, **9**, 59–64.

Goyder, J. C. (1982). Further evidence on factors affecting response rates to mailed questionnaires. *American Sociological Review*, **47**, 550–3.

Goyder, J. (1985). Face-to-face interviews and mailed questionnaires: The net difference in response rate. *Public Opinion Quarterly*, **49**, 234–52.

Groves, R. M. (1978). On the mode of administering a questionnaire and responses to open-ended items. *Social Science Research*, **7**, 257–71.

Groves, R. M. and Kahn, R. L. (1979). *Surveys by telephone. A national comparison with personal interviews*. Academic Press, New York.

Groves, R. M., Biemer, P. P., Lyberg, L. E., Massey, J. T., Nicholls, W. L., and Waksberg, J. (1988). *Telephone survey methodology*. John Wiley and Sons, New York.

Hartge, P., Brinton, L. A., Rosenthal, J. F., Cahill, J. I., Hoover, R. N., and

Waksberg, J. (1984). Random digit dialing in selecting a population-based control group. *American Journal of Epidemiology*, **120**, 825–33.

Haynes, S. G., Levine, S., Scotch, M., Feinleib, M., and Kannell, W. B. (1978). The relationship of psychosocial factors to coronary heart disease in the Framingham Study 1. Methods and risk factors. *American Journal of Epidemiology*, **107**, 362–83.

Herrman, N. (1985). Retrospective information from questionnaires II. Intrarater reliability and comparison of questionnaire types. *American Journal of Epidemiology*, **121**, 948–53.

Hochstim, J. R. (1967). A critical comparison of three strategies of collecting data from households. *Journal of the American Statistical Association*, **62**, 976–82.

Jekel, J. F. (1984). 'Rainbow Reviews': Publications of the National Center for Health Statistics. *Journal of Chronic Disease*, **37**, 681–8.

Jekel, J. F. (1986). 'Rainbow Reviews': II. Recent publications of the National Center for Health Statistics. *Journal of Chronic Disease*, **39**, 189–93.

Jekel, J. F. (1987). 'Rainbow Reviews' III. Recent publications of the National Center for Health Statistics. *Journal of Chronic Disease*, **40**, 439–43.

Jekel, J. F. (1990). 'Rainbow Reviews': IV. Recent publications of the National Center for Health Statistics. *Journal of Chronic Disease*, **43**, 261–6.

Jones, E. E. and Sigall, H. (1971). The bogus pipeline: A new paradigm for measuring affect and attitude. *Psychology Bulletin*, **76**, 349–64.

Jordan, L. A., Marcus, A. C., and Reeder, L. G. (1980). Response styles in telephone and household interviewing: a field experiment. *Public Opinion Quarterly*, **44**, 210–22.

Jussaume, R. A. and Yamada, Y. (1990). Viability of mail surveys in Japan and the United States. *Public Opinion Quarterly*, **54**, 219–28.

Karveti, R. L. and Knuts, L. R. (1985). Validity of the 24-hour dietary recall. *Journal of the American Dietetics Association*, **85**, 1437–42.

Kelen, G. D., DiGiovanna, T., Bisson, L., Kalainov, D., Sivertson, K. T., and Quinn, T. C. (1989). Human immunodeficiency virus infection in emergency department patients. *Journal of the American Medical Association*, **262**, 516–22.

Kiesler, S. and Sproull, L. S. (1986). Response effects in the electronic survey. *Public Opinion Quarterly*, **50**, 402–13.

Klesges, R. C., Klesges, L. M., Swensen, A. M., and Pheley, A. M. (1985). A validation of two motion sensors in the prediction of child and adult physical activity levels. *American Journal of Epidemiology*, **122**, 400–10.

Lepkowski, J. M. (1988). Telephone sampling methods in the United States. In *Telephone survey methodology*, (ed. R. M. Groves, P. P. Biemer, L. E. Lyberg, J. T. Massey, W. L. Nicholls, and J. Waksberg), pp. 73–98. John Wiley and Sons, New York.

Lowe, J. B., Windsor, R. A., Adams, B., Morris, J., and Reese, Y. (1986). Use of a bogus pipeline method to increase accuracy of self-reported alcohol consumption among pregnant women. *Journal of Studies on Alcohol*, **47**, 173–5.

Maklan, D. and Waksberg, J. (1988). Within-household coverage in RDD surveys. In *Telephone survey methodology*, (ed. R. M. Groves, P. P. Biemer, L. E. Lyberg, J. T. Massey, W. L. Nicholls, and J. Waksberg), pp. 51–69. John Wiley and Sons, New York.

McMichael, A. J., Jensen, O. M., Parkin, D. M., and Zaridze, D. G. (1984). Dietary and endogenous cholesterol and human cancer. *Epidemiologic Reviews*, **6**, 192–216.

NCHS (National Center for Health Statistics) (1980). *Environmental health: a plan for collecting and coordinating statistical and epidemiologic data.* Department of Health and Human Services, Washington. DHHS Publication No. (PHS) 80–1248.

NCHS (National Center for Health Statistics) (1981). *Facts at your fingertips. A guide to sources of statistical information on major health topics.* Dept of Health and Human Services, Washington. DHHS Publication No. (PHS) 81–1246.

Nelson, R. O. and Hayes, S. C. (1986). *Conceptual foundations of behavioral assessment.* The Guildford Press, New York.

O'Brien, J. W. and Wasserman, S. R. (1986). *Statistics sources. A subject guide to data on industrial, business, social, educational, financial and other topics for the United States and internationally*, (10th edn). Gale Research Company, Detroit.

O'Toole, B. I., Battistutta, D., Long, A., and Crouch, K. (1986). A comparison of costs and data quality of three health survey methods: mail, telephone and personal home interview. *American Journal of Epidemiology*, **124**, 317–28.

Patterson, T. L., Sallis, J. F., Nader, P. R., Rupp, J. W., McKenzie, T. L., Roppe, B., and Bartok, P. W. (1988). Direct observation of physical activity and dietary behaviours in a structured environment: Effects of a family-based health promotion program. *Journal of Behavioural Medicine*, **11**, 447–59.

Perera, F. P. and Weinstein, I. B. (1982). Molecular epidemiology and carcinogen-DNA adduct detection—new approaches to studies to human cancer causation. *Journal of Chronic Diseases*, **35**, 581–600.

Potter, J. D. and McMichael, A. J. (1986). Diet and cancer of the colon and rectum: a case-control study. *Journal of the National Cancer Institute*, **76**, 557–69.

Rolnick, S. J., Gross, C. J., Garrard, J., and Gibson, R. W. (1989). A comparison of response rate, data quality, and cost in the collection of data on sexual history and personal behaviours. Mail survey approaches and in-person interview. *American Journal of Epidemiology*, **129**, 1052–61.

Rothman, K. J. (1981). Induction and latent periods. *American Journal of Epidemiology*, **114**, 253–9.

Siemiatycki, J., Campbell, S., Richardson, L., and Aubert, D. (1984). Quality of response in different population groups in mail and telephone surveys. *American Journal of Epidemiology*, **120**, 302–14.

Stewart, D. W. (1984). *Secondary research: information sources and methods.* Applied Social Research Methods Series, Vol. 4. Sage Publications, Beverley Hills, California.

Stover, R. V. and Stone, W. J. (1974). Hand delivery of self-administered questionnaires. *Public Opinion Quarterly*, **38**, 284–7.

Sudman, S. and Bradburn, N. (1984). Improving mailed questionnaire design. In *Making effective use of mailed questionnaires*, (ed. D. C. Lockhart), pp. 33–47. Jossey-Bass, San Francisco.

Thornberry, O. T. and Massey, J. T. (1988). Trends in United States telephone coverage across time and subgroups. In *Telephone survey methodology*, (ed. R. M. Groves, P. P. Biemer, L. E. Lyberg, J. T. Massey, W. L. Nicholls, and J. Waksberg), pp. 25–49. John Wiley and Sons, New York.

Trewin, D. and Lee, G. (1988). International comparisons of telephone coverage. In

Telephone survey methodology. (ed. R.M. Groves, P.P. Biemer, L.E. Lyberg, J.T. Massey, W.L. Nicholls, and J. Waksberg), pp. 9–24. John Wiley and Sons, New York.

Verbrugge, L.M. (1980). Health diaries. *Medical Care*, **18**, 73–95.

Waksberg, J. (1978). Sampling methods for random digit dialing. *Journal of American Statistical Association*, **73**, 40–6.

Weeks, M.F., Kulka, R.A., Lessler, J.T., and Whitmore, R. (1983). Personal versus telephone surveys for collecting household health data at the local level. *American Journal of Public Health*, **73**, 1389–94.

3

Exposure measurement error and its effects

The most elegant design of a clinical study will not overcome the damage caused by unreliable or imprecise measurement. (Fleiss 1986)

INTRODUCTION

Measurement error is one of the major sources of bias in epidemiological studies. It can lead to spurious conclusions about the relationship between exposure and disease. In this book we confine our attention to error in the measurement of exposure.

The *exposure measurement error* for an individual can be defined as the difference between the measured exposure and the true exposure. The *true exposure* is the agent of interest, for example the exposure hypothesized to cause the disease, and would include a specified time period of interest, such as a period in which the exposure could have caused the disease. *Validity* refers to the capacity of an exposure variable to measure the true exposure in a population of interest. Measures of validity are measures of the exposure measurement error in a population.

Error in measurement of the exposure can be introduced during almost any phase of a study. Possible causes include:

- faulty design of the instrument
- errors or omissions in the protocol for use of the instrument
- poor execution of the protocol during data collection
- limitations due to subject characteristics (e.g. poor memory of past exposures, or day-to-day variability in biological characteristics)
- errors during data entry and analysis

Examples of each of these are given in Table 3.1.

A particular concern is *differential exposure measurement error*, which occurs when exposure measurement error differs according to the disease or outcome being studied. One source of differential measurement error is *recall bias*, that is, when cases, for example, report exposures differently from controls because of their knowledge or feelings about the disease. Other sources of differential error include:

- the data collector's knowledge of the subject's disease status

Table 3.1 Examples of sources of measurement error

Errors in the design of the instrument
  Lack of coverage of all sources of the exposure on a questionnaire
  Inclusion of exposures that do not have the actual active agent
  Time period assessed by instrument not the true time period of interest
  Phrasing of questions that lead to misunderstanding or bias

Errors or omissions in the protocol for use of the instrument
  Failure to specify protocol in sufficient detail
  Failure to specify a method to handle unanticipated situations consistently
  Failure to include standardization of instrument periodically throughout
    data collection

Poor execution of the study protocol
  Failure of data collectors to follow protocol in same manner for all
    subjects
  Failure of subjects to read instructions in self-administered questionnaire
  Improper handling and/or analysis of biological specimens
  Influence of the personality, sex, race, or age of interviewer on subject's
    responses

Limitations due to subject characteristics
  Memory limitations of subjects including poor recall of exposures and
    influence of recent exposures on memory of past exposures
  Limitations of proxy respondents' knowledge and memory of subject's
    exposures
  Tendency of subjects to over-report socially desirable behaviours and
    under-report socially undesirable behaviours
  Short-term (e.g. day-to-day) variability in biological characteristics

Errors during data entry and analysis
  Data entry errors
  Errors in conversion tables used to convert subject responses to units of
    active agent
  Programming errors in creating variables for analysis

- the biological effects of the disease or treatment
- the biological effects or symptoms of the prediagnostic phase of the disease
- the subject's awareness of his risk of the disease (e.g. family history).

While differential exposure measurement error is a major concern when studies involve retrospective collection of exposure data, the latter two sources of differential error can occur in prospectively collected data as well.

One effect of measurement error in a study is that it leads to bias in the odds ratio (or other measure of association between the exposure and outcome); this is called *misclassification bias* or *information bias*.

This chapter is divided into two main sections, the first on measurement error in continuous exposure variables and the second on measurement error (misclassification) in categorial exposure variables. Within each of these sections, an approach to quantifying the measurement error is presented. In practice, validity usually cannot be ascertained, because a perfect exposure measure is generally not available. However, it is assumed that such a true measure does exist, at least in theory. Each section also includes a discussion of the effects of exposure measurement error on the odds ratio in epidemiological studies, and on power and sample size. To make possible an explicit analysis of the effects of measurement error, certain assumptions are made about the form of the measurement error. The purpose is to give the reader some insight into the effects of measurement errors of varying degrees.

Further ways of estimating measurement error, including techniques that do not require a perfect measure of the true exposure, are given in Chapter 4.

CONTINUOUS EXPOSURE MEASURES

The theory of measurement error in a continuous variable and its effects on studies of a continuous outcome were developed in the fields of psychometrics, survey research, and statistics (Hansen *et al*. 1961; Lord and Novick 1968; Cochran 1968; Nunnally 1978; Allen and Yen 1979; Bohrnstedt 1983; Fuller 1987). More recently, the effects of measurement error have been derived in the context of epidemiological studies of a continuous exposure variable and a dichotomous disease outcome (Prentice 1982; Whittemore and Grosser 1986; Armstrong *et al*. 1989).

A model of measurement error

A simple model of measurement error in a population is

$$X_i = T_i + b + E_i,$$

where $\mu_E = 0$ and $\rho_{TE} = 0$. This model is illustrated in Figure 3.1. In it, the observed measure X_i for a given individual i differs from the true value T_i for that individual as a consequence of two types of measurement error. The first is systematic error or *bias*, b, that would occur (on average) for all measured subjects. The second, E_i, is the additional error in X_i for subject i. *E* is referred to as the *subject error*, to indicate that it varies from subject to subject. It does not refer to error due to subject characteristics, but may rather include all of the sources of error outlined in Table 3.1.

For the population of potential study subjects, X, T, and E are variables with distributions; for example, the distribution of E is the distribution of subject measurement errors in the population of interest. X, T, and E have expectations (population means over an infinite population) denoted by

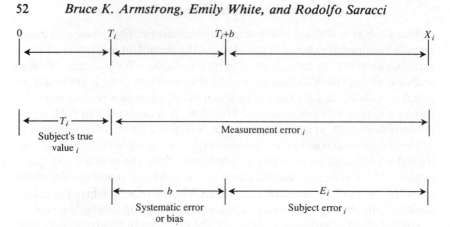

Figure 3.1   Measurement error in the measurement of X_i.

μ_X, μ_T, and μ_E, respectively, and variances denoted by σ_X^2, σ_T^2, and σ_E^2. Because the average measurement error in X in the population is expressed as a constant, b, it follows that μ_E, the population mean of the subject error, is 0. The assumption of the model that the correlation coefficient of T with E, ρ_{TE}, is 0 implies that the true values of exposure are not correlated with the subject errors in the population. In other words, subjects with high true values are assumed not to have systematically higher (or lower) errors than subjects with lower true values.

Example.   Suppose a portable scale is used to weigh subjects for a study of weight and hip fracture among a population of elderly women. Although current weight (X) will be measured, the true exposure of interest (T) is the subject's average weight over the previous 5 years. (The true exposure could be measured in theory by averaging multiple weighings over the 5-year period.) Measures of weight in the population of interest would yield observations for X that would differ from each subject's true weight T because of measurement error, as shown in the example in Table 3.2.

The measurement error can be broken down into two components:

the systematic bias, b, that would affect all members of the study population

the remainder of the error, E, that varies from subject to subject.

In this example, suppose the bias in X (in the population to be studied) is 1 kg. The sources of systematic bias in X might be:

the scale is miscalibrated so that it reads on average 0.5 kg too heavy

Table 3.2 Example of measurement error in observations of body weight in a series of subjects where X_i represents the observed weight, T_i the true weight, b the bias, and E_i the remainder of the error

	Subject (i)			
	1	2	3	4 ...
X_i(kg)	61	50	70	63
T_i(kg)	59	52	69	60
Measurement error	2	−2	1	3
b(kg)	1	1	1	1
E_i(kg)	1	−3	0	2

subjects currently weigh on average 0.5 kg more than their average weight over the previous five years.

The sources of subject error might include:

randomness in the mechanics of the scale beyond the scale's usual 0.5 kg overestimation

the difference between each individual's current weight and her average five-year weight (beyond the average 0.5 kg increase).

Other sources of error that could contribute to bias and subject error include:

the weight of the subjects' clothes

misreading of the scale by the interviewer

random hour-to-hour and day-to-day fluctuations in 'current' weight.

Measures of measurement error

Two measures of measurement error are used to describe the validity of X, that is, the relationship of X to T in the population of interest, based on the above model and assumptions. One is the bias or the average measurement error in the population, which in the difference between the population mean of X and the population mean of T, $b = \mu_X - \mu_T$.

The other is a measure of the *precision* of X, that is, a measure of the variation in the measurement error in the population. One measure of precision is the variance of E, σ_E^2. (Note that the model is formulated in such a way that the variance of E, σ_E^2, is the variance of the measurement error; b, a constant, does not contribute to the variance.)

To further understand the concepts of bias and precision, consider a situation in which X only has a systematic bias, with $E_i = 0$ for all subjects (i.e. $\sigma_E^2 = 0$). For example, suppose that the only source of error in a measurement of weight (X) is that the scale weighs each subject exactly 1 kg too heavy. Then, despite this systematic bias, the variable X could be used to order each person correctly in the population by his or her value of T. X would be perfectly precise. However, if E_i varied from person to person (around the mean $\mu_E = 0$), the ordering would be lost. The greater the variance of E, relative to the variance of X, the less precise is X as a measure of T.

The measure of precision we adopt here is the correlation of T with X, ρ_{TX}, termed the *validity coefficient* of X. Under the above model, it can be shown that the square of ρ_{TX} is 1 minus the ratio of the variance of E to the variance of X (Allen and Yen 1979):

$$\rho_{TX}^2 = 1 - \frac{\sigma_E^2}{\sigma_X^2} = \frac{\sigma_T^2}{\sigma_X^2}. \qquad [3.1]$$

ρ_{TX}^2 is also the proportion of the variance of X explained by T. From Equation 3.1 it can be seen that the smaller the error variance, the greater ρ_{TX}^2. ρ_{TX} can range between 0 and 1, with a value of 1 indicating that X is a perfectly precise measure of T. ρ_{TX} is assumed to be 0 or greater; that is, for X to be considered to be a measure of T, X must be positively correlated with T.

Example. Continuing the preceding example, the bias would be measured as the difference between the population mean of X and the population mean of T, which was 1 kg. The precision could be measured by the correlation of T with X. Suppose ρ_{TX} were 0.8, this would mean that only 64 per cent (0.8^2) of the variance in X is explained by T, with the remainder of the variance being due to error.

Measurement error is not an inherent property of an instrument, but rather a property of the instrument applied in a particular manner to a specific population. Therefore, the error can vary not only between two instruments which measure the same exposure, but also for a single instrument when applied differently or when applied to different population groups which vary by, say, level of education. Measurement error could also differ between the population of cases and the population of controls in a case-control study. In addition, the validity coefficient is dependent on the variance of the true exposure in the population (σ_T^2). Therefore, even if the error variance, σ_E^2, were the same for two populations, ρ_{TX} would differ if σ_T^2 differed.

The terminology used in measurement error varies between fields of study. We will use the terms validity, accuracy, and measurement error as general terms describing the accuracy of X as a measure of T, including both the concepts of bias and precision. Some authors use the terms validity and accuracy to refer to lack of bias only. In addition, 'true value' can have various meanings. We define T as the underlying variable of interest. Our definition of the 'true value' is similar to what is termed a 'construct' or 'latent variable' in other fields, although these terms imply that the true value is unmeasurable.

Effects of measurement error on the population mean and variance of exposure

In a study population, both the mean and variance of the measured exposure X differ from the true exposure mean and variance because of measurement error. Under the above model, the population mean of X differs from the true mean (the population mean of T) by b:

$$\mu_X = \mu_T + b.$$

The population variance of X, based on the model and assumptions, is (Allen and Yen 1979):

$$\sigma_X^2 = \sigma_T^2 + \sigma_E^2 = \frac{\sigma_T^2}{\rho_{TX}^2}. \tag{3.2}$$

Thus the variance of X in the population is greater than the variance of T, due to the addition of the variance of the measurement error. From the example given above, if the validity coefficient (ρ_{TX}) were 0.8, then the variance of measured weight X would be 56 per cent greater than the variance of $T (\sigma_X^2 = \sigma_T^2/0.8^2 = 1.56\,\sigma_T^2$ by Equation 3.2).

Figure 3.2 demonstrates the effect of measurement error on the distribution of X in a population assuming, for the purposes of the example, a

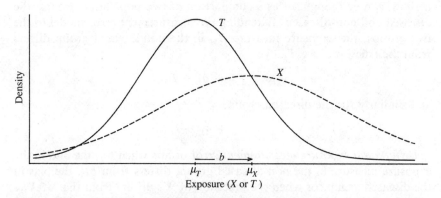

Figure 3.2 The effect of measurement error on the distribution of a normally distributed exposure. T, true exposure; X, exposure measured with error; μ_T, population mean of T; μ_X, population mean of X.

normally distributed exposure and normally distributed error. The bias in the measure causes a shift in the distribution of X compared with T. The imprecision of X (measured by ρ_{TX}) causes a greater variance or dispersion of the distribution of X compared with that of T. Even if a measure were correct on average $(b = 0)$, there could still be substantial effects of measurement error due to lack of precision which would lead to a greater dispersion in the measured exposures.

Effects of differential measurement error on the odds ratio

Measurement errors have an effect on the observable mean and variance of an exposure variable within a population, but of greater concern is the effect of exposure measurement error on the measure of association (e.g. an odds ratio or a correlation) between an exposure and an outcome in a study. In the next few sections of this chapter, examples of such effects of measurement errors will be given.

The equations given in this chapter are based on the assumption that the only source of error in the measure of association between the exposure and disease is measurement error in the exposure. The other sources of bias, including measurement error in the disease, selection bias, confounding, or the error due to sampling a finite number of subjects, are assumed to be absent.

It is common in epidemiological studies to measure the exposure as a continuous variable, and for the outcome to be a dichotomous disease state. The commonly used measure of association is the *odds ratio*, the odds of disease at one level of exposure relative to the odds of disease at another (usually lower) level of exposure; it is an estimate of the rate ratio.

Studies of dichotomous outcomes, whether they are case-control or cohort designs, can be thought of as a comparison of two population groups, the diseased and non-diseased. Extending the measurement error model to the two groups, the exposure measure X_N in the non-diseased group differs from the true exposure T_N by

$$X_{iN} = T_{iN} + b_N + E_{iN}$$

and similarly for the diseased group,

$$X_{iD} = T_{iD} + b_D + E_{iD}.$$

Differential exposure measurement error occurs when b_N, the bias in the exposure measure in the non-diseased group, differs from b_D, the bias in the diseased group, or when the precision of X_N differs from that of X_D.

Figure 3.3 gives a graphical presentation of an example of differential measurement error, specifically differential bias between cases and controls. In the figure, the true mean exposure in the diseased group, μ_{T_D}, is greater

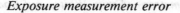

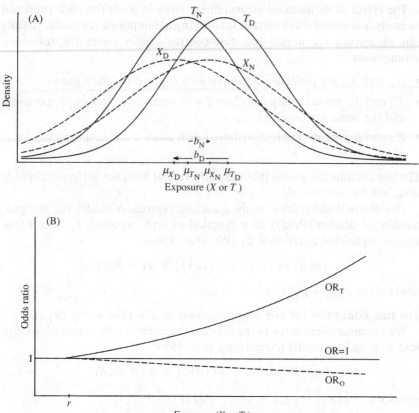

Figure 3.3 The effects of differential measurement error (differential bias) on the distributions of exposure among the non-diseased and diseased groups (A) and on the odds ratio curve (B). T_N and T_D are the true exposures among non-diseased group and diseased group respectively, X_N and X_D are the exposures measured with error among non-diseased group and diseased group respectively, OR_T is the true odds ratio for exposure versus reference level r, and OR_O is the observable odds ratio for exposure versus reference level r.

than the true mean exposure in the non-diseased group, μ_{T_N}. This leads to a positive slope in the true odds ratio curve (OR_T). (The odds ratio curve is shown as the odds ratio for disease among those with exposure level X or T versus an arbitrary reference point (r).) In this example, the bias for the non-diseased group is positive so the distribution of X_N is shifted to the right relative to T_N, and the bias among those with disease is negative so that the distribution of X_D is shifted to the left relative to T_D. This leads the observable odds ratio curve (OR_O) to cross over the null value of 1: it slopes downwards from 1 rather than upwards as X gets larger.

The effect of differential measurement error in X on the odds ratio can be easily quantified when certain simplifying assumptions are made. Results can be derived for unmatched case-control studies under the following assumptions:

- X_N and X_D are modelled as above with $\rho_{TE} = 0$ for each group
- T_N and T_D are normally distributed with means μ_{T_N} and μ_{T_D} respectively and the same variance, σ_T^2
- E_N and E_D are normally distributed with mean 0 and common variance, σ_E^2.

The last assumption means that only differential bias, not differential precision, will be considered.

The above assumptions imply a logistic regression model for the probability of disease $(\Pr(d))$ as a function of true exposure T, with a true logistic regression coefficient β_T (Wu *et al.* 1986):

$$\log \left[\Pr(d)/(1 - \Pr(d)) \right] = \alpha_T + \beta_T T,$$

where $\beta_T = (\mu_{T_D} - \mu_{T_N}) / \sigma_T^2$.

The true odds ratio for any u unit increase in T is $OR_T = \exp(\beta_T u)$.

With measurement error in the exposure variable X, the assumptions also lead to a logistic model (Armstrong *et al.* 1989):

$$\log \left[\Pr(d)/(1 - \Pr(d)) \right] = \alpha_O + \beta_O X,$$

where $\beta_O = [(\mu_{T_D} - \mu_{T_N}) + (b_D - b_N)] / (\sigma_T^2 + \sigma_E^2)$.

The observable logistic regression coefficient, β_O, differs from β_T because of the measurement error in X. β_O can be expressed in terms of β_T (if $\beta_T \neq 0$) as follows:

$$\beta_O = \left(1 + \frac{b_D - b_N}{\mu_{T_D} - \mu_{T_N}} \right) \rho_{TX}^2 \beta_T. \qquad [3.3]$$

β_O differs from β_T by two factors. The effect of the second factor (ρ_{TX}^2), which can range from 0 to 1, is predictable; it has the effect of diminishing the size of β_O in relation to β_T. However, the first factor, which depends on the ratio of $b_D - b_N$ to $\mu_{T_D} - \mu_{T_N}$, can be any magnitude and either positive or negative, so β_O could be greater than or less than the true coefficient β_T, or even have a different sign. Thus the observable odds ratio for any u unit increase in X, $OR_O = \exp(\beta_O u)$, could be closer to the null value of 1, further from the null value, or cross over the null value in comparison with the true odds ratio.

Example. Suppose the study of weight and hip fracture had a case-control design and that the true average weight among cases was 2 kg less than the weight among controls. If the bias of the weight measure among controls (b_N) was 1 kg, but cases had gained an additional 2 kg ($b_D = 3$ kg) between their hip fracture and their participation in the study because of their immobility, then (assuming non-differential precision), by Equation 3.3:

$$\beta_O = \left(1 + \frac{3-1}{-2} \right) \rho^2_{TX}\beta_T = 0.$$

This shows that a differential bias between cases and controls of 2 kg would completely obscure a true difference of −2 kg, leading to no observable association between weight and hip fracture in the study.

The above equations and Figure 3.3 were based on the assumption of an equal error variance, σ^2_E, for the diseased and non-diseased groups, but differential measurement error will also occur if σ^2_E differs between groups. If the biases were equal but if σ^2_E differed (and σ^2_T were equal for the two groups), the shape of the odds ratio function could change. For example, the observable curve could be U-shaped when, in reality, disease frequency increases consistently with increasing exposure (Gregorio *et al.* 1985). These effects of differential precision are generally less of a problem in interpretation of the exposure–disease association than the effects of differential bias described above. Therefore, the assessment of differential bias is generally of greater concern.

Effects of non-differential measurement error on the odds ratio

When the assumptions made in the above section hold, there is *non-differential exposure measurement error* if there is equal bias and equal error variance (or equivalently equal ρ_{TX}) between the diseased and non-diseased groups. Figure 3.4 illustrates the effects of non-differential measurement error. Under non-differential measurement error, the two distributions may shift, but they are not shifted with respect to each other, because there is equal bias for the two groups. Thus, based on the model presented, the observable difference in the mean values of X between cases and controls ($\mu_{X_D} - \mu_{X_N}$) is equal to the true difference ($\mu_{T_D} - \mu_{T_N}$). However, the lack of precision in X widens each distribution and leads to more overlap and less distinction between the distributions of X_N and X_D compared with the true distributions. The odds ratio curve is flattened towards the horizontal line of odds ratio equal to 1 for all X.

When there is non-differential measurement error, and the assumptions of the last section hold, Equation 3.3 can be simplified to (Whittemore and Grosser 1986; Wu *et al.* 1986):

$$\beta_O = \rho^2_{TX}\beta_T. \qquad [3.4]$$

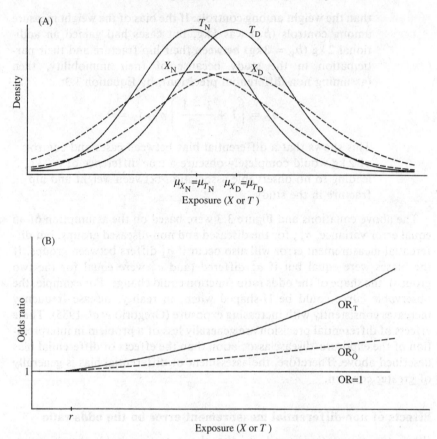

Figure 3.4   The effects of non-differential measurement error on the exposure distributions of the non-diseased and diseased groups (A), and on the odds ratio curve (B). T_N and T_D are the true exposures among non-diseased group and diseased group respectively, X_N and X_D are the exposures measured with error among non-diseased group and diseased group respectively, OR_T is the true odds ratio for exposure versus reference level r, OR_O is the observable odds ratio for exposure versus reference level r.

This states that the observable logistic regression coefficient, β_O, from analyses with X measured with non-differential error is closer to the null value of 0 than the true β_T, by the factor ρ_{TX}^2. Equation 3.4 is referred to as an *attenuation equation*, because it shows that the observable association is attenuated towards the null hypothesis of no association.

While the difference in bias of X between cases and controls ($b_D - b_N$) can play a major role in the bias in the odds ratio under differential measurement error (Equation 3.3), Equation 3.4 shows that the bias in the odds ratio (the attenuation) under non-differential measurement error is a function of the precision of X (measured by ρ_{TX}) but not of the bias in X.

Prentice (1982) has shown that under similar assumptions, Equation 3.4 also approximately applies to estimates of β obtained from the proportional hazards model for data from cohort and matched case-control studies.

There are two ways to interpret attenuation formula 3.4 in terms of the odds ratio. First, if $OR_T = \exp(\beta_T u)$ is the true odds ratio for a u-unit increase in T, and $OR_O = \exp(\beta_O u)$ is the observable odds ratio for a u unit increase in X, then:

$$OR_O = OR_T^{\rho_{TX}^2}. \qquad [3.5]$$

This states that the observable odds ratio for any fixed difference in units of X is equal to the true odds ratio for the same fixed difference in units of T to the power ρ_{TX}^2. Since $0 \le \rho_{TX}^2 \le 1$, the observable odds ratio will be closer to the null value of 1 (no association) than the true odds ratio. The observable odds ratio does not cross over the null value if X and T are, at least, positively correlated.

Example. In a study of coffee intake and myocardial infarction, suppose an intake of five cups per day doubles the risk of disease: $OR_T = 2$ for each increase of five cups per day. If the correlation of the reported 'usual' coffee consumption with the true intake is 0.7, then the observable odds ratio for a five-cup intake is $2^{0.49} = 1.4$ (from Equation 3.5). Thus even when the association between X and T is moderately strong, the resulting attenuation in the odds ratio can be large.

The attenuation formula can also be looked at in another important way. Since one effect of measurement error is to increase the variance of X compared with T (Equation 3.2), there would be a greater spread of misclassified exposures than true exposures within the groups of cases and controls (as in Figure 3.4). Rather than comparing OR_T to OR_O based on some fixed difference in *units* of T or X, one might compare OR_T for a difference in terms of the standard deviation of T to OR_O for the same difference in terms of the standard deviation of X. The true odds ratio of disease for an increase in T of s standard deviations of T is

$$OR_T = \exp(\beta_T s \sigma_T).$$

The observable odds ratio of disease for an increase in X of s standard deviations of X is (de Klerk *et al.* 1989)

$$OR_O = \exp(\beta_O s \sigma_X) = OR_T^{\rho_{TX}}. \qquad [3.6]$$

This states that the observable odds ratio for a difference of s standard deviations of X is equal to the true odds ratio for a difference of s standard deviations of T to the power ρ_{TX}. Comparing Equation 3.6 with Equation 3.5, it is apparent that the atttenuation is less when the observable odds ratio is *interpreted* in terms of the standard deviation (or more generally, the distribution) of X, rather than interpreting the odds ratio in actual units of X.

Example. Using the coffee consumption and myocardial infarction example again, suppose that the true standard deviation of coffee intake per day is 2.5 cups and the true odds ratio for an increase of two standard deviations of T (five cups), OR_T, is 2. If $\rho_{TX} = 0.7$, the standard deviation of X is 3.57 (2.5/0.7 from Equation 3.2). Then, from Equation 3.6, the observable odds ratio for an increase of two standard deviations of X is $2^{0.7} = 1.6$. The interpretation of the observable odds ratio of 1.6 as the odds ratio for a difference of two standard deviations in exposure is more accurate than interpreting the observable odds ratio of 1.4 (from the previous example) as a measure of the odds ratio for a five-cup difference in exposure.

Further examples of the effects of non-differential measurement error on the odds ratio, based on Equations 3.5 and 3.6, are given in Table 3.3 (columns 3 and 4). The table shows that exposures with a validity coeffi-

Table 3.3 Effect of non-differential measurement error in a normally distributed exposure X on the observable odds ratio (OR_O)

ρ_{TX}^a	OR_T^b	u unit difference in X OR_O	$s\sigma_X$ difference in X OR_O	Upper versus lower quarter of X OR_O
0.5	1.5	1.11	1.22	1.19
0.7	1.5	1.22	1.33	1.29
0.9	1.5	1.39	1.44	1.39
0.5	2.0	1.19	1.41	1.35
0.7	2.0	1.40	1.62	1.54
0.9	2.0	1.75	1.87	1.76
0.5	4.0	1.41	2.00	1.81
0.7	4.0	1.97	2.64	2.35
0.9	4.0	3.07	3.48	3.11

[a] ρ_{TX} is the validity coefficient of X.
[b] OR_T represents the true odds ratio for a u unit difference in T for comparison to OR_O for a u-unit difference in X, OR_T represents the true odds ratio for an $s\sigma_T$ difference in T for comparison to OR_O for an $s\sigma_X$ difference in X, and OR_T represents the true odds ratio for the upper versus lower quarter of T for comparison to OR_O for the upper versus lower quarter of X.

cient, ρ_{TX}, near 0.5 would obscure all but the strongest associations, while measures so accurate as to have ρ_{TX} of 0.9 still lead to appreciable attenuation.

Effects of non-differential measurement error on power and sample size

Measurement error in X also affects the power of a study, or the sample size needed. For example, unmatched case-control studies often employ a sample size calculation based on the normality assumption for the exposure variable as follows:

$$n = 2[(Z_{\alpha/2} + Z_\beta)^2 \sigma^2]/d^2,$$

where $Z_{\alpha/2}$ denotes the upper 100 $(1 - \alpha/2)$ centile of the standard normal distribution, d is the magnitude of the difference to be detected between the mean exposure of the cases and controls, σ^2 is the common variance of the exposure in each group, α is the significance level for a two-sided test of the hypothesis, β is 1 minus the required power, and n is the sample size needed in each group (Kelsey *et al.* 1986).

The effect of non-differential measurement error under the model used in this chapter is to increase the variance of X such that $\sigma_X^2 = \sigma_T^2/\rho_{TX}^2$, while d would remain the same. Then n_X, the sample size needed to detect a difference of d in a study with non-differential measurement error, with reference to n_T, the sample size needed in a study in which the exposure is measured without error, is (Fleiss 1986)

$$n_X = n_T/\rho_{TX}^2. \qquad [3.7]$$

This formula may be of theoretical interest only, since an empirical estimate of σ_X^2 is usually available for the calculation of sample size. However, it can be used to show the potentially dramatic effects of poor exposure measurement on the sample size required. For example, if the correlation between T and X is 0.7 $(\rho_{TX}^2 = 0.49)$, then the sample size required when the imperfect measure is used is twice that required if a perfect measure were available.

Measurement error can also have adverse effects on the power of a study. The power of a case-control study involving a normally distributed exposure with common standard deviation σ and mean difference d can be derived from the following equation (Kelsey *et al.* 1986):

$$\text{power} = 1 - \Phi\left(\frac{d}{\sigma}\sqrt{\frac{1}{2}n} - Z_{\alpha/2}\right)$$

where $\Phi(z)$ is the probability that a standard normal variable is above z. As noted above, the effect of non-differential measurement error is to increase the standard deviation in the formula, such that $\sigma_X = \sigma_T/\rho_{TX}$. If an empirical estimate of σ_X is not available during the planning of a study, and if the sample size is miscalculated based on the variance of a more precise measure of exposure (as may be the case for measurements in a small-scale, well-controlled pilot study), the power of the study will be less than predicted.

Example. Suppose a sample size for a study is calculated to be able to detect a difference between cases and controls of 10 months in the mean exposure to a certain drug. An estimated standard deviation of 40 months for duration of exposure was based on medical record reviews. Then the sample size for a two-sided α of 5 per cent and 80 per cent power would be:

$$n = 2[(1.96 + 0.84)^2 40^2]/(10)^2$$
$$= 251 \text{ per group.}$$

Suppose that the record review gave nearly perfect measurements of the exposure, but the study exposure will actually be measured by self-report which has non-differential error such that $\rho_{TX} = 0.7$. Then the standard deviation of the study measure would be σ_T/ρ_{TX} or 57 months, and the study power would not be the calculated 80 per cent but instead only 50 per cent:

$$\text{power} = 1 - \Phi\left(\frac{10}{57}\sqrt{\frac{251}{2}} - 1.96\right)$$
$$= 50\%.$$

Effects of measurement error on measures of association between a continuous exposure and a continuous outcome

The effect of measurement error on the relationship of a continuous exposure with a continuous outcome also deserves mention. Suppose the relationship between a continuous exposure X and a continuous outcome Y is to be studied, and their association is to be assessed by correlation and regression. Suppose the measurement error in X is given by the model described on page 51, and Y is measured without error. There is non-differential measurement error in X with respect to the outcome Y when E is uncorrelated with Y. The observable correlation coefficient of X with Y in these circumstances is given by (Allen and Yen 1979)

$$\rho_{XY} = \rho_{TY}\rho_{TX}. \tag{3.8}$$

This equation states that the observable correlation ρ_{XY} is weaker than the true correlation ρ_{TY} by a factor equal to the validity coefficient of X.

Example. Suppose that the true correlation of physical activity over the preceding 5 years and current body mass index (ρ_{TY}) is 0.7. Assume that body mass index (weight/height^2) is measured without error, but the correlation of true activity level with physical activity as ascertained by a self-administered questionnaire in the study population (ρ_{TX}) is 0.6. Also assume that the error in the assessment of physical activity is not correlated with body mass index. Then the observable correlation coefficient (ρ_{XY}) in the study is (by Equation 3.8) $0.7 \times 0.6 = 0.4$, a considerable attenuation from the true association of 0.7.

If β_T is the true regression coefficient from the regression equation

$$Y = \alpha_T + \beta_T T,$$

then the observable regression coefficient β_O from the regression equation

$$Y = \alpha_O + \beta_O X,$$

is (Allen and Yen 1979)

$$\beta_O = \rho_{TX}^2 \beta_T. \tag{3.9}$$

Note that Equation 3.9 is identical to Equation 3.4. Also note that the attenuation formulas 3.8 and 3.9 are functions of ρ_{TX} but not of the bias in X. This is because adding a constant to a variable does not change its coefficient of correlation with another variable, or its regression coefficient.

Differential measurement error can have any effect on the correlation or regression coefficients. Depending on the nature of the relationship between E and Y, the association between X and Y could be stronger or weaker than the true association, or even have the opposite sign.

Violations of the assumptions

In this chapter, several simplifying assumptions have been made. First, the model states that X is a measure of T with a simple additive error E, and that ρ_{TE} is 0. In other words, large positive errors are not more (or less) common for large values of T. However, it is likely that in some situations the size of the error would depend on T. For example if X were a measure of the lifetime number of X-ray procedures, the under-ascertainment might become greater with increasing true lifetime numbers of procedures. A related violation may come about if X is a measure of T, but on a different scale of measurement. These violations are examples of a model in which X is a linear function of T (or equivalently, part of the error is proportional to T) as follows:

$$X_i = cT_i + b + E_i.$$

Only Equations 3.6, 3.7, and 3.8 still hold under this model. These equations do not change under a linear transformations of X.

Several other assumptions have been made, including the normality of T and E in equations expressing the effect of measurement error on logistic regression, and the assumptions of no sampling error, no confounding, and no error in ascertainment of disease. The purpose of the equations presented above is to permit estimation of the effects of varying degrees of measurement error in a simplified situation, to aid in the interpretation of the effects of measurement error. In actual studies of a continuous exposure, the distribution of the true exposure among cases and controls and the distribution of errors can take on almost any form. Unlike the simple model presented, the shape of the odds ratio curve could change under non-differential measurement error, and for some levels of exposure, the odds ratio could be biased away from the null or cross over the null value of 1 (Dosemeci *et al*. 1990). Further discussion of these limitations, as well as references to results derived under less restrictive assumptions, are given in Chapter 5.

CATEGORICAL EXPOSURE MEASURES

Measurement error in categorical variables is usually referred to as misclassification. Categorical variables, including dichotomous, nominal categorical or ordered categorical variables, are subject to all the sources of measurement error outlined in Table 3.1.

Measures of misclassification in categorical variables

Misclassification of exposure implies that a certain proportion of subjects who truly fall into a specific exposure category will be correctly classified, but the remainder will be misclassified into other categories. For all types of categorical variables, the measurement error for a population can be described in a *misclassification matrix*. This is a matrix of the proportions, C_{ij}, of those with true exposure category j, who will be classified into category i. This matrix can be represented as follows:

$$
\begin{array}{cc}
 & \text{True exposure } j \\
\end{array}
$$

$$
\begin{array}{cc}
\text{Classified} \\
\text{exposure } i
\end{array}
\quad
\begin{array}{c}
1 \\ 2 \\ \vdots \\ k
\end{array}
\begin{bmatrix}
C_{11} & C_{12} & \dots & C_{1k} \\
C_{21} & C_{22} & \dots & C_{2k} \\
\vdots & \vdots & & \vdots \\
C_{k1} & C_{k2} & \dots & C_{kk}
\end{bmatrix}
$$

$$
\text{Total} \quad 1 \quad\quad 1 \quad\quad\quad 1
$$

where k is the number of categories. Note that the C_{ij} sum down each column to 1 (the sum over true exposure j). The diagonal elements quantify the proportions correctly classified; a measure is perfect when the diagonal elements are all 1. As noted for measures of measurement error in continuous variables, the misclassification matrix depends on the instrument, the operational procedures, and the population to which the instrument is applied, and can differ by disease status and between different population groups.

For a dichotomous exposure ($k = 2$), only two classification probabilities are needed: the sensitivity and the specificity of the exposure measure. (The terms sensitivity and specificity are more commonly used to define the accuracy of a diagnostic test for disease, but the terms apply equally to accuracy of a dichotomous exposure measurement.) The *sensitivity* of the exposure measure is the proportion of those who truly have the exposure who will be correctly classified as exposed, and the *specificity* is the proportion of those who are truly unexposed who will be classified as unexposed. If category 1 is 'exposed' and 2 'unexposed' the misclassification matrix would be:

$$\begin{bmatrix} \text{sensitivity} & 1 - \text{specificity} \\ 1 - \text{sensitivity} & \text{specificity} \end{bmatrix}$$

The probability of misclassifying a truly exposed person as unexposed is $(1 - \text{sensitivity})$ and the probability of misclassifying a truly unexposed person is $(1 - \text{specificity})$.

Even though both sensitivity and specificity can range from 0 to 1, it is assumed that

$$\text{sensitivity} + \text{specificity} \geq 1.$$

In other words, for the instrument to be considered a measure of the exposure, it should classify a truly exposed person as exposed with greater (or at least equal) probability than it classifies a truly unexposed person as exposed.

Effects of misclassification on the observable distribution of exposure in a population

The misclassification matrix relates the true distribution of exposure in a population to the misclassified distribution. For a population whose true distribution into the k categories of exposure (expressed as proportions) is $[P_1, P_2,...,P_k]$, the observable (misclassified) distribution would be $[p_1, p_2,...,p_k]$ acording to this matrix equation:

$$\begin{bmatrix} C_{11} & \cdots & C_{1k} \\ \cdot & & \cdot \\ \cdot & & \cdot \\ \cdot & & \cdot \\ C_{k1} & \cdots & C_{kk} \end{bmatrix} \times \begin{bmatrix} P_1 \\ \cdot \\ \cdot \\ \cdot \\ P_k \end{bmatrix} = \begin{bmatrix} p_1 \\ \cdot \\ \cdot \\ \cdot \\ p_k \end{bmatrix} \qquad [3.10]$$

or in non-matrix form:

$$p_i = \sum_j C_{ij} P_j.$$

This equation shows that some proportion of people in each of the true categories may fall into each of the observable categories. Applying it to a dichotomous exposure, the observable proportion of the population who are exposed, p, is composed of a proportion (sensitivity) of those truly exposed (P) and a proportion ($1 -$ specificity) of those unexposed ($1 - P$):

$$p = \text{sensitivity} \times P + (1 - \text{specificity}) \times (1 - P). \qquad [3.11]$$

Effects of differential misclassification of a dichotomous exposure on the odds ratio

While the above equations express the effect of misclassification within one population, a more common situation in epidemiology is the comparison of exposure between two populations: those with the disease of interest and those without. The effects of misclassification of categorical exposure measures are straightforward for two types of studies: studies of the association between a dichotomous exposure and a dichotomous disease outcome (Bross 1954; Newell 1962; Gullen *et al.* 1968; Goldberg 1975; Copeland *et al.* 1977; Barron 1977; Fleiss 1981; Kleinbaum *et al.* 1982) and, under certain assumptions, studies of an ordered categorical exposure and a dichotomous disease outcome (Walker and Blettner 1985; de Klerk *et al.* 1989).

In an unmatched case-control study of a dichotomous exposure, under the assumption that the disease is measured without error, the effect of misclassification of exposure is to rearrange individuals in the true 2×2 table into an observable 2×2 table. Individuals in the diseased group remain in the diseased group but may be misclassified as to exposure status, and the non-diseased group is also rearranged as shown in Fig. 3.5. P_D and P_N are the true proportions exposed in the diseased and non-diseased groups respectively, and similarly p_D and p_N refer to the observable proportions exposed in the two groups.

There is *differential misclassification* when the sensitivity of the exposure measure for the diseased group (sens_D) differs from that for the non-diseased group (sens_N), or the specificity of exposure for the diseased group

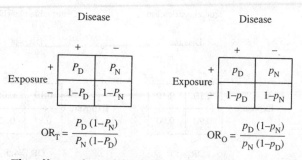

$$OR_T = \frac{P_D(1-P_N)}{P_N(1-P_D)} \qquad\qquad OR_O = \frac{p_D(1-p_N)}{p_N(1-p_D)}$$

Figure 3.5 The effects of misclassification of a dichotomous exposure on the distribution of exposure and the odds ratio. (P_D and P_N are the true proportions exposed in the diseased and non-diseased groups respectively, p_D and p_N are the observable proportions in each group, OR_T is the true exposure and OR_O is the observable odds ratio).

($spec_D$) differs from that for the non-diseased group ($spec_N$), or both. The observable odds ratio can be calculated by applying Equation 3.11 separately to the diseased and non-diseased groups (Goldberg 1975):

$$\left.\begin{aligned}
p_D &= sens_D P_D + (1 - spec_D)(1 - P_D) \\
p_N &= sens_N P_N + (1 - spec_N)(1 - P_N) \\
OR_O &= [p_D(1 - p_N)] / [p_N(1 - p_D)].
\end{aligned}\right\} \qquad [3.12]$$

As with continuous exposures, differential misclassification can have any kind of effect on the odds ratio; in comparison with the true odds ratio, the observable odds ratio can be closer to the null hypothesis of $OR = 1$, be further from the null, or cross over the null.

Example. In a case-control study of the relationship between maternal use of illegal drugs during pregnancy and infant birth defects, suppose all of the exposed mothers of the children with birth defects felt committed to accurately disclose any illegal drug use ($sens_D = 1.0$), while only half of exposed mothers of control children were inclined to admit drug use ($sens_N = 0.5$). Similarly, suppose that some (10 per cent) unexposed mothers of cases reported using illegal drugs during pregnancy ($spec_D = 0.9$) out of concern about the effects of use before pregnancy, while the unexposed control mothers accurately reported no use ($spec_N = 1.0$). Then if the true classification is as shown, the observable classification and observable odds ratio would be as follows (from Equations 3.12):

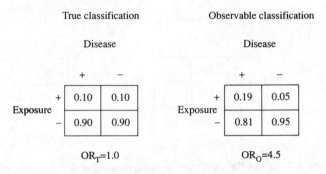

	True classification				Observable classification	
	Disease				Disease	

Thus, a true odds ratio of 1.0, that is, no association between the disease and exposure, could appear as a strong association because of differential misclassification.

Effects of non-differential misclassification of a dichotomous exposure on the odds ratio

Non-differential misclassification occurs when the sensitivity and specificity of the exposure measurement for the diseased group are equal to those for the non-diseased group. The effect of misclassification of disease on the odds ratio can be computed as in Equations 3.12, except that there is a common sensitivity and a common specificity for the diseased and non-diseased groups.

Table 3.4 gives examples of the effect of non-differential misclassification on the odds ratio. The observable odds ratio depends not only on the true odds ratio, the sensitivity, and the specificity, but also on the probability of exposure among the non-diseased. Non-differential misclassification leads to an attenuation of the odds ratio towards the null value of 1 (Gullen *et al.* 1968). As can be seen from the table, the attenuation can be appreciable even with a high sensitivity and specificity. For example, a true odds ratio of 4 is attenuated to 2.85 when sensitivity is 0.9, specificity is 0.9, and P_N is 0.5. The observable odds ratio does not 'cross over' the null value of 1 if, at least, the measurement classifies a truly exposed person as exposed with the same or greater probability as it classifies a truly unexposed person as exposed (i.e. sensitivity + specificity $\geq$ 1).

The results in Equations 3.12 for differential and non-differential misclassification of exposure in case-control studies also apply to cohort studies. However, for cohort studies in which exposed persons are over-sampled in comparison with unexposed persons, the sensitivity and specificity of the exposure measurement change after the sampling. In such cohort studies, the true 2 × 2 table can be considered to represent the entire population

Table 3.4 Effect of non-differential misclassification of a dichotomous exposure on the observable odds ratio (OR_O)

| | | | True odds ratio | | |
| | | | $OR_T = 1.5$ | $OR_T = 2.0$ | $OR_T = 4.0$ |
Exposure sensitivity	Exposure specificity	P_N^a	OR_O	OR_O	OR_O
0.6	0.9	0.1	1.17	1.34	1.93
0.6	0.9	0.5	1.24	1.42	1.86
0.6	0.99	0.1	1.40	1.79	3.20
0.6	0.99	0.5	1.30	1.54	2.12
0.9	0.9	0.1	1.24	1.48	2.41
0.9	0.9	0.5	1.38	1.73	2.85
0.9	0.99	0.1	1.45	1.89	3.61
0.9	0.99	0.5	1.43	1.82	3.11

^{a} P_N is the proportion exposed in the non-diseased group. P_D, the proportion exposed in the diseased group, is by definition

$$P_D = P_N OR_T / (1 + P_N(OR_T - 1)).$$

(before sampling), stratified by future disease status. Before one can sample by exposure, the population must be 'measured' as to exposure, leading to the misclassified 2 × 2 table and the resulting observable (future) odds ratio. The cohort sampling is based on the *misclassified* population, and that sampling does not change the observable odds ratio. However, *within* the cohort study after sampling, the sensitivity of the exposure measure is greater than the population sensitivity because exposed individuals who were correctly classified are more likely to enter the study than exposed individuals who were incorrectly classified as unexposed. The specificity also changes, as do the probabilities of exposure in the diseased and non-diseased groups.

Effects of non-differential misclassification of a dichotomous exposure on sample size and power

Non-differential misclassification leads to an increase in the sample size required for a study, because the observable odds ratio is attenuated. Sample size calculations for case-control studies usually depend on the hypothesized odds ratio and the proportion of the non-diseased group exposed. For cohort studies they depend on the odds ratio and the probability of disease among the non-exposed group. In planning a study, the sample size calculations should be based on estimates of the observable study parameters rather than estimates based on studies in which the exposure is measured with greater accuracy. If the increased sample size requirement due to misclassification is not taken into consideration in planning the study, non-differential misclassification results in a fall in study power (Bross 1954; Mote and Anderson 1965; Quade *et al.* 1980).

Example. Suppose animal experiments suggest that breast cancer risk is dependent on selenium intake. A case-control study of this relationship may classify case and control women into two exposure categories: those above the control median of selenium intake, and those below. The results of animal studies, which could measure selenium intake accurately, are extrapolated to yield a study hypothesis that those in the upper half of intake will have 0.6 times the risk as those in the lower half (OR = 0.6). The sample size based on this hypothesized odds ratio, equal-sized study groups, $\alpha = 0.05$, and 80 per cent power is (Kelsey *et al.* 1986):

$$n = \frac{2(Z_{\alpha/2} + Z_{\beta})^2 \bar{P}(1 - \bar{P})}{(P_D - P_N)^2} = 247 \text{ per group,}$$

where

$$P_D = \frac{P_N OR}{1 + P_N(OR - 1)} = 0.375$$

is the probability of exposure in the diseased group, P_N is the probability of exposure in the control group (0.5 in this example), and $\bar{P}$ is the mean exposure of the two groups. Suppose selenium intake over the etiologically relevant time period is difficult to measure in the study population, such that the sensitivity of the measure is 0.7 and the specificity 0.7 for both cases and controls. Then the observable odds ratio would equal 0.8 (by Equations 3.12). If the sample size of 247 for each group were used, the actual study power would only be 20 per cent.

Effects of non-differential misclassification in an ordered categorical exposure on the odds ratio

The effects of differential and non-differential misclassification can also be predicted for categorical exposure variables other than dichotomous variables. If the misclassification matrix for cases and controls were known and the true distribution of exposure among cases and non-cases were known, then Equation 3.10 could be applied separately to cases and controls. The resulting observable distribution of exposure among cases and controls could be used to calculate the observable odds ratios for a comparison of disease risk for each category of exposure versus the reference category.

When there are more than two categories of exposure, general conclusions cannot be drawn about the effect of non-differential misclassification on the odds ratio for each category (Dosemeci *et al.* 1990).

One special case of interest is non-differential misclassification of an ordered categorical exposure variable, when, as is common in epidemiology, the exposure variable is derived by dividing a continuous variable X into discrete categories. X is assumed to be measured with error as in the measurement error model presented for continuous variables, with X, T, and E normally distributed. Under these assumptions, the joint distribution of X and T is bivariate normal with correlation coefficient ρ_{TX}. This joint distribution can be used to quantify the misclassification matrix for an ordered categorical variable in which X is divided into categories (e.g. quarters or fifths) based on quantiles of X in the non-diseased group (Walker and Blettner 1985; de Klerk *et al.* 1989).

The last column of Table 3.3 gives examples of the attenuation of the odds ratio for those in the upper quarter of exposure versus the lowest quarter for several values of ρ_{TX} and of OR_T, the true odds ratio for those in the upper quarter versus the lowest quarter. The attenuation appears to be somewhat *more* (by about 10 per cent of OR_T) than that which would be predicted based on the attenuation formula for the odds ratio in the logistic model interpreted in terms of the distribution of the measured exposure (last column versus fourth column of Table 3.3) (de Klerk *et al.* 1989).

This indicates that classifying a continuous exposure into a small number of categories is not a useful approach to reducing the effects of measurement error. Classifying subjects into broad categories of exposure may appear to lessen the chance of measurement error in comparison with attempting to classify subjects more finely (e.g. a 'continuous' measure), because small errors may not be sufficient to misclassify a subject. However, this apparent protection from error is lost as a consequence of the fact that when a subject does move from one broad category to another the error is larger than when a finer categorization is used.

Categorizing a continuous variable does, however, have an advantage. It generally leads to an interpretation of the odds ratio in terms of the distribution of exposure, an approach that lessens the consequences of measurement error in comparison with interpreting the odds ratio in terms of units of exposure (last column compared with third column of Table 3.3).

EFFECT OF MEASUREMENT ERROR IN THE PRESENCE OF COVARIATES

In analysing the relationship between an exposure and an outcome, it is usually necessary to adjust for confounding factors. These factors, often exposures of interest themselves, are also subject to the sources of measurement error discussed in this chapter. For example, in a study with body weight as a primary exposure, it may be necessary to adjust for the potentially confounding effects of dietary intake of energy, an exposure which would be more difficult to assess accurately than the primary exposure.

The effects of measurement error in the primary exposure and covariates has been explored for a range of study designs and assumptions (Greenland 1980; Prentice 1982; Kupper 1984; Kelsey *et al*. 1986; Liu 1988; Prentice *et al*. 1989; Armstrong *et al*. 1989; Chen 1989). The effects can be quantified with reference to the multivariate distribution of the true and misclassified exposure and covariates. The effects of non-differential measurement error are similar for studies in which both the primary exposure and confounder are continuous bivariate normal variables (Armstrong *et al*. 1989), or the exposure and confounder are dichotomous (Greenland 1980), if the exposure error is independent of the confounder and the confounder error, and vice versa. When the confounding factor is measured with non-differential error, but the exposure is measured perfectly, residual confounding can remain after adjustment. Therefore the adjusted observed disease–exposure association could appear stronger (or weaker) than the true adjusted association. Adjustment by use of a poor measure of the confounder may be equivalent to no control of the confounder at all. When the exposure is measured with non-differential error and the covariate is measured perfectly, the attenuation toward the null of the adjusted disease–exposure association can be even greater than the attenuation of the crude association. When both the exposure and the confounder are measured with error, either of these effects can dominate so that the adjusted measure of association could be stronger or weaker than the true association.

Measurement error can also induce spurious effect modification. As noted earlier, the effect of measurement error on the odds ratio is dependent on the distribution of exposure (σ_T^2 for continuous variables and the true proportion exposed for dichotomous variables). Therefore when comparing, for example, the odds ratios across two or more groups categorized by the potential effect modifier, the observable odds ratios may differ even if the true odds ratios are identical, due to the differential effect of measurement error in these groups.

SUMMARY

Validity is not an inherent property of an instrument; it is a property of an instrument applied in a particular research context. For a continuous exposure X, the validity or measurement error in X can be represented by the bias ($\mu_X - \mu_T$) and by the validity coefficient, ρ_{TX}, the correlation of the true exposure T with the measured exposure X in the population. For categorical variables, the measurement error is quantified by the misclassification matrix, or equivalently, the sensitivity and the specificity for a dichotomous exposure measure. For studies comparing diseased and non-diseased groups, these measures should be assessed separately in the two groups.

Differential measurement error occurs when exposure measurement error varies by outcome status (e.g. diseased or non-diseased). It can cause the observed association between the measured exposure and the outcome to appear stronger or weaker than the true association, or can lead to an association in the opposite direction, thus completely invalidating the results of the study. For continuous exposures, differential bias is the major concern because it can lead to more untoward effects than differential precision.

Non-differential exposure measurement error can lead (although not invariably) to attenuation toward the null value of no association in the measure of association between the exposure and the outcome. This attenuation calls for a larger study sample size or, for a fixed sample size, gives less power to detect an association.

There are some important conclusions regarding the effects of non-differential measurement error:

- The magnitude of the bias in the odds ratio or the correlation coefficient does not depend on the sample size, so that increasing the sample size does not reduce the bias. However, increasing the sample size would increase the power to detect the attenuated association as significantly different from the null hypothesis.

- Interpreting the observed odds ratio in terms of the observed distribution of the exposure (e.g., the odds ratio for a one standard deviation increase in exposure, or for the upper quarter versus the lower quarter of exposure), rather than in terms of measured units of the exposure, provides a more accurate view of the odds ratio.

- A continuous exposure measurement that is 'good on average' (bias equal to 0 for both diseased and non-diseased) does not eliminate the effects of measurement error from the results of an analytical study. When there is non-differential measurement error in a continuous exposure measure X, it is not the bias in the measure but rather the degree of precision of X (measured by ρ_{TX}) that leads to bias in the measure of association between X and the outcome.

- Classifying individuals into ordered categories generally does not lessen the attenuation of the odds ratio due to measurement error.

The effects of measurement errors on measures of association between exposure and disease, on study sample size, and on study power can be estimated from simple equations under certain assumptions. These effects can be substantial and justify concern about the accuracy of exposure measurement in epidemiological studies. Elimination of differential measurement errors should be the highest priority and reduction of non-differential errors should be a major concern in the design and conduct of studies.

REFERENCES

Allen, M. J. and Yen, W. M. (1979). *Introduction to measurement theory*, pp. 1–117. Brooks/Cole, Monterey.

Armstrong, B.G., Whittemore, A.S., and Howe, G.R. (1989). Analysis of case-control data with covariate measurement error: Application to diet and colon cancer. *Statistics in Medicine*, **8**, 1151–63.

Barron, B.A. (1977). The effects of misclassification on the estimation of relative risk. *Biometrics*, **33**, 414–8.

Bohrnstedt, G.W. (1983). Measurement. In *Handbook of survey research*, (ed. P.H. Rossi, J.D. Wright, A.B. Anderson), pp. 70–121. Academic Press, Orlando, Florida.

Bross, I. (1954). Misclassification in 2 × 2 tables. *Biometrics*, **10**, 478–86.

Chen, T.T. (1989). A review of methods for misclassified categorical data in epidemiology. *Statistics in Medicine*, **8**, 1095–106.

Cochran, W.G. (1968). Errors of measurement in statistics. *Technometrics*, **10**, 637–66.

Copeland, K.T., Checkoway, H., McMichael, A.J., and Holbrook, R.H. (1977). Bias due to misclassification in the estimation of relative risk. *American Journal of Epidemiology*, **105**, 488–95.

de Klerk, N.H., English, D.R., and Armstrong, B.K. (1989). A review of the effects of random measurement error on relative risk estimates in epidemiological studies. *International Journal of Epidemiology*, **18**, 705–12.

Dosemeci, M., Wacholder, S., and Lubin, J.H. (1990). Does nondifferential misclassification of the exposure always bias a true effect toward the null value? *American Journal of Epidemiology*, **132**, 746–8.

Fleiss, J.L. (1981). *Statistical methods for rates and proportions*, (2nd edn), pp. 188–211. John Wiley and Sons, New York.

Fleiss, J.L. (1986). *The design and analysis of clinical experiments*, pp. 1,5. John Wiley and Sons, New York.

Fuller, W.A. (1987). *Measurement error models*. John Wiley and Sons, New York.

Goldberg, J.D. (1975). The effects of misclassification on the bias in the difference between two proportions and the relative odds in the fourfold table. *Journal of the American Statistical Association*, **70**, 561–7.

Greenland, S. (1980). The effect of misclassification in the presence of covariates. *American Journal of Epidemiology*, **112**, 564–9.

Gregorio, D.I., Marshall, J.R., and Zielenzny, M. (1985). Fluctuations in odds ratios due to variance differences in case-control studies. *American Journal of Epidemiology*, **121**, 767–74.

Gullen, W.H., Bearman, J.E., and Johnson, E.A. (1968). Effects of misclassification in epidemiologic studies. *Public Health Reports*, **83**, 914–8.

Hansen, M.H., Hurwitz, W.N., and Bershad, M. (1961). Measurement errors in censuses and surveys. *Bulletin of the International Statistical Institute*, **38**, 359–74.

Kelsey, J.L., Thompson, W.S., and Evans, A.S. (1986). *Methods in observational epidemiology*, pp. 254–308. Oxford University Press, New York.

Kleinbaum, D.G., Kupper, L.L., and Morgenstern, H. (1982). *Epidemiologic Research*, pp. 183–93, 220–41. Lifetime Learning Publications, Belmont, California.

Kupper, L.L. (1984). Effect of the use of unrealiable surrogate variables on the validity of epidemiologic research studies. *American Journal of Epidemiology*, **120**, 643–8.

Liu, K. (1988). Measurement error and its impact on partial correlation and multiple linear regression analyses. *American Journal of Epidemiology*, **127**, 864–74.

Lord, F.M. and Novick, M.R. (1968). *Statistical theories of mental test scores*. Addison-Wesley, Reading, Massachussetts.

Mote, V.L. and Anderson, R.L. (1965). An investigation of the effect of misclassification on the properties of χ^2-tests in the analysis of categorical data. *Biometrika*, **62**, 95–109.

Newell, D.J. (1962). Errors in the interpretation of errors in epidemiology. *American Journal of Public Health*, **52**, 1925–8.

Nunnally, J.C. (1978). *Psychometric theory*, (2nd edn), pp. 190–225. McGraw-Hill, New York.

Prentice, R.L. (1982). Covariate measurement errors and parameter estimation in a failure time regression model. *Biometrika*, **69**, 331–42.

Prentice, R.L., Pepe, M., and Self, S.G. (1989). Dietary fat and breast cancer: A quantitative assessment of the epidemiological literature and a discussion of methodological issues. *Cancer Research*, **49**, 3147–56.

Quade, D., Lachenbruch, P.A., Whaley, F.S., McClish, D.K., and Haley, R.W. (1980). Effects of misclassification on statistical inferences in epidemiology. *American Journal of Epidemiology*, **111**, 503–15.

Walker, A.M. and Blettner, M. (1985). Comparing imperfect measures of exposure. *American Journal of Epidemiology*, **121**, 783–90.

Whittemore, A.S. and Grosser, S. (1986). Regression methods for data with incomplete covariates. In *Modern statistical methods in chronic disease*, (ed. S.H. Moolgavkar and R.L. Prentice), pp. 19–34. John Wiley and Sons, New York.

Wu, M.L., Whittemore, A.S., and Jung, D.L. (1986). Errors in reported dietary intakes: I. Short-term recall. *American Journal of Epidemiology*, **124**, 826–35.

4

Validity and reliability studies

One must go seek more facts, paying less attention to techniques of handling the data and far more to the development and perfection of the methods of obtaining them. (Hill 1953)

INTRODUCTION

The serious adverse effects of the use of invalid exposure measurements have been described in Chapter 3. Selecting or developing an accurate measurement instrument is obviously a critical step in designing an epidemiological study. First, the available literature on the validity and reliability of instruments which measure the exposure of interest should be reviewed. Then, if a new instrument is to be developed which differs substantially from other methods, its reliability or, preferably, its validity should be assessed.

The term *reliability* is generally used to refer to the reproducibility of a measure, that is, how consistently a measurement can be repeated on the same subjects. Reliability can be assessed in a number of ways, of which only two are covered in this chapter. *Intramethod reliability* is a measure of the reproducibility of an instrument, either applied in the same manner to the same subjects at two or more points in time (test–retest reliability) or applied by two or more data collectors to the same subjects (inter-rater reliability). For example, a comparison could be made of exposure information from two data abstractors who extracted information from the medical records of the same group of subjects. *Intermethod reliability* is a measure of the ability of two different instruments which measure the same underlying exposure to yield similar results on the same subjects. Generally an intermethod reliability study compares a measurement method to be used in an epidemiological study with a more accurate but more burdensome method. For example, a questionnaire might be compared to an exposure diary for a group of subjects. Intermethod reliability studies of this type are sometimes called *validity studies*. Technically, however, an error-free comparison method of measurement is needed to directly measure validity, so the term intermethod reliability has been preferred. In most fields of study, the term reliability refers to intramethod reliability, and less work has been done on the design and interpretation of intermethod reliability studies. Intermethod reliability studies are dealt with in detail in this chapter because of their potential importance in epidemiology.

The first topic to be covered in this chapter is the relationship of measures of reliability to measures of validity. Measures of reliability are primarily important for what they reveal about the validity of a measurement, for, as shown in Chapter 3, the bias in an epidemiological study is a function of the validity of the exposure measure. The second section covers additional issues in the design of reliability and validity studies, and the third covers the statistical analysis of reliability and validity studies.

Many of the examples in this chapter are based on real data. Most are focused on dietary measurements, in particular the reliability of a food frequency estimate of fat intake. Part of this focus is a reflection of the increased interest in reliability studies, which is due to interest in assessing diet and the difficulties it presents. Additionally, by focusing on a single exposure, the reader can observe how measures of reliability are a function of the design of the reliability study, as well as of the accuracy of the instrument itself.

THE INTERPRETATION OF MEASURES OF RELIABILITY

This section covers the interpretation of measures of reliability in terms of measures of validity, and is meant to provide some general concepts for the interpretation of reliability studies. It is limited to continuous exposure measures. The results presented assume measures are obtained from an infinite population; that is, issues of sampling error are ignored.

A model of reliability and measures of reliability

Suppose each person in a population of interest is measured twice, either with one instrument or two instruments that purport to measure the same exposure. If two instruments are used, X_1 will denote the measure of interest, that is, the one to be used in the epidemiological study, and X_2 the comparison measure. For a given subject i, two (continuous) exposure measurements, X_{i1} and X_{i2}, are obtained. A simple model that could apply to intermethod or intramethod reliability studies is

$$X_{i1} = T_i + b_1 + E_{i1}$$
$$X_{i2} = T_i + b_2 + E_{i2}$$

where $\mu_{E_1} = \mu_{E_2} = 0$. The model can also be written

$$X_{ij} = T_i + b_j + E_{ij},$$

where X_{ij} is the observation on subject i of measure X_j.

This model states that subject i's first measure, X_{i1}, is equal to the true value of exposure for subject i, T_i, plus the constant bias of the first instrument in the population, b_1, plus the error for subject i on measure 1, E_{i1}. The second measure, X_{i2}, is equal to the same true value, T_i, plus the bias of the second instrument, b_2, plus a second error, E_{i2}.

In the population, X_1, X_2, T, E_1, and E_2 are random variables with distributions. The population mean of X_1 is denoted by μ_{X_1}, the variance by $\sigma^2_{X_1}$, etc. Because the bias of X_1 in the population is expressed as a constant b_1 and the bias of X_2 as b_2, it follows that the population means of the subject error terms, E_1 and E_2, are 0.

In a reliability study, information is available on X_1 and X_2 for each subject, but not on T. A reliability study can yield estimates of μ_{X_1}, μ_{X_2}, and the correlation between the two measures, $\rho_{X_1 X_2}$, termed the *reliability coefficient*.

In Chapter 3, two measures of the validity of a continuous exposure measure were shown to be important in assessing the impact of measurement error: the bias and the validity coefficient. The primary question is, if X_1 is the measure of interest, what can the estimates of μ_{X_1}, μ_{X_2} and $\rho_{X_1 X_2}$ from a reliability study tell us about the bias in X_1, b_1, and its validity coefficient, ρ_{TX_1}?

The measurement and interpretation of the bias in a measure

Reliability studies often cannot provide information on the bias in X_1 or X_2. In a reliability study based on the above model, only the *difference* between the biases of X_1 and X_2 can be observed:

$$(b_1 - b_2) = \mu_{X_1} - \mu_{X_2}. \qquad [4.1]$$

This equation states that the difference between the population means of the two measures is equal to the difference between their biases. This difference is often not very informative. If a similar degree of bias is present in both measures — for example, if the same miscalibrated scale is used to weigh each subject twice — the difference between the means of the two measures can be close to 0 even when there is considerable bias in both measures. However, if X_2 is an unbiased measure of $T (b_2 = 0)$, then

$$b_1 = \mu_{X_1} - \mu_{X_2}. \qquad [4.2]$$

Thus, only when the comparison measure X_2 is a perfect measure or when X_2 can be assumed to be unbiased (e.g. a well-calibrated scale), can a reliability study yield information about the bias in X_1.

As discussed in Chapter 3, differential bias in the exposure measure between cases and controls can have undesirable effects in an epidemiological study. (Differential precision may also be a concern, but is not discussed in this chapter.) To assess differential bias, a reliability study would need to measure X_1 and X_2 in a population of cases and a population of controls to yield estimates of the means of X_1 and X_2 among those with disease ($\mu_{X_{1D}}, \mu_{X_{2D}}$) and among the non-diseased group ($\mu_{X_{1N}}, \mu_{X_{2N}}$). The difference between the bias in X_1 between cases and controls, $b_{1D} - b_{1N}$, can be measured *only* if there is non-differential bias in the comparison measure X_2 ($b_{2D} = b_{2N}$). Then, if the simple additive model given above holds for both cases and controls,

$$(b_{1D} - b_{1N}) = (\mu_{X_{1D}} - \mu_{X_{2D}}) - (\mu_{X_{1N}} - \mu_{X_{2N}}). \qquad [4.3]$$

Example. To assess differential bias between colon cancer cases and controls in a retrospective food frequency estimate of fat intake (X_1), a reliability study could be conducted within an existing cohort study of colon cancer. X_1 could be compared to prospective information on fat intake (X_2) with reasonable certainty that any bias in X_2 is equal for cases and controls. If cases reported 40 per cent energy from fat on average prospectively and 42 per cent retrospectively, and controls reported 39 per cent prospectively and 38 per cent retrospectively, then the differential bias could be estimated from Equation 4.3 as

$$(\widehat{b_{1D} - b_{1N}}) = (42 - 40) - (38 - 39)$$

$$= 3\% \text{ energy.}$$

The inability of many reliability study designs to yield information on bias or differential bias is a major limitation. It should be recalled, however, that under non-differential measurement error (and certain other assumptions), the attenuation equations depend only on the validity coefficient and not on the bias. Thus, measures of reliability may be used to estimate at least some of the effects of measurement error in the absence of a measure of bias. When non-differential measurement error can be assumed, reliability can be assessed in a single population representative of the population in which the epidemiological study is to be conducted.

Relationship of reliability to validity under the parallel test model

When certain assumptions are met, reliability studies can yield information about the validity coefficient. One such set of assumptions is the *model of parallel tests* (Lord and Novick 1968; Nunnally 1978; Allen and Yen 1979; Carmines and Zeller 1979; Bohrnstedt 1983). The model is the same as the general model above, but with some additional assumptions:

$$\rho_{TE_1} = \rho_{TE_2} = 0$$

$$\sigma_{E_1}^2 = \sigma_{E_2}^2 = \sigma_E^2$$

$$\rho_{E_1 E_2} = 0.$$

The first assumption of the parallel test model is that the error variables, E_1 and E_2, are not correlated with the true value T. It is further assumed that E_1 and E_2 have equal variance, σ_E^2. This also implies that X_1 and X_2 have equal variance and that X_1 and X_2 are equally precise ($\rho_{TX_1} = \rho_{TX_2}$) (see Equation 3.2). This is usually a reasonable assumption in intramethod studies, since X_1 and X_2 are measurements from the same instrument. Finally, it is assumed that E_1 is not correlated with E_2. This important (and restrictive) assumption implies, for example, that an individual who has a positive error, E_1, on the first measurement is equally likely to have a positive or a negative error, E_2, on the second measurement. These assumptions are often summarized by saying that two measures are parallel measures of T if their errors are equal and uncorrelated. The parallel test model generally includes the assumption that $b_1 = b_2 = 0$, but this assumption is not needed for the results in this chapter.

Under the assumptions of parallel tests it can be shown that (Allen and Yen 1979):

$$\rho_{X_1 X_2} = \frac{\sigma_T^2}{\sigma_{X_1}^2} = 1 - \frac{\sigma_E^2}{\sigma_{X_1}^2} = \rho_{TX_1}^2 = \rho_{TX_2}^2$$

or equivalently [4.4]

$$\rho_{TX_1} = \rho_{TX_2} = \sqrt{\rho_{X_1 X_2}} \,.$$

These equations state that the reliability coefficient, $\rho_{X_1 X_2}$, is equal to the square of the validity coefficient for X_1 or X_2. This result is important, because it shows that if the assumptions are correct, the reliability coefficient, which is a measure of the correlation between two imperfect measures, can be used to estimate the correlation between T and X_1, *without* having a perfect measure of T. The correlation of X_1 with X_2 is less than the correlation of X_1 with T, due to the error in X_2.

Example. In a test–retest reliability study, serum cholesterol concentration was measured twice, one year apart (Shekelle *et al.* 1981). Suppose the 'true measure' of interest was each subject's average serum cholesterol over the year separating the two measurements. The two methods were identical, so that the assumptions of equal variances would be appropriate. The other assumptions are also considered to be met, including the assumptions of no correlation between the errors and the true measure or between the errors on the two measures. The correlation of X_1 with X_2 in the reliability study was 0.65. Then, by Equation 4.4 the correlation of X_1 with T (or the correlation of X_2 with T) can be estimated as 0.8.

The definition of the reliability coefficient of X_1 as the correlation between X_1 and X_2, two parallel measures of T, is one definition of reliability.

Based on Equation 4.4, the results in the last chapter which were expressed in terms of ρ_{TX}^2 could have been (and often are) expressed in terms of $\rho_{X_1 X_2}$. These expressions apply only when the meaning of the reliability coefficient is restricted to the correlation between parallel measures of T. However, we use the term reliability coefficient to refer to the correlation between measures of the same exposure, $\rho_{X_1 X_2}$, even when the assumptions of parallel tests do not hold. This means, for a given instrument, X_1, applied to a given population, that the reliability coefficient will vary with the choice of X_2, depending on the extent to which the assumptions of parallel tests do or do not apply, for a given X_2.

In real reliability studies, the assumptions of parallel tests are often incorrect. Two common violations will be discussed: unequal variances of E_1 and E_2, and correlated errors. Even when these assumptions are violated, the correlation between X_1 and X_2 can still provide some information about the validity coefficient of X_1.

Relationship of reliability to validity under unequal variances of E_1 and E_2

In the model of parallel tests, the variances of E_1 and E_2 are assumed to be equal, which implies that X_1 and X_2 are equally precise ($\rho_{TX_1} = \rho_{TX_2}$). This assumption is incorrect for certain reliability studies, particularly for many intermethod reliability studies. First consider a true validity study where X_1, the exposure measure of interest, is compared to a perfect measure of exposure, termed $X_2 (X_2 = T)$. Then, by definition,

$$\rho_{X_1 X_2} = \rho_{TX_1}. \qquad [4.5]$$

However, a perfect measure is often not available, so the exposure measure of interest, X_1, is often compared with an imperfect but more precise measure, X_2. This implies that $\rho_{TX_2} > \rho_{TX_1}$. If the other assumptions of the parallel tests model hold, including the assumption of uncorrelated errors, then

$$\rho_{X_1 X_2} < \rho_{TX_1} < \sqrt{\rho_{X_1 X_2}}. \qquad [4.6]$$

This equation states that when X_2 is more precise than X_1, and the errors in X_1 and X_2 are not correlated, the reliability coefficient $\rho_{X_1 X_2}$ can be used to yield an upper and lower bound for the validity coefficient of X_1. The lower bound for the validity coefficient of X_1 is the interpretation as if X_2 were a perfect measure (Equation 4.5), and the upper bound is the interpretation as if X_2 had equal error variance (Equation 4.4). The more accurate X_2 is, the closer the *lower* bound is to ρ_{TX_1}.

Example. Willett *et al.* (1985) conducted an intermethod reliability study to evaluate a food frequency questionnaire estimate of average daily fat intake over the preceding year (X_1). The comparison measure was an estimate of average daily fat intake from four 1-week diet diaries spread over the year (X_2). The observed correlation between the food frequency estimate and the diary estimate (energy adjusted) among 173 subjects was $\rho_{X_1 X_2} = 0.5$.

One might argue that the errors in the estimate of fat from a diet diary are not correlated with those on the food frequency questionnaire. The primary source of error on a food frequency questionnaire may be poor recall, while on the diet diaries it may be whether 4 weeks are fully representative of yearly intake. It was assumed that the four diaries yielded a more accurate measure of fat and, in fact, the variance from the diary estimate appeared to be smaller than the variance from the food frequency estimate. Then Equation 4.6 might apply:

$$0.5 < \hat{\rho}_{TX_1} < 0.7,$$

which suggests that the validity coefficient for X_1 would be between 0.5 and 0.7. Willett argued that the use of four 1-week diaries is a near-perfect criterion (e.g. there was little increase in $\rho_{X_1 X_2}$ when X_2 was based on four diaries rather than two). This suggests that ρ_{TX_1} is near the lower limit 0.5.

In an effort to find a comparison measure, X_2, with error uncorrelated with the error in X_1, the comparison measure may be less accurate than X_1 ($\rho_{TX_2} < \rho_{TX_1}$). Then if the other assumptions of the parallel tests model hold:

$$\rho_{TX_1} > \sqrt{\rho_{X_1 X_2}}. \qquad [4.7]$$

If it is not known whether X_1 or X_2 is more accurate, it can still be assumed that (Allen and Yen 1979)

$$\rho_{TX_1} \geq \rho_{X_1 X_2}. \qquad [4.8]$$

In other words, the correlation of X_1 with even a poor measure X_2 with uncorrelated errors gives a lower limit for the correlation of X_1 with the true measure. For example, if a blood measure of fat intake is available and the correlation of a food frequency measure of fat intake (X_1) with the blood measure (X_2) is 0.2, then Equation 4.8 shows that if there were no sources of correlated errors between X_1 and X_2 a lower limit for P_{TX_1} would be 0.2.

A model of reliability allowing for correlated errors

One assumption of the model of parallel tests that is often violated is the assumption of uncorrelated errors. Often $\rho_{E_1 E_2} > 0$. In other words, the error in one measure is positively correlated with the error in the other. Correlated errors occur when the sources of error in the first measurement on a subject tend to repeat themselves in the second. For example, weight may be consistently under-reported by some subjects on re-administration of a questionnaire.

A model for reliability that makes explicit the correlated errors is

$$X_{ij} = T_i + b_j + E_{ij},$$

where $E_{ij} = B_i + F_{ij}$. The error terms E_{i1} and E_{i2} for a given subject are the sum of two parts: a part that repeats itself on each measure of subject i, B_i, termed the *within-subject bias*; and a part that varies between measures (around a mean of 0 for subject i), F_{ij}, termed the *random error* (see Figure 4.1). E_1 and E_2 are correlated because they both include the within-subject bias.

To simplify the reliability coefficient under this model, let S_i be that part of X_1 and X_2 that is consistently measured for subject i on both instruments. S_i would be the sum of T_i plus B_i (plus the average bias across measures). Then the model of reliability can be rewritten as

$$X_{ij} = S_i + m_j + F_{ij},$$

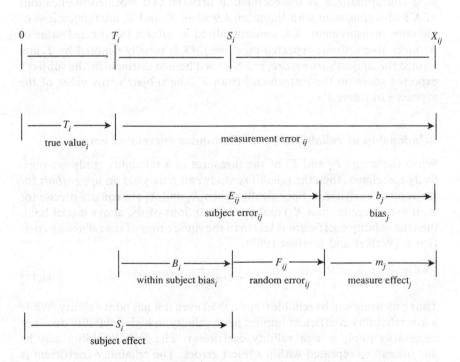

Figure 4.1 Measurement error in X_{ij}, the jth measure on subject i.

where S_i represents the effect of subject i and m_j the effect of measure j on X_{ij} (the m_j are the b_j minus the average bias across measures, such that $\Sigma m_j = 0$). If X_1 and X_2 are equally precise (and $\rho_{TF_1} = \rho_{TF_2} = 0$), then X_1 and X_2 meet the assumptions of parallel measures of S (not T). The reliability coefficient under this model is the proportion of the variance of X_1 explained by S, the part that is common to the repeated measures. That is, (Allen and Yen 1979)

$$\rho_{X_1 X_2} = \frac{\sigma_S^2}{\sigma_{X_1}^2} = \frac{\sigma_S^2}{\sigma_{X_2}^2} = 1 - \frac{\sigma_F^2}{\sigma_{X_1}^2}. \qquad [4.9]$$

The right-hand side of this equation shows that when there are correlated errors, the reliability coefficient reflects only the random component of error in X_1.

Equation 4.9 is essentially identical to the classical definition of the *reliability* of a measure X (Allen and Yen 1979; Dunn 1989):

$$\rho_X = \frac{\sigma_S^2}{\sigma_X^2}. \qquad [4.10]$$

ρ_X is conceptualized as the correlation between two repeated applications of X and is consistent with Equation 4.9 when X_1 and X_2 are replications of the same measurement. S_i is conceptualized as subject i's expected value of X (mean over infinite repeated measures). (S_i is usually denoted by T_i and termed the subject's *true score*, but S is used here to distinguish 'the subject's expected score on the instrument' from T, 'the subject's true value of the exposure of interest').

Relationship of reliability to validity under correlated errors

When the errors E_1 and E_2 of the measures in a reliability study are positively correlated, then the reliability study can only yield an *upper limit* for the validity coefficient. Specifically, when X_1 and X_2 are equally precise (or X_2 is more precise than X_1) and the assumptions of the above model hold, then the validity coefficient is less than the square root of the reliability coefficient (Walker and Blettner 1985):

$$\rho_{TX_1} < \sqrt{\rho_{X_1 X_2}}. \qquad [4.11]$$

Thus a measure can be reliable (repeatable) even if it has poor validity. While a low reliability coefficient implies poor validity, a high reliability does not necessarily imply a high validity coefficient. The high reliability may be due instead to repeated within subject errors. The reliability coefficient is only diminished by the random component of error, whereas the validity coefficient is a measure of both the random error and the within subject bias.

To interpret a reliability study, one should evaluate whether there are potential sources of correlated errors between the two measures. As outlined in Table 3.1, there is a wide range of sources of measurement error, and most of these could be sources of correlated errors.

Example. A test–retest reliability study was also conducted in the study by Willett *et al.* (1985) presented in the previous example. The observed correlation between the estimates of average daily fat intake from two administrations of the food frequency questionnaire, 1 year apart, was 0.6.

Sources of correlated errors between two administrations of a food frequency questionnaire include the following:

(a) Some subjects may consistently tend to report their 'best' diet rather than their usual diet.

(b) Certain high-fat foods eaten frequently by a few subjects may have been omitted from the questionnaire. Those subjects would have their fat intake consistently underestimated.

(c) The nutrient database used to convert foods to grams of fat may be incorrect for certain subjects. For example, those subjects who reduce the fat content of standard recipes such as stews, lasagna, etc., would have the fat content of their diet consistently overestimated.

(d) The time period assessed by the instrument (diet in last year) may differ from the true time period of interest (e.g. diet over the last 5 years). Then, those who have lowered the fat in their diet in recent years will have their fat intake underestimated on both administrations of the instrument compared with their true 5-year average fat intake.

Under this strong likelihood of correlated errors, Equation 4.11 would apply in interpreting this reliability study,

$$\rho_{TX_1} < 0.8,$$

so only an upper limit on the validity coefficient of the measurement can be estimated. This outcome clearly provides less information about the validity of the food frequency measure of fat than did the outcome of the intermethod reliability study described in the last example.

Correlated errors commonly occur in intramethod studies, but they could occur in intermethod studies as well. In the example of an intermethod study of a food frequency estimate of fat intake compared with a diet diary estimate, it was argued that the errors on the two instruments were unlikely to be significantly correlated. However, of the four sources of correlated errors noted in the above example, at least two could lead to correlated errors between a food frequency measure and a diet diary measure (the tendency of some subjects to report their best diet, and the issue relating to the time period of measurement). Reliability studies in which the errors of the measures are correlated cannot provide estimates of a lower bound for ρ_{TX_1}. Estimates of a lower bound depend on uncorrelated errors, so lower bounds should be interpreted cautiously.

Interpretation of the value of the reliability coefficient

Some authors have provided guidance on whether to consider the reliability of a measure poor, fair, or good from the value of the reliability coefficient. It may be more appropriate first to consider what information the reliability study yields about the validity of the measure, as discussed above. Then consideration could be given to the effect of the estimated measurement error in the exposure on the epidemiological study which will use the measure, based on the tables and equations in the last chapter.

For example, suppose a reliability study which complied with the parallel test model yielded $\rho_{X_1 X_2} = 0.64$, leading to an estimate of the validity coefficient, $\hat{\rho}_{TX} = 0.8$. If the true odds ratio were 2.0, and if the assumptions of non-differential measurement error and the other assumptions of Equation 3.6 were reasonable, then the estimated observable odds ratio would be

$$\hat{OR}_O = OR_T^{\hat{\rho}_{TX}} = 2^{0.8} = 1.7.$$

This might be considered to be acceptable attenuation. On the other hand, if a reliability study of a different instrument produced the same reliability coefficient (0.64) but, due to correlated errors between the measures, only an upper bound for ρ_{TX} of 0.8 could be estimated, then applying Equation 3.6 would yield

$$\hat{OR}_O < 1.7.$$

This estimate of the attenuated odds ratio includes only the attenuation due to the random error in X, and the actual attenuation would be greater. This instrument might not be acceptable.

Other violations of the assumptions of the model

In some situations the assumption of the basic model, which states that both X_1 and X_2 measure T with additive errors E_1 and E_2, is incorrect. One alternative to this model is that X_1 and X_2 or both may be a linear function of T:

$$X_{ij} = c_j T_i + b_j + E_{ij}.$$

(In intramethod studies it is assumed that c_1 and c_2 are equal, i.e. X_1 and X_2 have the same scale.) Reliability studies such as these can still yield information about the validity coefficient, but not about bias. The results presented so far in this chapter for interpreting the reliability coefficient $\rho_{X_1 X_2}$ in terms of the validity coefficient ρ_{TX_1} would also apply to the above model, because $\rho_{X_1 X_2}$ is not affected by linear transformations of X_1 or X_2. For example, a food frequency questionnaire measure of β-carotene (X_1) could be compared with serum β-carotene (X_2) and interpreted by Equations 4.7 or 4.8 (if there were no sources of correlated errors) even though serum β-carotene is not measured in the same units as β-carotene intake.

Further violations of the assumption that T and E are uncorrelated are beyond the scope of this book, but several practical points should be noted. First, a transformation of X, such as the logarithmic transformation, may reduce the dependence of E on T (Altman and Bland 1983). Second, when T and E are negatively correlated, the measure X will have a variance less than $\sigma_T^2 + \sigma_E^2$, possibly even a smaller variance than T: therefore the variances of two measures should not be compared to determine which is more precise.

Finally, the equations given so far have assumed a population of infinite size. In practice, there will be sampling error in the estimate of $\rho_{X_1 X_2}$. The confidence interval around estimates of $\rho_{X_1 X_2}$ should be taken into consideration when using the equations in this section to interpret reliability in terms of validity.

Interpretation of reliability studies of categorical variables

Most of the concepts presented for continuous variables apply in a qualitative way to interpretation of reliability studies of categorical variables. For example, when two imperfect categorical measures of exposure are being compared, part of the agreement between them could be due to repeated error. Mathematical relationships between measures of reliability and measures of validity for categorical variables are not straightforward. However, some reliability study designs can yield estimates of the sensitivity and specificity of each measure or can be used to estimate the bias in the odds ratio that would result from the misclassification (Hui and Walter 1980; Walter 1984; Clayton 1985; Kaldor and Clayton 1985; Walter and Irwig 1988; Dunn 1989).

ISSUES IN THE DESIGN OF VALIDITY AND RELIABILITY STUDIES

There are several issues that need to be considered in the design of reliability studies (Fleiss and Shrout 1977; Carmines and Zeller 1979; Dunn 1989;

Willett 1990). Most of these issues are also important in interpreting reliability studies carried out by others.

Purpose and timing of the reliability study

When a new instrument is to be developed for an epidemiological study, or when an existing one is to be applied in a substantially different population, a validity or reliability study of the instrument should be carried out first. Estimates of the validity or reliability coefficient and, when possible, the bias of the instrument can then be used to decide whether it is necessary to develop a more accurate instrument. If the measure is shown to be reasonably reliable, and by inference reasonably valid, this will increase confidence in the outcome of the epidemiological study.

Reliability studies conducted before the main epidemiological study, or early in its course, can be used not only to evaluate but also to improve the instrument. For example, an inter-rater reliability study could identify interviewers, abstractors, or laboratory personnel who need more training or should be dropped from the study. Such a study could be done by comparing three or more raters who collect data on the same subset of subjects. Computation of reliability coefficients for each pair of raters may reveal an individual rater who compares poorly with the others. In addition, the researcher should investigate the situations in which discrepancies between the repeated measurements have occurred. This can often lead to improvement of the instrument or the protocol for its use. For example, if disagreements on the variable marital status of subjects usually involved divorced subjects being erroneously classified as 'single', the category 'single' might be clarified by the label 'never married'.

An additional use of reliability studies is to estimate the impact of exposure measurement error on the results of a study after the parent epidemiological study has been completed. Information from a reliability study conducted on a subset of subjects concurrently with the epidemiological study can yield information about the validity of the exposure measure. This information can be used to adjust the observed odds ratio for the effects of measurement error. Adjustment procedures are discussed in Chapter 5.

Choice of comparison measures

Many types of comparison measures have been used in reliability studies. An instrument can be compared with a re-administration of the same instrument at a different time, by a different rater, or with variation of some other condition of interest, for example proxy respondent versus index subject. For intermethod studies, questionnaire data have been compared with medical records (Harlow and Linet 1989), physical or biochemical measures of exposure (Jarvholm and Sanden 1987; Siconolfi *et al.* 1985; Willett *et al.* 1983), interviews by experts such as nutritionists, industrial hygienists, or physicians (Eskenazi and Pearson 1988), exposure diaries (Willett *et al* 1985; Williams *et al.* 1989), and with direct observation (Klesges *et al.* 1985; Decker *et al.* 1986). Information from medical records has been compared with physician interviews and direct observation (Gerbert *et al.* 1988).

How is an appropriate comparison method selected? The issues discussed in the section on interpretation of measures of reliability (page 79–89) should provide some guidance in selecting a comparison measure. Ideally, measurements from the instrument whose accuracy is to be determined are compared with those provided by a perfect, or near perfect, measure of exposure. This type a study, a *validity study* allows one to estimate both dimensions of measurement error, the bias and the validity coefficient (Equations 4.2 and 4.5).

If a validity study is not possible, then one should consider comparing the instrument of interest to a measure of exposure with uncorrelated errors. A good choice is a comparison measure, X_2, that is more precise than the measure of interest, X_1, and has error unlikely to be correlated to X_1. Intermethod studies comparing questionnaire measures to records (e.g. comparing a questionnaire on oral contraceptive use to complete medical or pharmacy records) or to multi-week diaries (e.g. comparing a questionnaire on leisure physical activty over the last year to six 1-week diaries), often meet these criteria. Equations 4.1 and 4.6 can aid in interpreting such studies. If a comparison measure can be selected with equal error as well as error uncorrelated to the instrument of interest, this can yield good information on the validity coefficient of the instrument (Equation 4.4). Test–retest studies of biochemical measures can often be assumed to have equal and uncorrelated errors if the replicates are sampled over the entire time period to which the exposure measure is intended to relate. Often questionnaire measures of behaviours can be compared with relevant physical or biochemical measures under the assumption of uncorrelated errors (e.g. a questionnaire on physical activity can be compared to a treadmill test), but such comparisons are often limited because the physical or biochemical measure may be a poor measure of the behaviour. Equations 4.7 or 4.8 can be useful in interpreting such studies. However, if both the questionnaire and the biochemical test reflect recent exposure, and the instrument is intended to represent exposure over a longer period of time, the errors could be correlated.

When a comparison measure with uncorrelated error is not available, then only part of the measurement error can be assessed in the reliability study. The part of the error that is repeated cannot be measured. The researcher can attempt to select the comparison measure, X_2, so that the main sources of error in the measure of interest, X_1, are not repeated in X_2. For example, in assessing a questionnaire covering diet 10 years in the past, long-term recall might be the greatest concern. One reliability study of this issue selected subjects who had answered a diet questionnaire years earlier and compared their measurements from the questionnaire of interest with those on the earlier version (Wu *et al*. 1988). This design would permit assessment of the main sources of error, that due to poor recall and that due to random variation, even though some sources of error (e.g. omission of certain foods on both questionnaires) could be repeated on both questionnaires. By careful selection of X_2, correlated errors between X_1 and X_2 can be minimized and the reliability study may then yield more information about the validity of X_1.

Finally, a simple test–retest reliability study is often quick and inexpensive to undertake. If there are sources of correlated error, the study will yield only an upper limit for validity (Equation 4.11). Nonetheless, if the reliability coefficient proves to be *low*, the instrument should probably be abandoned or extensively revised.

In reviewing reliability studies by others, the same issues should be considered. The key questions are:

- Was the comparison method used close to perfect?
- Was there an imperfect comparison measure but with uncorrelated errors?
- If two or more measures with correlated errors were used, were the errors likely to be strongly or weakly correlated?

The answers to these questions will guide the interpretation of the reliability study.

Separate studies on diseased and non-diseased groups

The researcher must decide whether or not to attempt to measure differential error. To assess differential measurement error, the reliability study needs to be conducted on a sample of cases and a sample of controls, and the comparison measure needs to be carefully selected.

Differential *bias* is a particular concern (Chapter 3), therefore a comparison of the bias in the measure of interest, X_1, between cases and controls would be of major interest. For reliability studies to assess differential bias in X_1, a comparison measure X_2 needs to be selected that is unbiased or that can be assumed to have non-differential bias. Then the differential bias in X_1 can be estimated by Equation 4.3. For example, comparison of recall of a specific medication (X_1) with an abstract of medical records (X_2) among cases versus a similar comparison among controls may be a good way to assess differential bias: any bias in records is unlikely to be related to the disease under study, provided that a sufficient period prior to diagnosis is excluded. On the other hand, a test–retest reliability of recall of medications (assessed separately on cases and controls) would not reveal any differential bias between cases and controls, because the bias would occur in both measures.

Selection of subjects for reliability studies

Ideally, subjects in a reliability study should be a random sample of those in the population in which the epidemiological study will be carried out. This is because there are problems in generalizing reliability studies conducted on one population to another. These problems include the following:

- Reliability or validity studies which use self-selected volunteers might find the instrument to be more valid than it would be in the intended population, due to the higher level of motivation among the volunteers.
- Differences between populations in education, age, sex, and other factors could influence the validity and reliability of the instrument.
- Differences in the *distribution* of the true exposure between populations can influence the validity and reliability coefficients. Recall that ρ_{TX}^2 (also $\rho_{X_1 X_2}$ under parallel tests) is equal to

$$\frac{\sigma_T^2}{\sigma_X^2} = \frac{\sigma_T^2}{\sigma_T^2 + \sigma_E^2} = \frac{1}{1 + \sigma_E^2/\sigma_T^2}.$$

Thus even if the same instrument had the same error variance, σ_E^2, in two populations, the validity coefficient (or reliability coefficient) would be smaller in the population with least variation in true exposure, σ_T^2. For this reason, the use of the validity coefficient (and the reliability coefficient) to express measurement error has been criticized (Altman and Bland 1983). However, these are appropriate statistics in that they can be used to estimate the effect of measurement error on the bias in the observed odds ratio in the population of interest, which depends on the ratio σ_T^2/σ_X^2. Nonetheless, a validity or reliability coefficient assessed in one population may not apply to another with a different distribution of exposure.

Timing and order of measures

Correlated errors between measures in a reliability study may occur when subjects recall at the second or later testing the responses they gave on earlier tests. This recall can be minimized by separating the measures over time, usually by a month at least. However, when the two periods of testing are well separated, the two measures of exposure may refer to different time periods. Thus some lack of correlation between them may be due to true change in exposure over time. For example, a test–retest reliability study of a food frequency questionnaire estimate of fat intake over the last year, with the two administrations separated by a year, would not yield a perfect correlation even if the instrument was perfect, because of the one-year shift in the time period covered. However, this issue may not be a problem; depending on the true exposure of interest, it may be appropriate to include the variation in a measure over time as a source of measurement error.

In intermethod reliability studies, the instrument to be evaluated is generally given first because the comparison measure is usually less prone to error and may, therefore, be less affected by recall of the prior measurement. Knowledge that a measure is to be validated can influence subjects' responses (e.g. self-report of weight may be influenced by knowledge that they will be weighed), so the invitation to subjects to participate in the second measure should be given after the first measurement has been completed. In intramethod reliability studies, the order of measures (e.g. raters) should be randomized (although X_1 would always be the measure by rater 1, X_2 by rater 2, etc.).

Review of studies using the instrument

There is an addtional approach to assessing the validity of an instrument, which is similar to the concept of *predictive validity* from psychology (Nunnally 1978; Carmines and Zeller 1979). If an exposure measure has been shown to be associated with a disease or other outcome in several epidemiological studies, this provides some evidence that it is a valid measure. Specifically, it can be seen from Equation 3.8 that $\rho_{TX} > \rho_{XY}$. That is, the correlation between a continuous exposure variable X and a continuous outcome Y is a lower limit for the validity coefficient of X. The assumption is that the errors in the outcome Y and exposure X are uncorrelated. This approach of reviewing other epidemiological studies can also be applied in a qualitative way to studies with dichotomous disease outcomes. For example, if an estimate of vitamin A from a dietary questionnaire was significantly associated with disease in several studies, in agreement with prior hypotheses, this provides some evidence for the validity of the instrument. However, caution should be exercised in this approach; the disease–exposure association may be due to confounding between the exposure measure and some other risk factor for disease, or to other sources of bias in the study.

ANALYSIS OF VALIDITY AND RELIABILITY STUDIES

Selecting the appropriate measures of validity or reliability

This section covers some common approaches to the statistical analysis of validity and reliability studies.

The selection of the appropriate analysis depends on certain aspects of the design of the study (Fleiss 1981, 1986; Kelsey *et al.* 1986; Maclure and Willett 1987; Dunn 1989). First, is the exposure measure a continuous variable, a nominal (including dichotomous) categorical variable, or an ordered categorical variable? All of the statistical techniques to be discussed are for reliability and validity studies in which the two or more measures of exposure are on the same type of scale.

Second, is the study an intermethod reliability/validity study or an intramethod reliability study? In an intermethod reliability study or a validity study, the instruments usually differ, the variances of the measures may not be equal, and even the units of measure may not even be the same, for example a measure of β-carotene intake may be compared with serum β-carotene concentration. Further, our discussion of intermethod reliability is limited to the comparison of only two measures at one time. In the intramethod type of study the instruments used are essentially the same, possibly with some difference in administration; for example, two interviewers. Intramethod reliability studies can be performed using more than two measures per subject. One assumption of the analytical methods for intramethod studies is that the variances of the measures, $X_1, X_2, \ldots, X_k$, are equal for continuous measures, or that the measures are 'equally precise' (Fleiss 1986) for categorical exposures.

The issue of correlated errors does not influence the choice of analytical method for reliability studies, only the interpretation of the results.

Table 4.1 gives an overview of methods for the analysis of validity and reliability studies. The upper half gives methods for intermethod studies, and the lower half approaches for intramethod studies. These techniques will be described in this section, with emphasis on intramethod reliability. It is assumed that the reader is already familiar with the assumptions and computations of the Pearson product-moment correlation coefficient, the one- and two-sample t-test, and the analysis of variance (ANOVA) (Armitage and Berry 1987).

The emphasis in the analysis of reliability and validity studies is on parameter estimation; for example, estimation of $\rho_{X_1 X_2}$. Confidence intervals also add useful information. Statistical tests are less important, for it should almost be a 'given' that X_1 and X_2 are not related by chance.

Except for the evaluation of differential bias between cases and controls, the statistical techniques given in this section are for a single population. Many could be extended to the comparison of cases and controls, but these extensions are beyond the scope of this book.

Validity and intermethod reliability studies of continuous measures

Intermethod reliability studies and validity studies can be analysed using common statistical techniques.

In the analysis of continuous exposure variables under the model of

Table 4.1   Analysis of validity and reliability studies

Type of exposure measures	Statistical measure of reliability or validity	Condition under which statistic equals 1
Intermethod reliability and validity studies		
Continuous	Pearson correlation coefficient and $\bar{X}_1 - \bar{X}_2$	$X_{i1} = cX_{i2} + d$
Nominal or binomial	misclassification matrix	(not a summary measure)
Ordered categorical	misclassification matrix	(not a summary measure)
	or	
	Pearson correlation coefficient and $\bar{X}_1 - \bar{X}_2$	$X_{i1} = cX_{i2} + d$
	or	
	Spearman correlation coefficient	ranking by X_1 same as ranking by X_2
Intramethod reliability studies		
Continuous: $X_1, \ldots, X_k$ are essentially the same measure	intraclass correlation coefficient: one-way (R_1)	$X_{i1} = X_{i2} = \ldots = X_{ik}$
Continuous: $X_1, \ldots, X_k$ are the k measures (e.g. raters) to be used in the epidemiological study	intraclass correlation coefficient: two-way fixed effects (R_2)	$X_{i1} = X_{i2} = \ldots = X_{ik}$
Continuous: $X_1, \ldots, X_k$ represent k of many measures (e.g. raters) that will be used in the study	intraclass correlation coefficient: two-way random effects (R_3)	$X_{i1} = X_{i2} = \ldots = X_{ik}$
Continuous: same as two-way fixed effects except difference between means of measures not a source of error in parent study	intraclass correlation coefficient with difference in means excluded in variance of $X(R_4)$	$X_{i1} = X_{i2} + d_2 = \ldots$ $X_{ik} + d_k$
Nominal or binomial	Cohen's κ	$X_{i1} = X_{i2}$
Ordered categorical	weighted κ	$X_{i1} = X_{i2}$

additive independent errors, the difference between the biases of the two measures can be estimated as the difference between the sample means of X_1 and X_2 (from Equation 4.1):

$$\widehat{(b_1 - b_2)} = \bar{X}_1 - \bar{X}_2.$$

For a validity or reliability study in which X_2 is unbiased, $\bar{X}_1 - \bar{X}_2$ is an estimate of b_1, the bias in X_1. The value of t computed through a one-sample t-test on the variable $(X_{i1} - X_{i2})$ computed for each subject can be used to compute a confidence interval.

For reliability studies in which cases are compared with controls, if X_2 has non-differential bias then the difference in bias in X_1 between cases and controls can be estimated as (from Equation 4.3):

$$\widehat{(b_{1D} - b_{1N})} = (\bar{X}_{1D} - \bar{X}_{2D}) - (\bar{X}_{1N} - \bar{X}_{2N}).$$

The value of t from a two-sample t-test on the variable $(X_{i1} - X_{i2})$ can be used to compute a confidence interval for the difference in b_1 between the two groups.

The Pearson product-moment correlation and its confidence interval can be used to estimate $\rho_{X_1 X_2}$ for intermethod or validity studies. If X_1 and X_2 are, at least, positively associated, then the Pearson correlation coefficient would range from 0 to 1. The correlation is equal to 1 when X_1 is a perfect linear transformation of X_2 for all subjects:

$$X_{i1} = cX_{i2} + d.$$

For example, if subjects in an epidemiological study were to be weighed on a portable scale which was validated against a highly accurate scale, a Pearson correlation coefficient close to 1 would suggest that the portable scale was highly precise. If there were a consistent difference between the two measures, (e.g. if the portable scale was miscalibrated 2 kg too heavy, or even if the portable scale weighed in pounds and the comparison scale was a kilogram scale), this would not reduce the correlation $\rho_{X_1 X_2}$.

Example. In an intermethod reliability study on 110 women, an estimate of percentage of energy intake from fat (X_1) from a food frequency questionnaire was compared with a four-day diet record (X_2). The results of the study were:

	mean (% energy)	standard deviation
X_1	39.1	6.6
X_2	37.5	6.0

Pearson correlation coefficient = 0.45

An estimate of the difference in the biases of X_1 and X_2 is:

$$\widehat{(b_1 - b_2)} = 39.1 - 37.5 = 1.6\% \text{ dietary energy.}$$

That is, the food frequency questionnaire overestimates percentage dietary energy from fat by 1.6 per cent compared with a food record. The estimated reliability coefficient is based on the Pearson correlation coefficient, $\hat{\rho}_{X_1 X_2} = 0.45$.

In assessing the relationship between X_1 and X_2, one might also consider adjustment for potentially confounding factors that may explain the association of X_1 and X_2, other than by way of their relationship with T.

Analysis of validity and intermethod studies of categorical measures

Several methods can be used to analyse validity or intermethod reliability studies of categorical exposure variables. For a nominal categorical variable the validity or intermethod reliability can be described by the misclassification matrix (or, for a dichotomous variable, by the sensitivity and specificity) as described in Chapter 3.

The misclassification matrix is also appropriate for ordered categorical variables. Depending on the distribution of the ordered categorical variable, the difference in means and the Pearson product-moment correlation coefficient between the two categorical measures or the Spearman rank correlation coefficient might be used. Recall from Chapter 3 that the effect of measurement error in an ordered categorical variable can also be described (under certain assumptions) in terms of the validity coefficient of the underlying continuous variable from which the categorical variable was created. This means that the difference in means and the correlation between the two underlying continuous variables could be appropriate.

Because the misclassification matrix is not a summary measure, κ (described below) is often used to analyse intermethod reliability studies of categorical variables. However, these methods were developed under assumptions more appropriate to intramethod reliability studies.

Analysis of intramethod reliability studies: the concept of inter-changeable measures

The primary distinction we have made between intermethod and intramethod reliability studies is that intermethod studies use two instruments and intramethod studies involve repeated applications of one instrument. However, the most important distinction in terms of selecting an analytic method is that in intermethod studies only one measure, X_1, is to be used in the full epidemiological study: we are interested in the reliability of X_1. In intramethod studies, the two or more measures compared are to be used interchangeably as a single exposure measurement in the epidemiological study. For example, in an intramethod reliability study, X_1 may refer to a measure by one interviewer and X_2 to one by a second interviewer, but in the parent epidemiological study each subject will be questioned by one or other of the two interviewers. In intramethod studies, we are interested not in the reliability of X_1 or X_2 but in the reliability of the interchangeable measure 'X', the measure to be used in the epidemiological study.

There is a key difference between intermethod and intramethod reliability. In intermethod reliability, any systematic difference between X_1 and X_2 reflects a consistent bias which affects all subjects in the parent study, and thus does not affect the precision of X_1. In intramethod reliability, on the other hand, a systematic difference between measures contributes to a lack of precision in X because it affects some subjects but not others. For example, if one interviewer weighs subjects on a correctly calibrated scale and a second rater's scale is miscalibrated 2 kg too heavy, this source of error will affect only the subjects measured by the second rater. Thus any consistent difference between study interviewers would increase the variance of the exposure measure (σ_X^2) in the full study and decrease the reliability compared with the use of only one interviewer. The Pearson product-moment correlation is not appropriate for intramethod studies, because systematic differences (in bias or scale) between X_1 and the comparison measure X_2 are not reflected in the Pearson correlation.

Special analytical methods have been developed for intramethod reliability studies, particularly in the context of inter-rater reliability studies. For continuous variables, the reliability of X, ρ_X, is estimated by a version of the intraclass correlation coefficient (R). The *intraclass correlation coefficient* is an estimate of ρ_X as defined in Equation 4.10. That is,

$$\hat{\rho}_X = R = \frac{\hat{\sigma}_S^2}{\hat{\sigma}_X^2}.$$

The variance of X in the full epidemiological study, σ_X^2, is estimated under the assumption that in the full study each subject will be *randomly* assigned one measure (e.g. one interviewer). The intraclass correlation is diminished by the error in X due to systematic differences between measures $X_1, \ldots, X_k$ as well as that due to random error. Thus the intraclass correlation (except for R_4 discussed below) is equal to 1 only when there is *exact* agreement between measures, that is, when $X_{i1} = X_{i2} = \ldots X_{ik}$ for each subject.

The intraclass correlation coefficient can be interpreted by Equation 4.4 or Equation 4.11, depending on whether there are correlated errors between X_1 and X_2 or not. The bias in X cannot be estimated in an intramethod study. The mean difference between measures, $(\bar{X}_1 - \bar{X}_2)$, can be used to reflect the systematic difference between measures, but any consistent difference between X_1 and X_2 beyond chance also contributes to a lower estimate of ρ_X by the intraclass correlation coefficient.

Four versions of the intraclass correlation coefficient are discussed here.

This discussion is followed by a presentation of an analogous statistic, κ, for intramethod reliability studies of categorical variables. Books by Fleiss (1981, 1986) and by Dunn (1989) contain excellent discussions of the intraclass correlation coefficient and κ.

Intraclass correlation for a simple replication study

Intramethod reliability studies of continuous exposure measures are analysed by analysis of variance (ANOVA) techniques. The selection of the appropriate version of the intraclass correlation coefficient depends on the reliability study design, within the context of ANOVA models.

First, consider a simple replication reliability study in which there is no characteristic that distinguishes the first and second measure across all subjects. Examples of this type of design include a study in which blood from each subject is analysed three times in the laboratory, or a study in which medical records are abstracted twice for each subject by two randomly selected abstractors from a pool of three or more abstractors. In studies of this type, the order of the measures can be considered arbitrary. This study design is analysed by a one-way random effects model ANOVA.

Each of n subjects is measured k times, with X_{ij} being the jth measure on subject i, $\bar{X}_i$ the mean for subject i, and $\bar{X}$ the overall mean. The computations for a one-way ANOVA appear in Table 4.2. The model is $X_{ij} = S_i + F_{ij}$, where S is the subject effect and F the random error as described on pages 85–6. The reliability coefficient of X can be estimated by the intraclass correlation coefficient from the one-way random effects model, termed here R_1:

$$\hat{\rho}_X = R_1 = \frac{\hat{\sigma}_S^2}{\hat{\sigma}_X^2} = \frac{\text{BMS} - \text{WMS}}{\text{BMS} + (k-1)\text{WMS}},$$

where BMS is the between-subjects mean square and WMS the within-subjects mean square.

Example. Table 4.3 presents a summary of the data and an analysis of variance for a test–retest study of a food frequency questionnaire measure of percentage energy from fat. The two measures were derived from two administrations of the questionnaire to 110 subjects 6 months apart. If this were considered to be a simple replication study, the reliability coefficient would be estimated as:

$$\hat{\rho}_X = R_1 = \frac{64.37 - 15.81}{64.37 + 15.81} = 0.61.$$

A lower $100\,(1 - \alpha)$ per cent confidence interval for R_1 can be estimated, under the assumption of normality of X and of the random error, from

Table 4.2 One-way analysis of variance and two-way analysis of variance for the computation of intraclass correlation coefficients

One-way ANOVA

Source of variance	Sum of squares (SS)	Degrees of freedom (df)	Mean square (MS = SS/df)	Expected mean square
Between subjects	$k\sum_i (\bar{X}_i - \bar{X})^2$	$n - 1$	BMS	$\sigma_F^2 + k\sigma_S^2$
Within subjects (random error)	$\sum_i\sum_j (x_{ij} - \bar{X}_i)^2$	$n(k - 1)$	WMS	σ_F^2
Total	$\sum_i\sum_j (x_{ij} - \bar{X})^2$	$nk - 1$		

Two-way ANOVA

Source of variance	Sum of squares (SS)	Degrees of freedom (df)	Mean square (MS = SS/df)	Expected mean square
Between subjects	$k\sum_i (\bar{X}_i - \bar{X})^2$	$n - 1$	SMS	$\sigma_F^2 + k\sigma_S^2$
Between measures	$n\sum_j (\bar{X}_j - \bar{X})^2$	$k - 1$	MMS	$\left\{ \sigma_F^2 + \dfrac{n}{k - 1}\sum_j m_j^2 \;(F)^a \atop \sigma_F^2 + no_M^2 \;(R)^b \right.$
Random error	by subtraction	$(n - 1)(k - 1)$	EMS	σ_F^2
Total	$\sum_i\sum_j (X_{ij} - \bar{X})^2$	$nk - 1$		

[a] Fixed effects model
[b] Random effects model

$$R_1 \geq \frac{\dfrac{\text{BMS}}{\text{WMS}} - f}{\dfrac{\text{BMS}}{\text{WMS}} + (k-1)f}$$

where f denotes the $(1 - \alpha)$ centile from tables of the F distribution with $n - 1$ and $n(k - 1)$ degrees of freedom.

Fleiss (1986) gives a method for the analysis of reliability studies in which the number of measures, k, can vary across subjects.

Intraclass correlation for subjects by measures (two-way) design

The remaining designs to be considered are intramethod reliability studies in which the two or more measures may have different characteristics; that is, the order of measures is not arbitrary. An example would be an inter-rater reliability study in which all subjects are interviewed by the same two interviewers, with X_1 being the measure by rater 1, X_2 by rater 2. When the k raters in the reliability study are the same as the k raters who will participate in the epidemiological study, the intraclass correlation coefficient from the two-way fixed effects ANOVA model (R_2) is appropriate. When the k raters in the reliability study are a *sample* from a population of raters to be used in the epidemiological study, the intraclass correlation coefficient from the two-way random effects ANOVA model (R_3) applies. An example of this would be when two interviewers participate in the reliability study as representative of the several interviewers who will participate in the full study.

The ANOVA table for this two-way (subjects by measures) design under the assumption of no interaction between subjects and measures, is given in the lower half of Table 4.2. X_{ij} is the jth measure on subject i, $\bar{X}_i$ is the mean for subject i, and $\bar{X}_j$ the mean for measure j. The computations of the mean squares given in the table are the same for the fixed and random effects models, but the estimate of σ_X^2 and therefore of R differs. SMS, MMS, and EMS are the mean squares for subjects, measures, and error respectively.

The two-way fixed effects model, where m_j is the fixed effect of measure j, is

$$X_{ij} = S_i + m_j + F_{ij}.$$

Under this model, the intraclass correlation coefficient (R_2) is estimated by

$$R_2 = \frac{\hat{\sigma}_S^2}{\hat{\sigma}_X^2} = \frac{n(\text{SMS} - \text{EMS})}{n\text{SMS} + (k-1)\text{MMS} + (n-1)(k-1)\text{EMS}}.$$

No simple method is available for a confidence interval.

Under the two-way random effects model $X_{ij} = S_i + M_j + F_{ij}$, where M_j, is the random effect of measure j, the intraclass correlation coefficient (R_3) is (Bartko 1966):

$$R_3 = \frac{\hat{\sigma}_S^2}{\hat{\sigma}_X^2} = \frac{n(\text{SMS} - \text{EMS})}{n\text{SMS} + k\text{MMS} + (nk - n - k)\text{EMS}}.$$

A lower $100(1 - \alpha)$ per cent confidence limit for R_3 has been derived by Fleiss and Shrout 1978 (see Fleiss 1986).

The estimates of the intraclass correlation for both fixed and random effects models include the variation between measures (e.g. between raters) as a source of variance in X. R_3 is generally less than R_2 when applied to the same data. This is because the error in X is estimated to be larger when the measures (e.g. raters) in the reliability study are only a sample of the measures to be used in the full study.

Example. Suppose that two interviewers administered a food frequency questionnaire to each subject in a reliability study, and the same two interviewers will be employed in the full study. Then the fixed effects model applies, and R_2 is an appropriate estimate of ρ_X. The computation is illustrated on the same data as in the previous example (Table 4.3). From the two-way ANOVA:

$$R_2 = \frac{110(64.37 - 13.81)}{110(64.37) + 233.81 + 109(13.81)} = 0.63.$$

Table 4.3 Example of an analysis of variance for a test–retest study of percentage energy from fat estimated from a food frequency questionnaire

Variable	N	Mean (% kcal)	Standard deviation
% energy at baseline (X_1)	110	37.5	5.96
% energy at 6 months (X_2)	110	35.5	6.53

	One-way ANOVA		
Source of variance	Sum of squares	Degrees of freedom	Mean square
Between subjects	7015.89	109	64.37
Within subjects (random error)	1739.52	110	15.81
Total	8755.41	219	39.98

	Two-way ANOVA		
Source of variance	Sum of squares	Degrees of freedom	Mean square
Between subjects	7015.89	109	64.37
Between measures	233.81	1	233.81
Random error	1505.71	109	13.81
Total	8755.41	219	39.98

Intraclass correlation which excludes the mean differences between measures

For some reliability study designs, the systematic differences between the measures, the differences between the $\bar{X}_j$, do not need to be included as a source of variance in X. This is the case when it is intended to adjust for the systematic difference between measures in the epidemiological study. For example, if interviewers produced different mean estimates of exposure, one might adjust in the epidemiological study for interviewer effects. Under these circumstances the intraclass correlation coefficient, R_4, is used. R_4 may also be appropriate for reliability studies in which the difference between X_1 and X_2 can be explained by a 'learning effect' or other factors that will not add error (variance) to the measure X in the full study.

When the measurement effects are to be excluded as a source of variance in X, the intraclass correlation coefficient for the fixed effects model is

$$R_4 = \frac{\text{SMS} - \text{EMS}}{\text{SMS} + (k-1)\text{EMS}}.$$

It has a lower $100(1 - \alpha)$ confidence limit:

$$R_4 > \frac{\dfrac{\text{SMS}}{\text{EMS}} - f}{\dfrac{\text{SMS}}{\text{EMS}} + (k-1)f}$$

where f denotes the $(1 - \alpha)$ centile of the F distribution with $(n-1)$ and $(n-1)(k-1)$ degrees of freedom.

R_4 will equal 1 when the measures are identical for each subject except for a constant difference between measures:

$$X_{i1} = X_{i2} + d_2 = \ldots X_{ik} + d_k.$$

(R_4 differs from the Pearson correlation coefficient, in that R_4 includes any differences in scale as a source of variance in X.)

When the k measures, $X_1, \ldots, X_k$, have identical distributions, all four versions of R are essentially the same and are equal to the Pearson product-moment correlation coefficient.

Cohen's κ for binary or nominal variables

The intramethod reliability of nominal categorical variables, including dichotomous variables, is measured by Cohen's κ (Cohen 1960). This can be computed from a reliability study in which n subjects have each been measured twice where each measure is a nominal variable with k categories. (Note that k here refers to number of categories, not number of measures

Table 4.4 Layout of data for computation of Cohen's κ and weighted κ

		Measure 2				
		1	2	.	.	k	Total
	1	p_{11}	p_{12}	.	.	p_{1k}	r_1
	2	p_{21}	p_{22}	.	.	p_{2k}	r_2
Measure 1	.	.	.	.	.	.	.
	.	.	.	.	.	.	.
	.	.	.	.	.	.	.
	k	p_{k1}	p_{k2}	.	.	p_{kk}	r_k
	Total	s_1	s_2	.	.	s_k	1

per subject.) It is assumed that the two measures are equally accurate. To compute κ the data are laid out as a $k \times k$ table as in Table 4.4. The p_{ij} are the proportions of subjects who fall into the ith category in measure 1 and the jth category in measure 2. Note that the p_{ij} proportions in the table sum to 1 over the entire table. The r_i and s_j are the marginal proportions for the first and second measure respectively.

An obvious measure of agreement between two measures is the proportion of subjects for whom there was agreement. The observed proportion of agreement, P_o, is the sum of the proportions on the diagonal:

$$P_o = \sum_{i=1}^{k} p_{ii}.$$

However, this simple measure does not take into consideration the agreement that would be expected by chance. For example, suppose one interviewer classified 5 per cent of subjects as exposed and 95 per cent as unexposed, but a second interviewer (who perhaps skipped the question) classified all subjects as unexposed. Then the percentage agreement would be 95 per cent, which does not reflect the poor reliability of the measure.

κ is a measure of agreement that corrects for the agreement that would be expected by chance. The expected agreement (on the diagonal), P_e, is:

$$P_e = \sum_{i=1}^{k} r_i s_i.$$

κ is estimated as the observed agreement beyond chance divided by the maximum possible agreement beyond chance:

$$\hat{\kappa} = \frac{P_o - P_e}{1 - P_e}.$$

$\hat{\kappa}$ is equal to 1 when there is exact agreement between the two measures for all subjects. It is greater than 0 when agreement is greater than chance, but can be less than 0 if agreement is less than expected by chance.

An approximate lower $100(1 - \alpha)$ per cent confidence bound for $\hat{\kappa}$ (if $\kappa \neq 0$) is (Fleiss *et al.* 1969; Fleiss 1981):

$$\hat{\kappa} - Z_\alpha \times \text{s.e.}(\hat{\kappa})$$

where Z_α is the value of the $(1 - \alpha)$ centile of the standard normal variable and s.e. $(\hat{\kappa})$ is the estimated standard error of $\hat{\kappa}$:

$$\text{s.e.}(\hat{\kappa}) = \sqrt{\frac{a + b - c}{(1 - P_e)^2 n}}$$

where

$$a = \sum_{i=1}^{k} p_{ii} [1 - (r_i + s_i)(1 - \hat{\kappa})]^2,$$

$$b = (1 - \hat{\kappa})^2 \sum_{i=1}^{k} \sum_{\substack{j=1 \\ i \neq j}}^{k} p_{ij}(r_i + s_j)^2,$$

and

$$c = [\hat{\kappa} - P_e(1 - \hat{\kappa})]^2.$$

Example. Consider the reliability study described above in the intraclass correlation examples, and suppose subjects were to be divided into only two categories of fat intake: those above the median in percentage energy from fat and those below. Cross-classifying the 110 subjects by the two measures yields the following table, with the proportions in brackets:

		2nd measure		
		Upper half	Lower half	
1st measure	Upper half	40 (0.364)	15 (0.136)	55 (0.5)
	Lower half	15 (0.136)	40 (0.364)	55 (0.5)
		55 (0.5)	55 (0.5)	110 (1.0)

Then

$$P_o = 0.364 + 0.364 = 0.727,$$

$$P_e = (0.5 \times 0.5) + (0.5 \times 0.5) = 0.50,$$

$$\hat{\kappa} = \frac{0.727 - 0.5}{0.5} = 0.45.$$

When the number of categories is greater than two, the source of unreliability may become clearer by computing a κ for each category compared with all other categories combined. When the number of measures per subject is greater than two, another version of κ has been derived, under the assumption that there is no order to the measures (Landis and Koch 1977; Fleiss 1986). The assumptions and resulting κ are similar to the one-way ANOVA intraclass correlation coefficient.

Weighted κ for ordered categorical variables

The κ presented above for nominal categories is a measure of exact agreement, with all disagreements considered to be equally serious. For example, if rater 1 categorizes a subject as falling into category 1, and rater 2 disagrees, κ will be the same whether the second rating is category 2, 3, 4, etc. When the measure of interest in an intramethod reliability study is an ordered categorical variable, the use of κ is not appropriate. Instead κ_w, *weighted κ*, (Cohen 1968) is used instead, as this measure yields a higher reliability when disagreements between raters are small compared with when they are large. In other words, weighted κ gives 'partial credit' for close but not exact agreement.

Weighted κ is estimated by

$$\hat{\kappa}_w = \frac{P_o - P_e}{1 - P_e},$$

where P_o is the weighted observed proportion of agreement (across the entire table):

$$P_o = \sum_{i=1}^{k} \sum_{j=1}^{k} w_{ij} p_{ij},$$

P_e is the weighted expected proportion of agreement (across the entire table):

$$P_e = \sum_{i=1}^{k} \sum_{j=1}^{k} w_{ij} r_i s_j,$$

and p_{ij}, r_i and s_j are the proportions shown in Table 4.4.

The usual weight applied for one measure yielding category i and the other category j is:

$$w_{ij} = 1 - \frac{(i - j)^2}{(k - 1)^2}.$$

This gives a weight of 1 for exact agreement and a weight of 0 when one measure yields the lowest category and the other the highest (kth) category.

A confidence interval for $\hat{\kappa}_w$ can be computed based on the large sample estimate of the standard error of $\hat{\kappa}_w$ (for $\kappa_w \neq 0$):

$$\text{s.e.}(\hat{\kappa}_w) = \sqrt{\frac{a - b}{(1 - P_e)^2 n}}$$

where

$$a = \sum_{i=1}^{k} \sum_{j=1}^{k} p_{ij} [w_{ij} - (\bar{w}_i + \bar{w}_j)(1 - \hat{\kappa}_w)]^2,$$

$$b = [\hat{\kappa}_w - P_e(1 - \hat{\kappa}_w)]^2,$$

$$\bar{w}_i = \sum_{j=1}^{k} s_j w_{ij},$$

and

$$\bar{w}_j = \sum_{i=1}^{k} r_i w_{ij}.$$

For the reliability study used in the previous examples, if percentage calories from fat were divided into four equal ordered categories, κ_w would be 0.57.

Ordered categorical variables are often created by categorizing a continuous variable. In these situations, the intraclass correlation coefficient could also be computed on the underlying variable.

Interpretation and limitations of κ and weighted κ

Certain similarities allow κ and κ_w to be interpreted as reliability coefficients. κ for binary variables and κ_w are equal to the intraclass correlation coefficient based on the two-way random effects model (R_3), except for a term that goes to 0 as n increases (Fleiss and Cohen 1973; Fleiss 1975; Dunn 1989), when the categories are numerically coded 1 for category 1, 2 for category 2, etc. κ_w is also equal to the Pearson product-moment correlation coefficient if the marginal distributions of the two measures are identical (Cohen 1968).

There are several limitations to the interpretation of κ and κ_w (Maclure and Willett 1987). The value of κ_w varies with the number of exposure categories. In the reliability study of percentage energy from fat used in the previous examples, κ was 0.45 when the measure was divided into two categories and κ_w was 0.57 when four categories were used. (The intraclass correlation was 0.61 when percentage energy from fat was treated as a continuous variable.)

In addition, the value of κ or κ_w depends on the distribution of exposure in the population. Thus κ cannot be used to compare the reliability of two instruments measuring the same underlying exposure if the two reliability studies were conducted in populations which may have different distributions of the true exposure. This is similar to the problem of comparing reliability coefficients across populations which differ in the variance of exposure. However, this dependence of κ on the prevalence of exposure may be a desirable property for, as noted in Chapter 3, the attenuation of the odds ratio depends on the exposure prevalence as well as the sensitivity and specificity of the measurement. When κ is derived from a study in which the two dichotomous measures compared have equal sensitivity, equal specificity and independent error probabilities (similar to the parallel test model), κ has been shown to be crudely related to the attenuation of the odds ratio under non-differential misclassification (for a limited range of parameters) (Thompson and Walter 1988):

$$OR_O \cong (OR_T - 1)\kappa + 1.$$

In addition, since κ_w could be interpreted as an intraclass correlation coefficient, the interpretations given for $\rho_{X_1 X_2}$ in terms of ρ_{TX_1} in this chapter (and subsequently in terms of the attenuation of the odds ratio given in the last chapter) might crudely apply to κ_w, depending on the degree of violation of the assumptions of the error model.

Neither κ nor weighted κ_w is sufficient to detect differential misclassification between cases and controls. κ is a single summary measure of the misclassification in the measure, while the assessment of differential misclassification requires estimates of sensitivity and specificity for cases and controls (or the misclassification matrices for $k > 2$). κ could be similar for cases and controls even when there is differential misclassification, that is when the underlying sensitivity and specificity of the exposure measurement differs substantially between the two groups. This is analogous to the problem that intramethod reliability studies of continuous variables can provide information only on precision but not on bias, and therefore cannot assess differential bias between cases and controls.

Other types of analysis of reliability studies

Some authors (Liu *et al.* 1978) present the reliability of a continuous measure X in terms other than the reliability coefficient ρ_X. The *ratio of the within-subject variance*, σ_W^2, *to the between-subject variance*, σ_S^2, is sometimes used, where S in the subject effect and σ_W^2 is defined as $\sigma_X^2 - \sigma_S^2$. This ratio is a simple transformation of ρ_X:

$$\frac{\sigma_W^2}{\sigma_S^2} = \frac{1 - \rho_X}{\rho_X},$$

where ρ_X is based on the appropriate measure of the reliability coefficient. Because the ratio of within- to between-subject variance provides the same information as the reliability coefficient, the equations presented in Chapters 3, 4 and 5 as functions of ρ_X (or of ρ_{TX}^2 when ρ_X can be considered as an estimate of ρ_{TX}^2) could be presented in terms of σ_W^2/σ_S^2 by substituting

$$\rho_X = 1/[(\sigma_W^2/\sigma_S^2) + 1].$$

One additional analytical technique for reliability studies of continuous measures deserves mention: the *coefficient of variation* (Garber and Carey 1984). For laboratory measures, reliability is often assessed by repeated analysis of a single reference material with known true measurement t. For example a fluid with a known concentration of retinol might be repeatedly analysed to yield measures of X, the measured retinol concentration. (This type of study only assesses the laboratory error, of course, and excludes errors due to storage and handling of specimens, and error due to the variation in the measure over time within individuals.) In such studies, the mean and variance of X can be used to assess the reliability of X. The bias of the measure can be estimated as

$$b = \bar{X} - t.$$

Because t is a constant, the variance of X in the reliability study is equal to the variance of the random error F:

$$\hat{\sigma}_F^2 = \hat{\sigma}_X^2.$$

A reliability coefficient cannot be estimated, because the comparison measure is constant (t) for each measurement of X. Instead a coefficient of variation, CV, defined as the estimated standard deviation divided by the mean of $X \times 100$, is often used:

$$CV\% = \frac{\hat{\sigma}_X}{\bar{X}} \times 100.$$

A small CV is considered to indicate a reliable measure. However, it may be more informative to relate the variance of the random error, $\hat{\sigma}_F^2$, to the expected variance of X in the population of interest (see right-hand side of Equation 4.9), to yield information closer to the reliability coefficient of X in the population of interest.

Reliability study designs may be more complex than those covered in this chapter, in order to yield more information about the measurement error. For example, an intramethod study could have two interviewers question each subject with each interview coded by two coders, or an intermethod study could be conducted of three or more instruments which measure the same exposure. Dunn (1989) provides other approaches to the analysis of simple intermethod and intramethod studies, and also gives methods for more complex designs.

In addition, reliability studies might include evaluation of several exposures simultaneously for, as noted in Chapter 3, the bias in the odds ratio for one exposure depends on the measurement error in the covariates as well as the primary exposure. Procedures have been developed that incorporate information from reliability studies of multiple exposures into the analysis of the parent epidemiological study; these are briefly described in Chapter 5. These procedures yield an estimate of the effect of the unreliability of the exposure measure(s) on the odds ratio in the particular research context of interest; this could be more informative than a reliability coefficient or κ.

Finally, reliability studies of some instruments do not require a comparison measure. In the social sciences, the reliability of a total score on a test is often assessed by the reliability of parts of the test, e.g. by the correlation between test items or the correlation between two halves of the test (Carmines and Zeller 1979; Dunn 1989). This is termed *internal consistency reliability*, and the Spearman–Brown formula given in Chapter 5 (Equation 5.3) or related equations are used to assess the reliability of the total score. This approach may be useful for some applications in epidemiology. (One note of caution: in some packaged programs, SPSS in particular, the term reliability is often used to refer to the reliability of the sum of the measures. If you are interested in the reliability of the individual measures X_1, X_2, etc., the reliability coefficient that is reported by the program may not be the statistic you are interested in.)

Sample size for reliability studies

The computation of the required sample size depends on the design and aim of the reliability study. For an intermethod reliability study conducted to assess differential bias between cases and controls, the required sample size could be based on a two-sample comparison of means (Kelsey *et al*. 1986), where the variable of interest is $(X_{i1} - X_{i2})$. For a validity or intermethod reliability study conducted to estimate $\rho_{X_1 X_2}$, the sample size should be that needed to evaluate the correlation between two variables (Willett 1990). Note that the null hypothesis to be tested is not $\rho_{X_1 X_2} = 0$ (for it should be assumed that X_1 and X_2 are at least positively correlated); rather the study should have sufficient power to detect whether $\rho_{X_1 X_2}$ is greater than some minimum value. For intramethod reliability studies, Donner and Eliasziw (1987) have presented methods for selecting the appropriate number of subjects and number of measurements per subject for studies which will be analysed using the intraclass correlation coefficient, and Jannarone *et al*. (1987) have given an approach for studies which estimate κ.

SUMMARY

Reliability studies can be designed to provide information about the validity of a measure if the comparison measure is carefully selected. If a comparison measure without differential bias between cases and controls is chosen, then a reliability study can yield estimates of differential bias in the measure of interest. Useful information about the validity coefficient can be obtained from a comparison of the measure of interest with an equally accurate or more accurate measure when the errors between the two measures are uncorrelated. When the measures in a reliability study have correlated errors, the reliability coefficient can provide only an upper limit to the validity coefficient.

The choice of an analytical technique for a validity or reliability study depends on whether the exposure is measured as a continuous variable, as a nominal categorical (or dichotomous variable), or as an ordered categorical variable. The choice also depends on whether the two or more measures in the reliability study will be used interchangeably in the full epidemiological study or only one will be used, and on other design issues. For example, for a reliability study in which a continuous exposure measure from proxy respondents was compared with the same measure from the subjects themselves, the Pearson correlation coefficient might be appropriate for the analysis if all interviews in the full study were to be from proxy respondents; a version of the intraclass correlation coefficient (R_2) might be used if both proxies and index cases were to be included in the full study; and another version (R_4) might be used if both were included but a factor indicating whether the interview was by index or proxy respondent was to be adjusted for in the full study. Versions of Cohen's κ are most commonly used to summarize the information obtained in reliability studies involving nominal or ordered categorical variables.

REFERENCES

Allen, M.J. and Yen, W.M. (1979). *Introduction to Measurement Theory*, pp. 1–117. Brooks/Cole, Monterey.

Altman, D.G. and Bland, J.M. (1983). Measurement in medicine: The analysis of method comparison studies. *The Statistician*, 32, 307–17.

Armitage, P. and Berry, G. (1987). *Statistical methods in medical research*, (2nd edn). Blackwell Scientific Publications, Oxford.

Bartko, J.J. (1966). The intraclass correlation coefficient as a measure of reliability. *Psychological Reports*, 19, 3–11.

Bohrnstedt, G.W. (1983). Measurement. In *Handbook of survey research*, (ed. P. Rossi, J. Wright, and A. Anderson), pp. 70–121. Academic Press, Orlando, Florida.

Carmines, E.G. and Zeller, R.A. (1979). *Reliability and validity assessment*. Sage, Beverly Hills, California.

Cohen, J. (1960). A coefficient of agreement for nominal scales. *Educational and Psychological Measurement*, 20, 37–46.

Cohen, J. (1968). Weighted kappa: nominal scale agreement with provision for scaled disagreement or partial credit. *Psychological Bulletin*, 70, 213–20.

Clayton, D. (1985). Using test-retest reliability data to improve estimates of relative risk: an application of latent class analysis. *Statistics in Medicine*, 4, 445-55.

Decker, M.D., Booth, A.L., Dewey, M.J., Fricker, R.S., Hutcheson, R.H., and Schaffner, W. (1986). Validity of food consumption histories in a foodborne outbreak investigation. *American Journal of Epidemiology*, 124, 859-63.

Donner, A. and Eliasziw, M. (1987). Sample size requirements for reliability studies. *Statistics in Medicine*, 6, 441-448.

Dunn, G. (1989). *Design and analysis of reliability studies*. Edward Arnold, London, and Oxford University Press, New York.

Eskenazi, B. and Pearson, K. (1988). Validation of a self-administered questionnaire for assessing occupational and environmental exposures of pregnant women. *American Journal of Epidemiology*, 128, 1117-29.

Fleiss, J.L. (1975). Measuring agreement between two judges on the presence or absence of a trait. *Biometrics*, 31, 651-9.

Fleiss, J.L. (1981). *Statistical methods for rates and proportions*, (2nd edn), pp. 188-236. John Wiley and Sons, New York.

Fleiss, J.L. (1986). *The design and analysis of clinical experiments*, pp. 1-32. John Wiley and Sons, New York.

Fleiss, J.L. and Cohen, J. (1973). The equivalence of weighted kappa and the intraclass correlation coefficient as measures of reliability. *Educational and Psychological Measurement*, 33, 613-9.

Fleiss, J.L., Cohen, J., and Everitt, B.S. (1969). Large sample standard errors of kappa and weighted kappa. *Psychological Bulletin*, 72, 323-7.

Fleiss, J.L. and Shrout, P.E. (1977). The effects of measurement errors on some multivariate procedures. *American Journal of Public Health*, 67, 1188-91.

Fleiss, J.L. and Shrout, P.E. (1978). Approximate interval estimation for a certain intraclass correlation coefficient. *Psychometrika*, 43, 259-62.

Garber, C.C. and Carey, R.N. (1984). Laboratory statistics. In *Clinical chemistry: theory, analysis, and correlation*, (ed. L. Kaplan and A. Pesce), pp. 290-2. C.V. Mosby, St. Louis, Missouri.

Gerbert, B., Stone, G., Stulbarg, M., Gullion, D.S., and Greenfield, S. (1988). Agreement among physician assessment methods. *Medical Care*, 26, 519-35.

Harlow, S.D. and Linet, M.S. (1989). Agreement between questionnaire data and medical records. The evidence for accuracy of recall. *American Journal of Epidemiology*, 129, 233-48.

Hill, A.B. (1953). Observation and experiment. *New England Journal of Medicine*, 248, 995-1001.

Hui, S.L. and Walter, S.D. (1980). Estimating the error rates of diagnostic tests. *Biometrics*, 36, 167-71.

Jannarone, R.J., Macera, C.A., and Garrison, C.Z. (1987). Evaluating inter-rater agreement through 'case-control' sampling. *Biometrics*, 43, 433-7.

Jarvholm, B. and Sanden, A. (1987). Estimating asbestos exposure: a comparison of methods. *Journal of Occupational Medicine*, 29, 361-3.

Kaldor, J. and Clayton, D. (1985). Latent class analysis in chronic disease epidemiology. *Statistics in Medicine*, 4, 327-35.

Kelsey, J.L., Thompson, W.D., and Evans, A.S. (1986). *Methods in observational epidemiology*, pp. 277, 285-308. Oxford University Press, New York.

Klesges, R.C., Klesges, L.M., Swenson, A.M., and Pheley, A.M. (1985). A validation of two motion sensors in the prediction of child and adult physical activity levels. *American Journal of Epidemiology*, **122**, 400–10.

Landis, J.R. and Koch, G.G. (1977). The measurement of observer agreement for categorical data. *Biometrics*, **33**, 159–74.

Liu, K., Stamler, J., Dyer, A., McKeever, J., and McKeever, P. (1978). Statistical methods to assess and minimize the role of intra-individual variability in obscuring the relationship between dietary lipids and serum cholesterol. *Journal of Chronic Diseases*, **31**, 399–418.

Lord, F.M. and Novick, M.R. (1968). *Statistical theories of mental test scores*, pp. 13–278. Addison-Wesley, Reading, Massachusetts.

Maclure, M. and Willett, W.C. (1987). Misinterpretation and misuse of the kappa statistic. *American Journal of Epidemiology*, **126**, 161–9.

Nunnally, J.C. (1978). *Psychometric theory*, pp. 190–255. McGraw-Hill, New York.

Shekelle, R.B., Shryock, A.M., Paul, O., Lepper, M., Stamler, J., Lui, S., and Raynor, W.J. (1981). Diet, serum cholesterol, and death from coronary heart disease: The Western Electric Study. *New England Journal of Medicine*, **304**, 65–70.

Siconolfi, S.F., Lasater, T.M., Snow, R.C.K., and Carleton, R.A. (1985). Self-reported physical activity compared with maximal oxygen uptake. *American Journal of Epidemiology*, **122**, 101–5.

Thompson, W.D. and Walter, S.D. (1988). Variance and dissent. A reappraisal of the kappa coefficient. *Journal of Clinical Epidemiology*, **41**, 949–58.

Walker, A.M. and Blettner, M. (1985). Comparing imperfect measures of exposure. *American Journal of Epidemiology*, **121**, 783–90.

Walter, S.D. (1984). Commentary on 'Use of dual responses to increase validity of case-control studies.' *Journal of Chronic Diseases*, **37**, 137–9.

Walter, S.D. and Irwig, L.M. (1988). Estimation of test error rates, disease prevalence and relative risk from misclassified data: a review. *Journal of Clinical Epidemiology*, **41**, 923–37.

Willett, W. (1990). *Nutritional epidemiology*, pp. 34–126. Oxford University Press, New York.

Willett, W.C., Stampfer, M.J., Underwood, B.A., Speizer, F.E., Rosner, B., and Hennekens, C.H. (1983). Validation of a dietary questionnaire with plasma carotenoid and alpha-tocopherol levels. *American Journal of Clinical Nutrition*, **38**, 631–9.

Willett, W.C., Sampson, L., Stampfer, M.J., Rosner, B., Bain, C., Witschi, J., Hennekens, C.H., and Speizer, F.E. (1985). Reproducibility and validity of a semiquantitative food frequency questionnaire. *American Journal of Epidemiology*, **122**, 51–65.

Williams, E., Klesges, R.C., Hanson, C.L., and Eck, L.H. (1989). A prospective study of the reliability and convergent validity of three physical activity measures in a field research trial. *Journal of Clinical Epidemiology*, **42**, 1161–70.

Wu, M.L., Wittemore, A.S., and Jung, D.L. (1988). Errors in reported dietary intakes. II. Long-term recall. *American Journal of Epidemiology*, **128**, 1137–45.

5

Reducing measurement error and its effects

In most statistical approaches to observer variability, . . . no efforts have been made to detect and remove sources of inconsistency. After noting the disagreements and quantifying them with kappa scores or other indices of concordance, investigators write the paper and depart from the analytic scene. (Feinstein 1983).

INTRODUCTION

In Chapters 3 and 4 we have described the effects of exposure measurement error and how the extent of measurement error can be assessed. The primary focus of exposure measurement, however, should not be on assessment but on the reduction of measurement error and its effects.

Several approaches to the reduction of measurement error and its effects are discussed in this chapter. The first is the use of multiple measures of exposure, an important method of reducing measurement error. Next, adjustment procedures are briefly covered; these are methods of 'correcting', study results for the effect of measurement error by using information from validity or reliability studies. Finally, minimization of error by means of quality control procedures is discussed. These procedures include a wide range of methods of reducing measurement error during each phase of a study, from instrument development through data collection and creation of the data set for analysis.

USE OF MULTIPLE MEASURES OF EXPOSURE

The use of the average (or sum) of two or more measures of the exposure for each subject in an epidemiological study can be an effective method of decreasing the measurement error, in comparison with the use of a single measurement. The measures can be repeated administrations of the same instrument, or measurements from two different instruments. For example serum cholesterol could be measured by use of an average of three measurements from samples collected over a year. Or, dietary fat could be assessed as an average of a food frequency measurement and a measurement from a 7-day diet diary.

The use of *multiple measures* refers to repeated measurement of all subjects in an epidemiological study to *reduce* measurement error; this differs from a reliability study, in which a sample of subjects would be repeatedly measured to *assess* measurement error. Nonetheless, many of the concepts introduced in the last chapter are important in understanding the benefits of multiple measures.

The use of multiple measures to increase validity under parallel test model

The improvement in the validity of an exposure variable resulting from the combination of multiple measures is easily demonstrated when the errors in the two or more measures to be averaged are equal and uncorrelated (the parallel test model) (Carmines and Zeller 1979; Bohrnstedt 1983; Fleiss 1986; Dunn 1989).

Suppose each individual in a population is measured k times, by use of parallel measures of the underlying true exposure T, yielding observations of continuous variables $X_1, \ldots, X_k$. Recall from Chapter 4 that, under the model of parallel tests, the errors of the measures $(E_1, \ldots, E_k)$ are uncorrelated with each other and with T, and the variances of the errors are equal (σ_E^2). This implies that the correlation of each X_j with T is identical, ρ_{TX}. The average measure for individual i, A_i, is computed as

$$A_i = \frac{X_{i1} + \ldots + X_{ik}}{k},$$

where X_{ij} represents the observation on subject i of variable X_j. Then the variable A has a validity coefficient:

$$\rho_{TA} = \sqrt{\sigma_T^2 / (\sigma_T^2 + \sigma_E^2/k)}. \qquad [5.1]$$

It can be seen from Equation 5.1. that, as k increases, the term σ_E^2/k goes to 0. This shows that the validity coefficient of A is greater than that of the individual measures, $X_1, \ldots, X_k$ (i.e. Equation 5.1 is greater for $k \geq 2$ than for $k = 1$), and that the validity coefficient of A approaches 1 as k increases.

Equation 5.1 can be rewritten as a function of the validity coefficient of the parallel measures, ρ_{TX}:

$$\rho_{TA} = \sqrt{\frac{k\rho_{TX}^2}{1 + (k-1)\rho_{TX}^2}}. \qquad [5.2]$$

If ρ_{TX} is known from a validity or reliability study, then the validity coefficient for A can be calculated from Equation 5.2. Table 5.1 gives examples of the improvement in validity one can achieve by using multiple parallel measures of T. For example, averaging two measures each with a validity

Table 5.1 Improvement in the validity of a measure by averaging k parallel measures[a]

Number of measures k	$\rho_{TX} = 0.5$ ρ_{TA}	$\rho_{TX} = 0.7$ ρ_{TA}
1	0.50	0.70
2	0.63	0.81
3	0.71	0.86
5	0.79	0.91
10	0.88	0.95

[a] ρ_{TX} is the validity coefficient of each parallel measure, X_j, of T; ρ_{TA} is the validity coefficient of A, the average of the parallel measures

coefficient of 0.7 can yield a new exposure measure with a validity coefficient of 0.8. Similarly, averaging five measures each with a validity coefficient of 0.5 can also yield a new measure with validity coefficient of 0.8.

The same concept expressed in terms of the reliability of A, ρ_A, as a function of the reliability of X is the Spearman–Brown formula (Spearman 1910; Brown 1910):

$$\rho_A = \frac{k\rho_{X_1 X_2}}{1 + (k - 1)\rho_{X_1 X_2}}.$$ [5.3]

$\rho_{X_1 X_2}$ represents the common correlation between any two of the k measures, and may be estimated from the average Pearson correlation coefficient of the pairs of measures (Carmines and Zeller 1979; Bohrnstedt 1983).

The advantage of using multiple, parallel exposure measures for each subject in an epidemiological study (assuming non-differential misclassification) is that it would result in less attenuation of the observed odds ratio (or other measure of association) due to measurement error. This also implies that a smaller sample size is required for a given power. For example, in a case-control study with equal numbers of cases and controls, the sample size required with k measures per subject, n_k, compared to the sample size needed when only one measure per subject is used, n_1, is (Fleiss 1986):

$$n_k = \frac{1 + (k - 1)\rho_{X_1 X_2}}{k} n_1.$$ [5.4]

Example. Suppose a case-control study is to be conducted on the relationship between serum cholesterol and colon cancer in a large health maintenance organization, where records of prediagnostic serum cholesterol levels are available. A test–retest reliability study of serum cholesterol levels over the time period of interest yields an estimate of the reliability coefficient $\hat{\rho}_{X_1 X_2} = 0.60$. Under the assumptions of parallel measures, the validity coefficient can be estimated as $\hat{\rho}_{TX} = \sqrt{0.60} = 0.77$ (from Equation 4.4). If three measures of serum cholesterol over the relevant time period were averaged per subject, the estimated validity of the average would be (from Equation 5.2):

$$\hat{\rho}_{TA} = \sqrt{\frac{3 \times 0.60}{1 + 2 \times 0.60}} = 0.90.$$

To interpret the effect of the use of three replicate measures on the bias in the odds ratio of the study of interest, Equation 3.6 might be used. With three measures per subject, if the true odds ratio were 2, the observable odds ratio would be $2^{0.90} = 1.9$, rather than $2^{0.77} = 1.7$ if only one measure per subject were used. Moreover, the number of subjects needed would be (from Equation 5.4):

$$\hat{n}_3 = \frac{1 + (3 - 1) \times 0.6}{3} n_1$$

$$= 0.73 n_1,$$

i.e. 27 per cent fewer subjects than would be required if one measure per subject were used.

Determining the number of measures under parallel tests

One method of determining k, the number of parallel measures per subject, is to select it so as to yield a desired level of the validity coefficient of A, ρ_{TA}. The number of measures can be calculated from Equation 5.2 (by use of $\rho_{X_1 X_2} = \rho_{TX}^2$ under parallel tests) as

$$k = \frac{\rho_{TA}^2 (1 - \rho_{X_1 X_2})}{\rho_{X_1 X_2} (1 - \rho_{TA}^2)}. \qquad [5.5]$$

Example. Continuing with the last example, suppose a measure of serum cholesterol with validity coefficient of 0.85 was wanted. Then it would be necessary to average k independent measures per subject, where

$$\hat{k} = \frac{0.85^2 (1 - 0.60)}{0.60 (1 - 0.85^2)} = 1.7,$$

or two measures per subject.

There are, of course, disadvantages to the use of multiple measures. One is the increased burden on respondents which may lead to a fall in the participation rate, particularly if more study visits are required. Another is the increase in cost per subject which, depending on the trade-off between this increase and the reduced sample size required, could increase the total cost of the study. The choice of the number of measures requires balancing the expected reduction in bias in the odds ratio against total study cost and respondent burden.

One approach is to select the number of measures per subject to minimize total study costs (Fleiss 1986). Costs are minimized by selecting k measures per subject, where

$$k = \sqrt{\frac{1 - \rho_{x_1 x_2}}{c \rho_{x_1 x_2}}} , \qquad [5.6]$$

and c is the ratio of the cost of one measurement to all other study costs per subject (recruitment costs, costs of other data collection). If k is not an integer, the total study cost, t, for the two integers around k can be estimated and the lowest cost selected, using

$$t \sim \left(\frac{1 + (k - 1)\rho_{x_1 x_2}}{k}\right)(1 + ck)$$

which states that total costs, t, are proportional to the number of subjects times costs per subject. A single measure is optimal when $c > (1 - \rho_{x_1 x_2})/\rho_{x_1 x_2}$.

Example. Suppose in the preceding example that the number of replicate measures were to be selected so as to minimize total study costs. If the cost of an additional cholesterol measurement was 0.25 in relation to all other costs, then:

$$\hat{k} = \sqrt{\frac{1 - 0.6}{0.25 \times 0.6}} = 1.6$$

which means the optimal number of replicates is between 1 and 2. For two measures per subject,

$$\hat{t} \sim \left(\frac{1 + (2 - 1) \times 0.6}{2}\right)(1 + 0.25 \times 2)$$

$$= 1.20.$$

For one measure per subject,

$$\hat{t} \sim (1)(1 + 0.25)$$

$$= 1.25.$$

Therefore using two measures would minimize study costs.

The use of multiple measures with unequal variances or correlated errors

The possibility of violation of the assumptions of the parallel test model must be considered when the use of multiple measures is evaluated (Kelsey *et al.* 1986). It may be that the two or more measures to be averaged do not have equal error variance. In this situation, averaging a precise measure with a less precise measure may result in a variable, A, which is less valid than the better measure alone. An obvious example is the use of the average of a perfect measure of exposure and an imperfect measure.

When the two or more measures to be averaged have correlated errors, but the other assumptions of parallel tests hold, the improvement in the validity of the exposure measure will be less than that predicted by Equations 5.1 or 5.2. Only the random error will be reduced by averaging, not the within-person bias (Liu 1988). If the errors are perfectly correlated (i.e. the measure is perfectly repeatable, even though it is not a perfect measure of exposure), the use of multiple measures will lead to no improvement in validity. Under correlated errors, as k increases the validity coefficient ρ_{TA} does not approach 1. The improvement in the reliability of A will be as predicted in Equation 5.3, but under correlated errors, the reliability will only yield an upper limit for validity (i.e. $\rho_{TA} < \sqrt{\rho_A}$).

The use of the sum

All of the equations presented above apply to using a sum,

$$S_i = X_{i1} + \ldots + X_{ik},$$

rather than an average. The sum has the same validity and reliability as an average, because the two differ only by a constant multiple, $1/k$.

Use of multiple measures when the exposure is a categorical variable

When the exposure measure is a dichotomous variable, there may be multiple measures indicating whether the subject was exposed or not. One example is exposure to human papilloma virus, which might be assessed by two different laboratory tests, each of which has measurement error. Dichotomous variables are usually summed, rather than averaged, to create an exposure score equal to the number of measures on which a subject was positive. If there are only two measures per subject, the summation leads to an exposure variable with three categories: exposed on both, exposed on one, exposed on neither. The resulting exposure variable could be treated as an ordered categorical variable; however, it is not a measure of dose (since the subject was either exposed or not), but rather an indicator of the measurement error in the exposure. Thus the odds ratio for those classified as exposed on both measures versus exposed on neither would generally have less attenuation than the odds ratio for those classified as exposed on one measure only. Marshall and Graham (1984) and Kelsey *et al.* (1986) discuss these and other approaches to using multiple binary exposure measures. A related approach incorporates information on multiple measures of the underlying (latent) categorical exposure to yield an estimate of the true odds ratio (see next section on adjustment procedures).

When the exposure is a nominal categorical variable or an ordered categorical variable, there is no simple approach to the combination of information from multiple measures of exposure. However, since many ordered categorical exposures are created by categorizing a continuous variable, the two or more continuous measures could be averaged and the subjects categorized by their average measure.

Further use of multiple measures to reduce measurement errors

There is another approach to the use of multiple measures to improve the validity of the exposure measure. In this approach, when the two or more measures are inconsistent beyond some tolerance level, further information is obtained to resolve the difference.

For example, in a study of the concentration of selenium in toenails, which may be technically difficult to measure, the specimen was divided into several samples (Hunter *et al.* 1990). If analysis of the first two did not yield consistent results, another analysis was performed and then the three measures, rather than two, were averaged. The tolerance could be set by requiring $|X_{i1} - X_{i2}|$ or the standard deviation for each subject (or the coefficient of variation for each subject) to be within some limit. Another example comes from a case-control study of breast cancer in relation to oral contraceptive use (Coulter *et al.* 1986; UK National Case-Control Study Group 1989). Subjects were interviewed concerning past oral contraceptive use, and their medical records were also abstracted. Inconsistencies were resolved by re-questioning the subjects. When this approach is possible, it may improve the validity of a measure more than simple averaging would.

ADJUSTMENT OF STUDY RESULTS FOR THE EFFECT OF MEASUREMENT ERROR

Another approach to accounting for the effect of measurement error is to estimate the impact of measurement error on the study results after the study has been conducted. By use of estimates of the exposure measurement error from a validity study, it is possible to adjust the observed exposure–disease association from the epidemiological study to yield an estimate of the true association. The equations given in Chapter 3, which give the observable measure of association as a function of the true measure and the measurement error, can be used to derive equations that yield estimates of the true measure of association given the observed measure of association and estimates of the measurement error. These 'adjustment' or 'de-attenuation' equations are given in Table 5.2. The reader is referred to Chapter 3 for the notation and assumptions used in the derivation of the equations.

Example. Suppose a cohort study of years of occupational exposure to rubber, assessed by self-report, in relation to bladder cancer yielded an odds ratio of 1.3 for each 10 years increase in reported exposure. Suppose also that a validity study among a subset of the subjects yielded an estimate of 0.6 for the validity coefficient, ρ_{TX}, between self-report of years of exposure and industrial records of exposure (assumed here to be a near-perfect measure). Then, information from these two studies can be used to adjust

Table 5.2   Equations for the true measure of association as a function of the observable measure of association and the exposure measurement error. (See Chapter 3 for the notation, the assumptions used in derivation of the equations, and the interpretation of equations.)

Equation	From equation	Differential or non-differential
Continuous exposure, dichotomous outcome		
$\beta_T = \left(1 - \dfrac{b_D - b_N}{\mu_{X_D} - \mu_{X_N}}\right) \dfrac{\beta_O}{\rho_{TX}^2}$	[3.3]	differential
$\beta_T = \beta_O/\rho_{TX}^2$	[3.4]	non-differential
$OR_T = OR_O^{1/\rho_{TX}^2}$	[3.5]	non-differential
$OR_T = OR_O^{1/\rho_{TX}}$	[3.6]	non-differential
Continuous exposure, continuous outcome		
$\rho_{TY} = \rho_{XY}/\rho_{TX}$	[3.8]	non-differential
$\beta_T = \beta_O/\rho_{TX}^2$	[3.9]	non-differential
Dichotomous exposure, dichotomous outcome		
$OR_T = \dfrac{P_D(1 - P_N)}{P_N(1 - P_D)}$	[3.12]	differential or non-differential

where $P_D = (p_D - 1 + spec_D)/(sens_D + spec_D - 1)$
and $P_N = (p_N - 1 + spec_N)/(sens_N + spec_N - 1)$

the observed odds ratio to yield an estimate of the true odds ratio (based on the equation in Table 5.2 derived from Equation 3.5, provided the assumptions hold):

$$\widehat{OR}_T = (1.3)^{1/0.6^2} = 2.1.$$

This suggests that poor exposure measurement may have led to the weak observed association between the exposure and disease, because the observed odds ratio is consistent with a true odds ratio of 2.1 for 10 years of exposure.

Information from reliability studies can also be used in adjustment procedures, to the extent that the reliability study provides information about the validity of the exposure variable (see Chapter 4). If the reliability study were of two parallel measures, $\sqrt{\rho_{X_1 X_2}}$ could be substituted for ρ_{TX} in the equations in Table 5.2. However, as discussed in Chapter 4, reliability studies may yield only an upper limit for the validity coefficient. This leads to a conservative estimate of the true odds ratio under non-differential measurement error, i.e. the estimate would only be corrected for the random component of measurement error.

Chapter 3 notes that for a cohort study in which sampling is by exposure status, the degree of misclassification changes after sampling. Adjustment procedures for cohort studies should be based on the estimates of exposure measurement error within the cohort(s) after any sampling by exposure status.

While adjustment procedures may aid in understanding the results of a study, caution should be exercised in interpreting the results. First, the assumptions used in the derivation of the equations in Table 5.2 may not be appropriate. In particular, an assumption of non-differential measurement error could be incorrect, so it is preferable if the exposure measurement error can be assessed separately for the diseased and non-diseased groups to account for non-differential misclassification. For continuous exposures, the assumptions of the simple measurement error model, normality of exposure and error, and the logistic model of disease–exposure relationship, often also fail to hold. Second, both the observed measure of association between the disease and exposure and the estimated measurement error have sampling error; this needs to be considered in estimation of the true association. Third, the estimates of the measurement error should be estimates from the same population(s) as the study to be corrected, yet such estimates may not be available. Finally, as noted in Chapter 3, the presence of covariates modifies the effect of exposure measurement error. Information on the multivariate measurement error structure of the primary exposure and covariates is required in order to correct fully for measurement error. Therefore, unless these issues have been accounted for, the emphasis of the adjustment procedure should be on interpretation of the observed estimate of effect, not on the corrected estimates.

A great deal of work has been done on adjustment procedures, or more generally, procedures which incorporate information from a validity or reliability study of the exposure in the statistical analysis of the disease-exposure relationship (Tenenbein 1970; Barron 1977; Copeland *et al.* 1977; Prentice 1982; Greenland and Kleinbaum 1983; Clayton 1985; Kaldor and Clayton 1985; Stefanski and Carroll 1985; Whittemore and Grosser 1986; Espeland and Hui 1987; Fuller 1987; Walter and Irwig 1988; Armstrong *et al.* 1989; Chen 1989; Carroll 1989; Pepe *et al.* 1989; Rosner *et al.* 1989; Qizilbash *et al.* 1991; Pepe and Fleming 1991). Many of these procedures take into consideration some of the issues discussed above; in particular, some make less restrictive assumptions about the error model, yield confidence intervals that incorporate sampling error from the reliability study, and/or allow a multivariate (exposure and covariate) measurement error structure. In addition, some are appropriate for the analysis of epidemiological studies which use multiple measures of exposure on each subject; this is equivalent to incorporating information from a reliability study that included all subjects from the full epidemiological study, rather than a subset of subjects. These methods may prove to be useful in accounting for measurement error.

OTHER METHODS

One method of taking into consideration the effects of measurement error on the power of a study was discussed in Chapter 3. In the design of an epidemiological study, the sample size calculations should be based on estimates of the observable parameters (the standard deviation of the exposure, the observable odds ratio, etc.) as they will be affected by measurement error, and not based on estimates from more accurate measures that may be available from pilot work. However, if the attenuated association is quite weak, increasing the sample size so that a weak association can be detected may lead to results that are difficult to interpret. Weak associations are often spuriously produced in epidemiological studies, through selection bias or inadequate control of confounding factors.

Another method for reducing the effects of measurement error was briefly mentioned in Chapter 4. In the analysis of an epidemiological study, adjustment for a covariate that is related to the exposure measurement error may reduce the effect of the error on the measure of association between the exposure and disease. For example, it may be necessary to adjust for interviewer effects if different interviewers (randomly assigned to subjects) yielded different mean exposure levels, or to adjust for the season in which a food frequency questionnaire was completed if season influenced the subjects' perception of their diet over the last year. While this is an established technique for studies of continuous outcomes (Fleiss 1986), its usefulness has not been fully evaluated for studies in which the outcome is a dichotomous variable, as is common in epidemiology (Greenland and Robins 1985).

QUALITY CONTROL PROCEDURES

Quality control procedures implemented at each stage of an epidemiological study can play an important part in reducing measurement error.

Quality control issues are discussed in the following chapters in relation to specific methods of exposure measurement. However, many quality control procedures are common to a number of methods of exposure measurement (see, for example, Dennis *et al.* 1980; Sudman and Bradburn 1983; Horwitz and Yu 1984; Hilsenbeck *et al.* 1985; Meinert 1986), and it is was thought useful to summarize them here (Table 5.3) because of their importance in reducing measurement error. These procedures relate particularly to the field collection of data from subjects themselves or from records, and the subsequent data processing up to the point of carrying out an analysis that makes use of orginal or derived variables. Quality control as it relates to the collection and processing of biological or environmental samples for laboratory-based measurements is dealt with in Chapters 9 and 10.

Table 5.3   General quality control procedures for the collection of data on exposure in epidemiological studies

---

DESIGN OF THE INSTRUMENT
Design of forms
  Include all items needed to compute dose, timing of exposure, etc.

  Include adequate subject identifiers—at least an identification number and a check digit or alphabetic code on all forms.

  Use separate forms for each method of exposure measurement.

  Make instructions clear and data collection items unambiguous.

  Use different typefaces for instructions, data collection items, and responses.

  Provide mutually exclusive and exhaustive response categories for closed-ended items.

  Make forms self-coding for simple items—e.g. data collector circles a number corresponding to the appropriate response category.

  Make response codes consistent within and across forms—e.g. 1 = no, 2 = yes.

  Provide for coding without loss of information—i.e. do not design forms so that continuous data are categorized at the coding stage.

Table 5.3   cont.

Do not require computation by data collectors, rather make provision on the form for entry of raw data into the computer.

Design forms for direct entry of data into the computer.

Study procedures manual
Always have a study procedures manual.

Include at least the following in the study procedures manual:
- description of the study in *general* terms
- sample selection, recruitment and tracking procedures
- informed consent and confidentiality procedures
- data forms
- general methods of data collection
- item-by-item clarification of questions and responses, including special cases
- editing procedures
- coding instructions for items not self-coded on form
- codebooks

Update manual and distribute updated pages whenever procedural changes are made.

PREPARING FOR DATA COLLECTION
Pre-testing instruments
Have instruments reviewed by other researchers.

Pre-test instruments on samples of convenience.

Train data collectors and pre-test instruments on samples similar to study subjects.

Identify problems through feedback from pre-test subjects and data collectors and by monitoring data collection (e.g. observing interviews, re-abstracting records) and make appropriate changes as early as possible.

Review frequencies of responses to identify items with little variation in responses.

Modify instrument.

Training of data collectors
Discuss importance of complete and accurate data.

Review study manual.

Practise data collection.

Monitor initial data collection by each data collector.

Resolve problems.

Table 5.3 cont.

QUALITY CONTROL DURING DATA COLLECTION

Supervision of data collectors

Assign cases and controls in a case-control study (or exposed and unexposed subjects, where this is known in advance, in a cohort study) in the same proportions to each data collector.

Maintain ignorance of data collectors to case-control (or exposed-unexposed) status of subjects, as far as possible.

Replicate some proportion of data collection (e.g. 10 per cent of subjects) to identify fictitious data, items with poor reliability, data collectors with errors on certain items, etc.

Compare the distribution of study variables among data collectors.

Compare distributions of study variables over time.

Address problems identified through monitoring immediately with the relevant data collector(s).

Conduct staff meetings for retraining, discussion of problems, and motivation.

Editing and coding

Have data collectors edit data forms immediately to clarify responses and check for missing items.

Have editor perform a second edit soon after data collection to check for missing items, inadmissible codes, inconsistencies among responses, illegible responses, etc.

Have editor code open-ended questions and query those inadequately answered.

Correct errors by call back to subjects (or check-back to records).

Have one staff member maintain an editor's log to ensure consistency of recording and coding of unanticipated responses, and to record comments and responses coded as 'other'.

QUALITY CONTROL DURING DATA PROCESSING

Key entry

Create a codebook with format and codes of 'raw' data items.

Enter data contemporaneously with data collection.

Double-enter (verify) all data.

Edit data by computer by performance of range and logic checks contemporaneously with data entry.

Correct errors and feed back findings of relevance to data collection.

Table 5.3   cont.

Creation of new variables

Check and recheck the programming code used to create new variables.

Check the correctness of new variables by manual computation from a sample of original records, whenever reasonably possible.

Review distributions of original and created variables.

Create a codebook with detailed descriptions of new variables created, including the original variables and programming code used to create them.

Design of the data collection instrument

In addition to questionnaires, data collection forms can include forms for abstraction of data from medical records, diaries to be kept by subjects, etc. In designing or reviewing the data collection forms to be used in a study, the first concern should be whether they include complete coverage of the items necessary to compute the exposure variables of interest (dose, time of commencement of exposure, duration of exposure, etc.) and the necessary covariates.

Generally, there should be one form per subject per method of exposure measurement. Colour coding of forms may help in studies with multiple forms per subject. A *check digit* on the subject identification (ID) number, an arithmetic combination of the other numbers in the ID (Anderson *et al.* 1974), allows identification of incorrect ID numbers (e.g. errors due to transposing two numbers). The check digit is computed as part of the ID before ID numbers are assigned, and can be checked after the data have been entered as part of computer editing of the data. An incorrect check digit implies an incorrect ID number. Alternatively, or in addition, an alphabetic code based on the subject's name, such as the first three letters of the last name, could be part of the subject ID. Check digits or an alphabetic code are particularly useful when data from several forms are merged.

Data forms should be designed for accuracy and ease of use during all stages of data collection and processing: the original data collection, coding and editing, and entry of data into the computer. *Coding*, that is, assigning numbers to responses that are given in words, is handled in one of two ways. For items with a small number of possible responses (e.g. marital status), the form should be pre-coded (e.g. 1 = married, . . ., 5 = never married). Codes used in the form (and preferably across all forms used in a study) should be consistent. For example, no = 1, yes = 2 should be the same on all forms. Circling the code number simplifies data entry, and is an unambiguous way of signifying the correct response. For items with a large number of possible responses (e.g. occupation), the responses should be recorded in words with space provided for coding at a later time.

The data collector or the subject should not carry out calculations unless they are necessary for the data collection. Instead, information should be sought as simple 'raw' data items, and calculations performed during data processing. Units of measurement should be specified on the form. Generally, numerical data should be recorded without loss of information; in other words, continuous data should not be categorized at the time of data collection.

A more detailed treatment of the formatting of questionnaires is given in Chapter 6, and additional information about record abstraction forms and diaries is given in Chapter 8.

A data collection instrument should include detailed instructions on its use. These instructions should form part of a study procedures manual and would include an explanation of every item, and the interpretation of each response to the item. The editing and coding procedures should also be included. This manual serves initially as a training manual, then as a reference for data collectors, and finally as a detailed record of the data collection procedures. Table 5.3 lists the contents of a typical study procedures manual. An interviewer's manual, a particular kind of study procedures manual, is outlined in Table 7.7. One staff member, usually the project director, should be responsible for any changes to the manual and for the distribution of those changes to other staff members.

Preparing for data collection

Before data collection can begin, the instrument must be pre-tested and the data collectors trained in the study procedures. Steps in pre-testing are listed in Table 5.3. A more detailed account of pre-testing in relation to questionnaires is given in Chapter 6. In addition, as noted in Chapter 4, reliability studies can be used during the pre-test phase to investigate and reduce sources of error. By identifying the sources of disagreements in repeated measures for a subject, the instrument can often be improved. Reliability studies of multiple data collectors who each collect data on the same subjects can identify those who need more training.

The study procedures manual can serve as the major training tool. Training begins with an overview of the study, and the importance of accurate data to the success of the study. Standardized execution of the protocol should be emphasized. To reduce differential bias introduced by the data collectors, the hypothesis should be presented in very general terms (e.g. 'we are looking at a range of lifestyle factors that may be associated with cancer of the colon'). After review of the procedures manual, the trainees practise the data collection tasks that they will perform, and have their work both observed and reviewed by the instructor. For large-scale studies, there is often a formal examination leading to '*certification*' in the procedures. This promotes uniform training, which is particularly necessary for multi-site studies. The initial data collection on study subjects by each new data collector should also be monitored closely, and any problems resolved.

The principal investigator of the study should be actively involved in this early phase of the study and in the early data collection, through observing or participating in pilot data collection and by discussing problems with data collectors. This often provides additional insights leading to improvements in the data collection instruments.

Quality control during data collection

Methods of quality control during data collection include assignment of equal proportions of cases and controls to each data collector in a case control study (or of exposed and unexposed subjects in a cohort study, if exposure status is known) and keeping the data collectors in ignorance of the case-control status (or exposure status) of subjects if possible.

Data collectors should edit their work immediately after data collection, to clarify responses and check for missing data. Missing or unclear data should be obtained or clarified by checking back with the subject (or with the record, for a record review study). Shortly after completion of the data collector's work on a subject, the forms should be reviewed again by an editor (the project director, or a person designated as the editor) to check for missing items, illegible responses, inadmissible codes (range checks), and logical inconsistencies among responses. (For example, in an abstract of a hospital birth record, it would be inconsistent for the type of birth to be reported as 'vaginal birth' but anaesthesia to be coded as 'general'.) The editor also checks for inadequate answers to questions requiring detailed coding (e.g. 'business owner' for occupation) and codes these items. The use of different coloured pens by different staff members makes it possible to track the additions and corrections made on a data form. Range and logic checks should also be carried out by computer. If this is done promptly it can reduce the amount of hand editing. Errors or problems identified by any of these editing procedures should be resolved by checking back with the subject or the original records, by improving the study procedures, by additional training for some or all data collectors, or a combination of these strategies.

Quality control during data collection can also include:

- replication of some proportion of each data collector's work by another or a senior data collector
- comparison of the distribution of variables among data collectors
- an analysis of trends in the variables over time.

Replication of data collection (e.g. telephone re-interview of a 10 per cent

Question A.5 Present Weight

Date	Subject ID	Problem	Date	Resolution	By Whom
10/15/89	10027	On steroid drugs gained 21 pounds	10/25/89	Leave weight as recorded--omit from analyses of weight	EW
1/27/90	10102	Had gallbladder problems, then surgery 3 weeks ago--lost 17 lbs.	2/5/90	Leave weight as recorded-- omit from analyses of weight	EW
2/17/90	10142	On weight loss diet--lost 15 pounds in 6 weeks	2/20/90	OK as recorded	EW

Figure 5.1 Example of an editor's log.

sample, covering a few key questions) at least detects the worst type of error — complete fabrication of answers. Analyses of trends over time might uncover interviewer fatigue, or drift in laboratory methods. For large studies, these analyses of key variables can yield periodic formal *quality control reports*. These, along with errors found during routine supervisory editing, can indicate which data collectors need additional training and which items need further clarification. Staff meetings can be useful for discussion of problems and for maintaining the interest of the staff in the quality of the data.

An additional quality control procedure is the keeping of an *editor's log*, a record of all problems in recording or coding answers and specimen handling or analysis, and subject comments that could affect the analysis or interpretation of the data. The log may include the date of the problem, the subject ID, the problem, the date the problem was resolved, who resolved it, and how. The editor's log is kept by one person only (e.g. the project director), and ensures uniform handling of problems. For example, a question on marital status may lead to unanticipated responses such as 'common law marriage' or 'married but husband has been in a nursing home for 5 years'. These responses should be coded consistently, or the question or responses clarified. The log may also include the wording of responses that were coded as 'other'. For example, a family history of breast cancer in a half-sister may have been coded as 'other relative', but the researcher would probably choose to include this response along with other second-degree relatives (aunts, grandmothers) during data analysis. It is much easier to do this by reference to an editor's log rather than having to refer back to the original forms. Organization of the log by question (in a computerized file, for example) allows easier reference to previous problems with the same item, and allows the investigator to review all problems item by item. Figure 5.1 shows a sample editor's log.

Quality control during data processing

Errors can be introduced in almost any phase of a study (Table 3.1), including the data processing stage. To minimize errors on data entry, data should be entered twice and a *verification* program used to signal disagreements. While errors introduced during data entry are not often considered to be a major source of measurement error, they can be quite important. In a study of macrosomic infants (4.5 kg or more at birth), Brunskill (1990) compared computerized birth certificate records with the actual birth certificates. Among the 39 high-birth-weight infants on the computerized records, the birth weight was wrong in 18. In nine cases, ounces on the birth certificate had been entered as pounds on the computer record (e.g. 12 oz entered as 12 lbs); in six, 1 lb (one pound) had been entered as eleven pounds (11 lb), and in three cases the decimal point had been misplaced (e.g. 510 g entered as 5100 g). As a result of this research, the birth certificates of the state in question now have the units of measurement pre-printed on the form; this change should eliminate some of the errors.

Errors in programming the calculation of exposure variables (such as dose) are another source of error in exposure measurement. These programming errors can easily occur as a consequence of not considering all possible combinations of the responses to the items that are used in creating the new variable. In particular, missing values need to be handled carefully. For example, suppose a new exposure variable was created equal to the number of the subject's second-degree relatives with a history of diabetes, where each of the subject's aunts, uncles, etc. were coded as *yes*, *no*, or *unknown*. Then for subjects with, say, two-second degree relatives, there are 9 (3^2) possible combinations of the two items, including difficult situations such as (*yes*, *unknown*) and (*no*, *unknown*). In most statistical packages, when two items are summed and one is 'missing', the sum is designated as 'missing'. However, if the new variable were well thought out, the researcher would probably override this standard handling of missing data by the statistical package. The programming of the computation of new variables should be checked by hand calculation on some cases and, when possible, by cross-classifying subjects by the items used to create the new variable and the new variable itself. Errors can also be identified by reviewing the frequency distributions of all raw and calculated variables (Stellman 1989).

CODEBOOK

Item No.	Variable Name	Description	Codes	Type[1]	Size[2]	Column Position
	ID	ID number	As given	I	5	1-5
1	SEX	Gender	1 = female 2 = male 9 = missing	I	1	6
2	AGE	Age of subject	As given 999 = missing	I	3	7-9
3	SMOKE	Subject smokes cigarettes?	1 = no 2 = yes 9 = missing	I	1	11
3a.	CIGNO	How many cigarettes a day?	As given 888 = N/A 999 = missing	I	3	12-14

[1] Type - identifies the length of the variable as defined in the database (text, integer, real)

[2] Size specifies the length of the variable in the database. For example, a text variable of 3 characters or an integer variable of 5 characters.

Figure 5.2   Example of a codebook.

Codebooks should be developed which describe the raw data as they were originally entered, as well as the new variables created during the course of analysis. A sample codebook is shown in Figure 5.2.

SUMMARY

The design and interpretation of an epidemiological study should take into account the effects of exposure measurement error, that is, that the observed odds ratio (or other measure of association) will be biased and, under non-differential measurement error, the power to detect an association will be reduced. For the study to have sufficient power, the sample size calculations should be based on parameters as they will be affected by measurement error. In addition, after a study has been completed, an estimate of the bias in the odds ratio can be calculated, based on estimates of the magnitude of the measurement error obtained from validity or reliability studies.

More importantly, the design and execution of a study should incorporate methods to reduce measurement error. One such method is the collection of multiple measures of the exposure for each subject in the study. If two or more measures of a single exposure have equal and uncorrelated errors, the average of the measures will be a more precise measure of the exposure than only one of the measures on its own. Use of the average or some other combination of the measures will lead to less bias in the measure of the effect of the exposure and a reduction in the required sample size. When the errors are not equal, or they are correlated, there may be less or even no reduction in measurement error. The use of multiple measures increases both the cost per subject and respondent burden, and these effects need to be taken into consideration when determining the number of measures to be used.

Systematic quality control procedures before, during, and after data collection are necessary to identify and correct measurement errors. Careful design of the data collection forms, complete documentation of study procedures, and pre-testing of the data collection instrument will eliminate some sources of error. The training and monitoring of data collectors should emphasize uniform execution of the study protocol. Review of the completed data forms by an editor and checks on the computerized data will uncover data items that need clarification or correction.

REFERENCES

Anderson, L.K., Hendershot, R.A., and Schoolmaker, R.C. (1974). Self-checking digit concepts. *Journal of Systems Management*, **25**, 36–42.

Armstrong, B.G., Whittemore, A.S., and Howe, G.R. (1989). Analysis of case-control data with covariate measurement error: application to diet and colon cancer. *Statistics in Medicine*, **8**, 1151–63.

Barron, B.A. (1977). The effects of misclassification on the estimation of relative risk. *Biometrics*, **33**, 414–8.

Bohrnstedt, G.W. (1983). Measurement. In *Handbook of survey research*, (ed. P. Rossi, J. Wright, and A. Anderson), pp. 70–121. Academic Press, Orlando, Florida.

Brown, W. (1910). Some experimental results in the correlation of mental abilities. *British Journal of Psychology*, **3**, 296–322.

Brunskill, A.J. (1990). Some sources of error in the coding of birth weight. *American Journal of Public Health*, **80**, 72–3.

Carmines, E.G. and Zeller, R.A. (1979). *Reliability and validity assessment*. Sage, Beverly Hills, California.

Carroll, R.J. (1989). Covariance analysis in general linear measurement error models. *Statistics in Medicine*, **8**, 1075–93.

Chen, T.T. (1989). A review of methods for misclassified categorical data in epidemiology. *Statistics in Medicine*, **8**, 1095–106.

Clayton, D. (1985). Using test-retest reliability data to improve estimates of relative risk: an application of latent class analysis. *Statistics in Medicine*, **4**, 445–55.

Copeland, K.T., Checkoway, H., McMichael, A.J., and Holbrook, R.H. (1977). Bias due to misclassification in the estimation of relative risk. *American Journal of Epidemiology*, **105**, 488–95.

Coulter, A., Vessey, M., and McPherson, K. (1986). The ability of women to recall their oral contraceptive histories. *Contraception*, **33**, 127–37.

Dunn, G. (1989). *Design and analysis of reliability studies*. Edward Arnold, London, and Oxford University Press, New York.

Dennis, B., Ernst, N., Hjurtland, M., Tillotson, J., and Grambsch, V. (1980). The NHLBI nutrition system. *Journal of the American Dietetic Association*, 77, 641–7.

Espeland, M.A. and Hui, S.L. (1987). A general approach to analyzing epidemiologic data that contain misclassification errors. *Biometrics*, 43, 1001–12.

Feinstein, A.R. (1983). An additional basic science for clinical medicine: IV. The development of clinimetrics. *Annals of Internal Medicine*, 99, 843–8.

Fleiss, J.L. (1986). *The design and analysis of clinical experiments*, pp. 1–32. John Wiley and Sons, New York.

Fuller, W.A. (1987). *Measurement error models*. John Wiley and Sons, New York.

Greenland, S. and Kleinbaum, D.G. (1983). Correcting for misclassification in two way tables and matched-pair studies. *International Journal of Epidemiology*, 12, 93–7.

Greenland, S. and Robins, J.M. (1985). Confounding and misclassification. *American Journal of Epidemiology*, 122, 495–506.

Hilsenbeck, S.G., Glaefke, G.S., Feigl, P., Lane, W.W., Golenzer, H., Ames, C., and Dickson, C. (1985). *Quality control for cancer registries*. US Department of Health and Human Services, Washington, DC.

Horwitz, R.I. and Yu, E.C. (1984). Assessing the reliability of epidemiologic data obtained from medical records. *Journal of Chronic Diseases*, 37, 825–31.

Hunter, D.J., Morris, J.S., Chute, C.G., Kusher, E., Colditz, G.A., Stampfer, M.J., Speizer, F.E., and Willett, W.C. (1990). Predictors of selenium concentration in human toenails. *American Journal of Epidemiology*, 132, 114–22.

Kaldor, J. and Clayton, D. (1985). Latent class analysis in chronic disease epidemiology. *Statistics in Medicine*, 4, 327–35.

Kelsey, J.L., Thompson, W.D., and Evans, A.S. (1986). *Methods in observational epidemiology*, pp. 285–308. Oxford University Press, New York.

Liu, K. (1988). Measurement error and its impact on partial correlation and multiple linear regression analyses. *American Journal of Epidemiology*, 127, 864–74.

Marshall, J.R. and Graham, S. (1984). Use of dual response to increase validity of case-control studies. *Journal of Chronic Diseases*, 37, 125–36.

Meinert, C.L. (1986). *Clinical trials: design, conduct, and analysis*. (Monographs in Epidemiology and Biostatistics, Vol. 8). Oxford University Press, New York.

Pepe, M.S. and Fleming, T.R. (1991). A non-parametric method for dealing with mismeasured covariate data. *Journal of the American Statistical Association*, 86, 108–113.

Pepe, M.S., Self, S.G., and Prentice, R.L. (1989). Further results on covariate measurement errors in cohort studies with time to response data. *Statistics in Medicine*, 8, 1167–78.

Prentice, R.L. (1982). Covariate measurement errors and parameter estimation in a failure time regression model. *Biometrika*, 69, 331–42.

Qizilbash, N., Duffy, S.W., and Rohan, T.E. (1991). Repeat measurement of case-control data: correcting risk estimates for misclassification due to regression dilution of lipids in transient ischemic attacks and minor ischemic strokes. *American Journal of Epidemiology*, 133, 832–8.

Rosner, B., Willett, W.C., and Spiegelman, D. (1989). Correction of logistic regression relative risk estimates and confidence intervals for systematic within-person measurement error. *Statistics in Medicine*, 8, 1051–69.

Spearman, C. (1910). Correlation calculated from faulty data. *British Journal of Psychology*, **3**, 271–95.

Stefanski, L. A. and Carroll, R. J. (1985). Covariate measurement error in logistic regression. *Annals of Statistics*, **13**, 1335–51.

Stellman, S. D. (1989). The case of the missing eights. An object lesson in data quality assurance. *American Journal of Epidemiology*, **129**, 857–60.

Sudman, S. and Bradburn, N. M. (1983). *Asking questions: a practical guide to questionnaire design*. Jossey-Bass, San Francisco, California.

Tenenbein, A. (1970). A doubling sampling scheme for estimating from binomial data with misclassification. *Journal of the American Statistical Association*, **65**, 1350–61.

UK National Case-Control Study Group (1989). Oral contraceptive use and breast cancer risk in young women. *Lancet*, **i**, 973–82.

Walter, S. D. and Irwig, L. M. (1988). Estimation of test error rates, disease prevalence and relative risk from misclassified data: a review. *Journal of Clinical Epidemiology*, **41**, 923–37.

Whittemore, A. S. and Grosser, S. (1986). Regression methods for data with incomplete covariates. In *Modern statistical methods in chronic disease*, (ed. S. H. Moolgavkar and R. R. Prentice), pp. 19–34. John Wiley and Sons, New York.

6

The design of questionnaires

I have been reported as having advocated, . . . 'that nobody should be subjected to more than five questions.' I am, indeed, in favor of shorter and brighter forms but not always to that extent. What I said on that occasion about the problems of making observations of any value, was this: 'broadly speaking, of any twenty questions asked in a field survey no more than five should be put to the surveyed, and no less than fifteen should be put to the surveyor by himself before he enters the field or, indeed, ventures to look over the gate.' In other words, I maintained, though doubtless somewhat clumsily, that one may ask as many questions as one believes useful — so long as the ratio one to the surveyed and three to the surveyor is maintained throughout. A basic query in the latter group will be in every case, 'is this question really necessary?' It is surprising how often that will effectively keep down the number incorporated. Hill (1953)

INTRODUCTION

For our purposes, a *questionnaire* can be defined as a tool designed to elicit and record, or guide the elicitation and recording of, recalled exposures from subjects of an epidemiological study. It contains questions to be put to the subject, and may also include answers to those questions from which the subject must choose those which are appropriate to him or her.

The objectives of questionnaire design are:

- to obtain measurements of exposure variables essential to the objectives of the study
- to minimize error in these measurements
- to create an instrument which is easy for the interviewer and subject to use, and for the investigator to process, and analyse.

These objectives are potentially in conflict, and any questionnaire usually represents a compromise among them. For example, it may be necessary to trade off some ease in processing and analysis against ease in completion by the interviewer or the subject. Similarly, the addition of some questions essential to the objectives of the study, for example questions about sexual behaviour in a study of the aetiology of cancer of the cervix, may make a questionnaire more difficult for an interviewer to administer and more threatening to the respondent. Judgement must be exercised in making decisions about the content and structure of questionnaires. Where compromise is necessary, the designer should favour decisions that maximize the usefulness of the questionnaire to the objectives of the study and minimize error in measurement.

In this chapter, we cover the major topics of importance in the design of questionnaires:

- choice of the items of data to be covered by the questionnaire
- the types of questions that can be used
- the material covered by each question
- the wording of questions
- physical format of questions
- the particular problem of collecting information on behaviours that vary with time
- question order
- aspects of structure of the questionnaire
- aids to recall
- practical aspects of pre-testing, producing and translating questionnaires.

More comprehensive accounts of the design of questionnaires can be found in Bennett and Ritchie (1975) and Sudman and Bradburn (1983).

CHOICE OF THE ITEMS TO BE COVERED

Questionnaire design usually begins with selection of the items of data that must be translated into questions. The ground to be covered is determined by two main factors: the objectives of the study and the limitations imposed by the burden that can be placed on respondents, including the feasible length of the questionnaire.

Objectives of the study

'The content of a questionnaire is generally designed to investigate the minimum amount of an individual's total experience that will provide sufficient information concerning the problem under study.' (Bennett and Ritchie 1975). Just as the objectives of the study determine the variables to be measured as a whole, they also determine the specific items to be covered in the questionnaire. If a question does not contribute to the achievement of the objectives, it has no place in the questionnaire.

Adequately detailed data should be sought for each essential exposure variable. A well-thought-out plan for data analysis, and a description of the algorithms that will be used to create exposure dose variables and covariates, will assist in determining the items and detail required. For each agent of interest, sufficient detail should be obtained to permit exposure to it to be distinguished from exposure to other agents that may cause the disease. In addition, it is usual to ask about the time exposure began, the time it ended, and the dose rate and its variation over time (see page 13).

Length of the questionnaire

The topics to be covered in a questionnaire and the detail in which they are covered are limited first and foremost by the length of time that subjects are willing to spend on the questioning process. While there are inevitable exceptions, it may be taken as a general rule that the maximum time that can be spent administering a questionnaire by face-to-face interview is 1–2 hours and, by telephone, 40 minutes to 1 hour. Self-administered questionnaires are at an added disadvantage in that the subject can gain an impression of the size of the response task before deciding whether to embark on it. Response rates among the general public appear not to be appreciably depressed by questionnaires of up to about 12 pages in length (Sudman and Bradburn 1983; Dillman 1978).

An illustration of the effect of questionnaire length on data quality was given by a study of the administration of long and short versions of the same questionnaire to high-school seniors. Respondents answering items that were included in large sets towards the end of long questionnaires were more likely to give identical answers to most or all items (a 'straight line' response pattern) than those answering items in small sets in short questionnaires (Herzog and Bachman 1981). One might reasonably suspect that a 'straight line' response pattern would be seen in long food-frequency questionnaires.

Other aspects of respondent burden

'Respondent burden concerns the level of demand placed on the respondent necessary to answer the survey instrument questions.' (Sudman and Andersen 1977). Length of the questionnaire is one aspect of respondent burden. Additional contributors to respondent burden are:

- length and distance (from the present) of the period over which recall is requested
- salience (or impact) to the subject of the topic of questioning, including its sensitivity
- frequency of the event
- complexity or detail of the data sought.

In general, recall over a long period of time or from the distant past, topics of low salience or impact, questioning regarding frequent events (such as eating), and complex questions (e.g. a full occupational history with details of exposure to hazards in each occupation) will all add to respondent burden. Being a proxy respondent for someone else is generally a further burden.

Increased burden on the respondent has several consequences:

- risk of termination of the interview or partial non-completion of a self-administered questionnaire increases

- quality of data obtained is reduced

- response rate is threatened

- the population may become alienated from survey research, and cooperation in future studies may be reduced. (Sudman and Andersen 1977).

The last effect is a particular problem for longitudinal studies requiring recurrent surveys in one population.

There is often a conflict between collecting information considered to be necessary to the objectives of the study, keeping the questionnaire to an acceptable length, and minimizing other aspects of respondent burden. In resolving this conflict, it is important not only to collect the *minimum* amount of information necessary to the objectives of the study, but also to ensure that questionnaire length and respondent burden are kept to levels that do not threaten participation by subjects or cause a material increase in error.

TYPES OF QUESTION

Questions are generally classified as either 'open-ended' or 'closed-ended'. *Open-ended questions* are questions to which no answers are provided by the investigator. Only the question is asked, and the respondent's answer is recorded verbatim. In an interview, extensive probing may be used to ensure that all relevant aspects of the topic are covered by the answer. *Closed-ended questions* are questions for which the range of possible answers is specified by the investigator and the respondent is asked to make a choice from among the answers provided.

Open-ended questions

Open-ended questions should be used in epidemiology for the eliciting and recording of *simple* facts to which there are a large number of possible answers—for example, age, occupation, country of birth, number of cigarettes smoked a day, amount of alcohol drunk in a particular period of time, etc. The use of closed-ended questions for these topics leads to loss of information and, when asking about a socially undesirable behaviour, a greater degree of error. Reporting of intake of beer, for example, was nearly

50 per cent less when a closed-ended rather than an open-ended question was used (Blair *et al.* 1977).

An additional advantage of open-ended questions is that the amount of a particular behaviour reported in closed categories may be influenced by the cut-off values chosen for the categories. Schwartz *et al.* (1985) found that when offered a range of categories from 'up to half an hour' to 'more than 2½ hours' for daily TV watching, 16.2 per cent of subjects estimated that they watched more than 2½ hours. When offered the range 'up to 2½ hours' to 'more than 4½ hours', 37.5 per cent estimated that they watched more than 2½ hours. It appears that the categories offered are seen as normative by the respondents and their responses are influenced away from the extremes, particularly if one or other extreme is viewed as socially undesirable.

The collection of data on income (used in epidemiology as a measure of socioeconomic status) may be an exception to the rule that simple factual data are best sought through open-ended questions. While there is probably no particular tendency for subjects to either over- or understate their income, they are sensitive about disclosing the exact amount. Thus a closed-ended question with income categories might be acceptable, where an open-ended question would not. It is also usual in self-administered questionnaires to ask questions with a limited range of categorical responses (such as 'What is your sex?' or 'What is your marital status?') as closed-ended questions to permit maximum use of self-coding responses.

When the likely answer to an open-ended question is neither simple nor factual, the use of such a question increases the burden on both respondent and interviewer and produces answers that are difficult both to code and to analyse.

Closed-ended questions

The use of closed-ended questions is comparatively uncommon in epidemiology for exposure measurement, and appropriately so for the reasons given above. Most data sought are both simple and factual and are best dealt with by open-ended questions. Even food-frequency questionnaires, which are traditionally closed-ended with categories such as *daily*, *4-6* times a week, *1-3* times a week, *1-3* times a month, less than once a month, and *never*, may be better in open-ended form. Thus, for example, the subjects might be asked to report the frequency with which each food is eaten over a specified recall period as the number of times per day, week, or month — depending on which is the most appropriate frequency unit for them. In self-administered questionnaires this flexibility can be achieved by providing columns for 'day', 'week', and 'month' and instructing the subject to enter a frequency number in one column only.

The alternative answers offered in a closed-ended question should be simple and brief, and mutually exclusive if only one is to be selected. If more than one response could be selected, it may be best to seek explicit 'yes/no' responses for each of the categories. If the response categories provided are not exhaustive of all possible responses, a final open category (e.g 'Other. Please give details . . .') should be given. A 'Don't know' option may also be offered if the possibility exists that some subjects will truly not know the answer. Recent research, however, has shown that, in approaching next-of-kin of dead subjects for data on demographic variables and aspects of health history and health-related behaviour, exclusion of the 'Don't know' option gave an appreciably higher proportion of usable responses for many items without adversely affecting response rate or intramethod reliability (Poe *et al.* 1988).

It is also important in closed-ended questions to limit the number of alternative response categories as far as is reasonably possible. A large number of alternative responses increases respondent burden, increases the probability of non-response to the question (Leigh and Martin 1987) and, for less sophisticated subjects, may increase the probability that one of the response options listed first will be selected (Krosnick and Alwin 1987).

QUESTION CONTENT

Questions may be about:

- *knowledge* (what people know)
- *attitudes* (what people say they want or think)
- *beliefs* (what people say is true)
- *experiences* (what has happened to people)
- *behaviours* (what people do, have done, or will do)
- *attributes* (what people are).

Only experiences, behaviours, and attributes are relevant to exposure measurement in epidemiology. Most of the research on question content and questionnaires, however, has related to questions about knowledge, attitudes, and beliefs. This research will be drawn on in what follows and, as far as possible, its relevance to exposure measurement through questionnaires outlined.

Like the subject matter as a whole, the content of individual questions is largely determined by the objectives of the study. It is therefore not possible to be prescriptive on this subject, but some general advice can be given.

Before developing questions on a particular topic, the investigator should become thoroughly familiar with the topic by reading and by discussions with experts. It is advisable to obtain copies of questionnaires that have been used previously by experts to cover the subject matter of the study, and to make prudent use of them, within the limits of any copyright restrictions that may apply and provided that due acknowledgement is given.

The use of standard questions has a number of advantages.

(a) The questions will usually have been used extensively and proved satisfactory in use.

(b) The questions may have been assessed for reliability and/or validity and, even if they have not, sufficient results may be available from their use to permit validity to be inferred.

(c) Their use will permit comparison among data sets and possibly the combining of data sets.

(d) It is an easy way of drawing on the expertise of others and it can substantially facilitate the task of questionnaire design.

All that said, it is important for the investigator to evaluate questions obtained from other sources in terms of the adequacy of their design, their appropriateness to the objectives of the current study, and their suitability for use in the population on which the study will be conducted. It should also be noted that questions developed for use in a face-to-face interview may require modification in their wording or format if they are to be used in a telephone interview or a mailed self-administered questionnaire.

Issues related to the use of 'standard' questions are dealt with in detail by Aday and Anderson (1979). Examples of standard questions that might be used in epidemiological studies are those recommended for the elicitation of demographic data by the Social Science Research Council (1975).

QUESTION WORDING

There are two important issues to be considered in question wording:

- How does one arrive at a suitable wording in the first place?
- Are small changes in wording likely to lead to differences in response?

The latter issue is particularly relevant to comparisons between populations and over time when the same basic data have been sought by slightly different questions.

Table 6.1 gives a list of questions that should be asked about the wording of each question in a questionnaire.

The words

The words used in a questionnaire should be the usual 'working tools' of the respondents. They should be neither too difficult (be suspicious of words more than seven letters in length) nor too simple. Difficult words may not

Table 6.1   Questions that should be asked about the wording of each question in a questionnaire (adapted from Dillman 1978)

- Will the words be uniformly understood by the subject population?
- Does it contain abbreviations, unconventional phrases, or jargon?
- Is it vague?
- Is it too precise?
- Is it biased?
- Is it threatening?
- Does it contain more than one concept?
- Does it contain a double negative?
- Are the answers mutually exclusive?
- Does it assume too much about the respondent's behaviour?
- Is an unambiguous time reference provided?
- Is the question cryptic?

be understood, and simple words (where better but more difficult words could have been used) may appear condescending, may not convey the right meaning, and may needlessly lengthen the questionnaire. Where doubt exists, however, there is a virtue in simplicity (Jobe and Mingay 1989). Abbreviations, unconventional phrases, and jargon present the same problems as difficult words; they may not be understood or, perhaps worse, they may be misunderstood.

These general principles may be illustrated by some examples. The question,

HAVE YOU EVER HAD AN ECG?

includes an abbreviation which is also technical jargon. In addition, the abbreviation used in *some* English-speaking countries is EKG, not ECG. Nonetheless, the abbreviation is likely to be familiar to many subjects, and perhaps more familiar than any alternative terms. The solution here is to offer some alternative terms in the question. For example:

HAVE YOU EVER HAD AN ECG, THAT IS, A 'HEART TRACING', EKG, OR ELECTROCARDIOGRAPH?

In the question:

HAVE YOU EVER HAD ELECTROLYSIS TO REMOVE BODY OR FACIAL HAIR?

'electrolysis' is a difficult word that would not be understood by some people. A possible alternative, however,

HAVE YOU EVER HAD BODY OR FACIAL HAIR REMOVED BY ELECTROLYSIS, THAT IS, BY AN INSTRUMENT THAT GIVES AN ELECTRIC SHOCK TO THE ROOT OF THE HAIR?

is longer, and probably not much more likely to be understood than the shorter question. It may, however, avoid some 'don't know', missed, or incorrect responses.

In one particular circumstance, the quantification of sensitive behaviour (e.g. sexual activity or the use of alcohol and illicit drugs), asking the respondent to supply words that he or she is accustomed to using to describe the behaviour may increase the accuracy of reporting (Blair *et al.* 1977). Two forms of question were asked about drunkenness:

IN THE PAST YEAR, HOW OFTEN DID YOU BECOME INTOXICATED WHILE DRINKING ANY KIND OF ALCOHOLIC BEVERAGE?

and

SOMETIMES PEOPLE DRINK A LITTLE TOO MUCH BEER, WINE OR WHISKEY SO THAT THEY ACT DIFFERENT FROM USUAL. WHAT WORD DO YOU THINK WE SHOULD USE TO DESCRIBE PEOPLE WHEN THEY GET THAT WAY, SO THAT YOU WILL KNOW WHAT WE MEAN AND FEEL COMFORTABLE TALKING ABOUT IT?

IN THE PAST YEAR, HOW OFTEN DID YOU BECOME (*RESPONDENT'S WORD*) WHILE DRINKING ANY KIND OF ALCOHOLIC BEVERAGE?

The second form of the question consistently increased the reporting of this and other sensitive behaviours. Because socially undesirable behaviours tend to be under-reported, an increase in reporting is assumed to mean reduction in error.

There are no data to suggest that the use of particular terms familiar to the subjects should be used for other than sensitive behaviours and, in general, slang or vulgar terms should not be used in questionnaires. Their use may lead to misunderstanding, the appearance of condescension and, for some subjects, offence.

Vague questions

Questions may contain vague words — words that vary substantially in their meaning among different people. 'Usually', 'normally', and 'regularly' are three commonly used vague descriptors of frequency. In many circumstances they can be replaced by more precise quantifiers. For example,

HOW OLD WERE YOU WHEN YOU FIRST BEGAN TO SMOKE CIGARETTES REGULARLY?

could be made more precise by asking,

HOW OLD WERE YOU WHEN YOU FIRST SMOKED ONE OR MORE CIGARETTES A DAY FOR ONE MONTH OR LONGER?

The latter wording eliminates uncertainty about the meaning of 'regularly'.

Similarly, it would be better to ask subjects about their 'usual' intake of alcoholic beverages over a specific period of time, e.g. the past 12 months, than to ask simply about their 'usual' intake.

Questions that are too precise

While precision is desirable, particularly when estimating amount or duration of exposure, respondent burden may be increased unduly if too much precision is requested. For example, in precisely quantifying dose rate and cumulative exposure to cigarette smoke, it might be tempting to ask smokers to estimate their average daily cigarette consumption for each year of their smoking life. This would be unreasonably burdensome and prone to substantial error in recall. A better approach would be to ask subjects about major changes in daily cigarette intake (e.g. an increase or decrease of five or more cigarettes a day), and document the extent and time of each of these changes.

Biased questions

Biased questions are questions that suggest to the respondent that a particular answer is preferred from among all possible answers. 'Leading' questions are well known, and should be easily avoided (see Dillman 1978). 'Loaded' questions are more likely to turn up in questionnaires seeking attitudes or beliefs than more factual data. The question,

DO YOU THINK THAT SMOKING SHOULD BE BANNED IN PLANES?

would be more likely to bias responses because of use of the strong negative word 'banned' than would the more neutral, and balanced,

DO YOU THINK THAT SMOKING SHOULD BE PERMITTED OR NOT PERMITTED IN PLANES?

A significant influence of question wording has been shown in surveys of attitudes to public assistance to the poor in the United States (Smith 1987). In six surveys spanning 17 years, the proportion of Americans in favour of more spending on welfare was substantially less when the word 'welfare' was used in the question than when the question referred to 'assistance to the poor'. Smith (1987) concluded that this difference was due to a connotation of 'welfare' with waste and bureaucracy that 'assistance to the poor' did not have, or not to the same degree.

Threatening questions

Threatening or sensitive questions are questions that '. . . ask respondents about behaviours that are illegal, contra-normative [deviant] or generally not discussed in public without tension, or relate to issues of self-preservation' (Blair *et al.* 1977). They fall into two distinct classes: those that ask about behaviours or attributes that are socially desirable, and those that ask about socially undesirable behaviours or attributes. The threat of questions about socially-desirable behaviours arises from the possibility that a person does not wish to admit that he or she does not practise the behaviour (e.g. giving to charity or — of more direct relevance to epidemiology — exercising regularly). These behaviours tend to be over-reported. Socially undesirable (or, at least, unmentionable) behaviours or attributes (such as past history of sexually transmitted disease, sexual activity, and alcohol drinking) tend to be under-reported. Questions about income, savings, and assets are threatening although they are not readily categorized as either socially desirable–or undesirable. A question can be considered as potentially threatening if subjects can possibly feel that there is a right or wrong answer to it (Sudman and Bradburn 1983).

A number of techniques have been used to maximize reporting of socially undesirable behaviours, two of which have already been mentioned: use of words familiar to the respondent and open-ended questions. Reporting of undesirable behaviours was also increased by use of a long introduction to the question (Blair *et al.* 1977). For example, the following introduction was added to the question on drunkenness:

OCCASIONALLY PEOPLE DRINK ON AN EMPTY STOMACH OR DRINK A LITTLE TOO MUCH AND BECOME (INTOXICATED *OR RESPONDENT'S WORD*). IN THE PAST YEAR, HOW OFTEN . . .

This introduction exemplifies another technique for dealing with question threat — deliberately loading the question. In this case the use of 'Occasionally', 'Drink on an empty stomach', and 'A little too much' all tend to minimize the significance of the behaviour so that the respondent will be more willing to report it. The threat may also be reduced by embedding the sensitive question in a list of questions on related topics, some of which are more threatening and some less so. Questions on past history of sexually transmitted disease, for example, can be asked in a series of questions on past disease history.

There is a difference between strategies appropriate to reduction in over-reporting of socially desirable behaviour and these appropriate to increased reporting of socially undesirable behaviour. Use of a long introductory statement, for example, is likely to encourage rather than discourage over-reporting unless it loads the question against reporting of the behaviour. A question on jogging might be asked as follows:

MANY PEOPLE FIND IT DIFFICULT TO GET REGULAR EXERCISE, LIKE JOGGING, THROUGH LACK OF TIME. HOW MANY TIMES DID YOU GO JOGGING IN THE PAST FOUR WEEKS

The significance of the behaviour may also be minimized by use of the phrase: 'Did you happen to . . .'

HOW MANY TIMES DID YOU HAPPEN TO GO JOGGING IN THE PAST FOUR WEEKS?

Socially desirable behaviours will also tend to be less over-reported if 'current' rather than 'usual' behaviour is asked about. It is reasonable to assume also, that the 'threat' of a question about a socially desirable behaviour, like that of a question about a socially undesirable behaviour, is reduced if it is embedded in a sequence of questions about non-threatening behaviours.

More than one concept

If a question contains more than one concept, the answer will be ambiguous. The following question was asked at interview in a case-control study of malignant melanoma:

HAVE YOU EVER USED HAIR DYES OR TEMPORARY COLOUR RINSES?

Yes   1

(*Go to question 10*) ← **No**   2

If yes

a. HOW MANY TIMES HAVE YOU USED PERMANENT AS OPPOSED TO TEMPORARY HAIR DYES?

_____ **times**

b. HOW MANY TIMES HAVE YOU USED TEMPORARY HAIR DYES OR COLOUR RINSES?

_____ **times**

Two out of the three parts of this question include two exposures. The failure to distinguish between hair dyes and colour rinses is comparatively unimportant in the first question, because it simply acts as a filter to the next two. The ambiguity in the third question, however, limited the interpretation of an unexpected positive finding; some temporary hair dyes, like permanent hair dyes, have contained potentially carcinogenic chemicals whereas colour rinses generally have not (Holman and Armstrong 1983). This question should have been separated into questions about number of uses of temporary hair dyes and number of uses of colour rinses.

Double negatives

A double negative can arise whenever a question that is phrased negatively can have a negative answer. Dillman (1978) gave the following example:

SHOULD THE CITY MANAGER NOT BE RESPONSIBLE TO THE MAYOR?

Yes   1

No   2

The question was asked because the city council was contemplating a change from the city manager being responsible to the mayor, to him or her not being responsible to the mayor. It is unnatural, however, to say 'yes' when the answer really means 'no' (that the city manager should *not* be responsible to the mayor), and so answers to this question would be ambiguous. The solution in this case was to ask who the city manager should be responsible to — the mayor or the city council. Double negatives are probably more common in questions on attitudes and beliefs than in questions likely to be asked in epidemiological studies.

Mutually exclusive answers

A subject could reasonably select more than one answer to the following question:

WHAT SPREAD DO YOU USE ON BREAD?
Circle the number beside your answer.

Butter	1
Low fat spread or	
Diet margarine	2
Regular margarine	3
Other spread	4
Please give details	

The subject is therefore uncertain about which alternative to choose, and there is a risk of non-response. The problem could be solved by asking 'What spread do you *usually* eat on bread?' or, preferably, by asking about the frequency of use of all the spreads individually.

Assumptions about the respondent

The following question assumes that the respondent eats steak:

HOW DO YOU LIKE YOUR STEAK TO BE COOKED
Circle the number beside your answer

Rare	1
Medium rare	2
Well done	3

If this assumption is wrong, at best the respondent will not answer the question (in a self-administered questionnaire) and, at worst, the respondent may find the assumption about his or her behaviour to be offensive. The solution is to add the response alternative, 'I don't eat steak', or to first ascertain whether or not the respondent eats steak and skip to a succeeding question if he or she does not.

An unambiguous time reference

Any period referred to in a question should be clear and unambiguous. The question described above on jogging 'in the past four weeks' could have been asked as follows:

HOW OFTEN DO YOU GO JOGGING?

This question, while most likely referring to the present, has no clear time reference. Different subjects would be likely to refer to different periods of time in the past in answering it.

In a case-control study, it is usually desirable to specify a time somewhat before onset of disease beyond which the exposure will not be recorded, to avoid eliciting behaviour that has been influenced by the onset of disease; or, for controls, that occurred after the date of diagnosis of the corresponding case. For example:

BEFORE 1989, HOW OFTEN DID YOU GO JOGGING?

A specific reference date, usually the date of diagnosis of the case or some date before onset of symptoms, may be assigned to each case and his or her matched controls. The use of this reference date is usually explained at the beginning of the interview or questionnaire, and questions relating to it usually begin: 'Before [reference date], how often . . .', etc.

One potential solution to problems of ambiguity in the time reference of a question is for the interviewer to have, or the questionnaire to include, a calendar on which the period referred to in that question, or a number of related questions, is marked out.

Cryptic questions

A cryptic question is a 'non-question'. For example,

1. SEX? _____

While the author of this question probably wanted to know whether the subject was male or female, and most subjects would have understood this, the 'question' is clearly open to alternative interpretations! Questions should be explicit, not implicit.

1. WHAT IS YOUR SEX?

Male	1
Female	2

QUESTION FORMAT

General principles

The principles of question formatting are summarized in Table 6.2. Examples of their application have been given in some of the questions shown in the preceding pages, the question on page 160, and in Figure 6.1.

These principles require little explanation. The different typefaces help to lead the interviewer or respondent to the correct parts of the question. The instructions eliminate the need for complex initial instructions and ensure, as far as possible, that they are being followed at all times. The vertical answer format avoids confusion over which answer relates to which number. Pre-coding of answer categories increases processing efficiency and does not add to respondent or interviewer burden. It is sometimes argued that code numbers for particular answers (e.g., 'yes' and 'no') in self-administered questionnaires should be varied to avoid response sets. However, a greater hazard is probably that, having associated a particular number with a particular answer, the respondent will inadvertently circle the wrong number when the pattern is changed. The circling of numbers is an unambiguous method of indicating response; the checking (ticking) of boxes is not. A check (tick), for example, may indicate that an item is the *right* one or the *wrong* one, depending on the culture and the individual. Some subjects

Table 6.2 Principles of formatting of individual questions

- Identify the separate parts of different questions with different type faces: e.g.
  CAPITAL LETTERS for the question
  bold face type for the alternative answers
  italics for instructions

- Include specific instructions and prompts (for interviewers) with each question.

- Use vertical answer formats.

- Pre-code all closed questions.

- Always associate the same code number with a particular response category.

- Record responses to closed-ended questions by circling the code number or the alternative answer.

- Provide spaces or boxes for coding open-ended questions.

- Consider ease of key entry of data when making design decisions (e.g. locate response codes against right-hand margin).

---

choose to use a cross instead of a check, with the same potential ambiguity. Coding boxes or spaces facilitate data entry without adding to respondent or interviewer burden.

Matrix formats

The collection of data about a number of exposures of interest to epidemiology is done most efficiently in the form of a matrix. For example, all places of residence, all occupations, or all uses of a particular medication may be recorded on one axis and, on the other, a number of specific details regarding each episode or period of exposure. The conversion of such matrices to a vertical, single-column format increases the length of questionnaires substantially and is tedious to both interviewer and respondent. It is therefore desirable to retain the form of the matrix in the questionnaire if possible. This can be done quite readily in interviewer-admininstered questionnaires where, if necessary, the matrix can extend over several pages. However, a matrix adds complexity to a self-administered questionnaire and this may increase respondent burden.

Figure 6.1 shows a matrix that was used to collect occupational information in a self-administered questionnaire. The data sought were limited in scope, and the matrix was kept small enough to fit on one page. The 'example' included in the question was intended to show the respondent the form and detail of response that was desired, in the hope that instructions for the question could be kept to a minimum.

In designing complex question formats, it is important to bear in mind the hypotheses that are to be tested in the data so obtained and the variables that will be derived from these questions for use in the analyses to test these hypotheses. This is best done by planning the analysis, including both database manipulation and statistical analysis, before the questionnaire is designed, and verifying that the variables needed for the analysis can be derived readily from the question formats proposed.

QUESTION ORDER

Beliefs about the order in which questions should appear in a questionnaire have been summarized by Sudman and Bradburn (1983).

General principles

Questions about a particular topic should be grouped together, and proceed from the general to the particular within a group. This approach, by focusing first in a general way on a particular behaviour or experience, assists and allows more time for recall of the specific details. It is sometimes suggested

12.   HAVE YOU EVER WORKED IN THE TIMBER OR WOODWORKING INDUSTRIES?

Circle the number beside your answer.

Yes   1

(go to question 13) ← No   2

If yes
Please describe your work with wood or timber in the spaces below.

Here is an example.

Jobs in timber or woodworking	Type of industry	Your job	Year job began	Year job ended
Last job	Furniture making	French polisher	19 5 7	19 7 4

Now please describe your work here.

Jobs in timber or woodworking	Type of industry	Your job	Year job began	Year job ended
Last job	_____	_____	19 __ __	19 __ __
	_____	_____		:_:_:_:_:_:_:
Job before that	_____	_____	19 __ __	19 __ __
	_____	_____		:_:_:_:_:_:_:
Job before that	_____	_____	19 __ __	19 __ __
	_____	_____		:_:_:_:_:_:_:
Job before that	_____	_____	19 __ __	19 __ __
	_____	_____		:_:_:_:_:_:_:
Job before that	_____	_____	19 __ __	19 __ __
	_____	_____		:_:_:_:_:_:_:
Job before that	_____	_____	19 __ __	19 __ __
	_____	_____		:_:_:_:_:_:_:

If there is not enough space, please detail the additional jobs on a separate sheet of paper and pin it here.

Figure 6.1   An open-ended question with matrix response intended for use in a self-administered questionnaire.

that questions using a particular response scale should be grouped together, but this is probably undesirable because it may tend to promote a *response set* — a tendency to give the same response to each question regardless of what the correct response should be.

The order in which questions are asked can influence the responses obtained. The evidence for this statement derives mainly from research into questions on attitudes and beliefs (see, for example, Helsing and Comstock 1975; McFarland 1981; and Schuman *et al.* 1981), but the possibility exists that similar effects could be observed for some questions relating to experiences, behaviours, or attributes. Thus for comparative studies between populations and over time, the order of the questions in the questionnaire should be kept constant as far as possible. Any new questions that are added should go at the end of the questionnaire. Alternatively, any change in question order might be evaluated by comparison of the old and new questionnaires in a single population. Apart from the guidance that it might give in the specific situation, such research would indicate whether or not order effects are common in epidemiological questionnaires.

The first question

It is common practice to place the demographic questions at the beginning, but this is not a good idea. These questions are of comparatively low interest to the respondents, and some of them are threatening (see below). Instead, the questionnaire should begin with a question or questions which relate directly to the topic of the research and will command the subject's interest. For example, in a study of sun exposure in relation to skin cancer, it is appropriate to begin with questions on recreational pursuits involving sun exposure.

Threatening questions

Threatening questions should be placed towards the end of the questionnaire, in order of increasing threat. This reduces the likelihood that they will precipitate early termination of the interview, or failure of completion of the questionnaire. The degree of threat presented by particular questions can be determined empirically by asking subjects 'how uneasy most people' would feel about particular topics of questioning in a questionnaire. In a questionnaire mainly about leisure and sporting activities, the degree of threat of particular topics, from greatest to least, was:

- masturbation
- use of marijuana
- sexual intercourse
- use of stimulants and depressants

- drunkenness
- petting and kissing
- income
- gambling with friends
- alcohol drinking
- general leisure and sporting activity (Blair *et al.* 1977).

Demographic questions (about race, religion, or income, for example) are sometimes threatening and usually boring, and therefore appropriately asked at the end of the questionnaire. If, for some reason (e.g. to select particular respondents), it is necessary to place them at the beginning, some explanation for their position should be given to the respondent.

Logical sequence

Within any topic, questions should follow a logical sequence; the sequence that the respondents might be expected to follow in thinking about the topic. Thus, for example, in collecting residential or job histories, it is usual to proceed chronologically beginning with the present residence or occupation and proceeding to successively earlier ones. The 'backwards' chronological approach gives the respondent more time to recall the events of the more distant past (Bradburn *et al.* 1987).

QUESTIONNAIRE STRUCTURE

In addition to the questions, every questionnaire should contain:

- an introduction
- instructions (for self-administered questionnaires)
- linking phrases between topics
- a final expression of appreciation to the respondent.
- space for comments from the respondent.

Introduction

In an interview, the introduction takes the form of a standard statement read by the interviewer. For a self-administered questionnaire it is given to the subjects to read, usually as part of the letter soliciting their co-operation. Table 6.3 lists items of information disclosed in the introductions to 108 surveys conducted by members of the American Association of Public Opinion Research in order of the frequency that they were disclosed (Sobal 1984). These items serve both to elicit co-operation and to discharge the

Table 6.3 Types of information disclosed in introductions to public opinion questionnaires in order of the frequency of disclosure (adapted from Sobal 1984). Items in **bold type** are considered the minimum that should be provided in an introduction

---

- **Research organization**
- **Interviewer (or study director for mail surveys)**
- **Research topic**
- Sponsor
- **Confidentiality**
- Anonymity
- **Purpose**
- Future use of the data
- Sampling technique
- **Survey length**
- Participation voluntary
- Sample size
- Request for consent signature

---

investigator's ethical obligations to the subject. The items in bold type in the list are probably the minimum that should be provided in any introduction.

There are some empirical data to guide the inclusion or exclusion of items from the introduction (Bradburn and Sudman 1979).

(a) Disclosure of the presence of potentially threatening topics in the questionnaire does not depress the response rate and, for ethical reasons, should be included in the introduction.

(b) Assurances of confidentiality have a positive effect on the subject's willingness to answer individual questions (although some data suggest otherwise; Frey 1986) and should be included.

(c) A request for signed consent to administration of the questionnaire reduces the participation rate.

Whether signed consent should be obtained for the administration of a questionnaire is arguable (see Chapter 12). If it is considered necessary, the request is best made after completion of the questionnaire. However, this approach may not be acceptable to some ethical review committees. In any case, full information should be provided to subjects before administration of the questionnaire, even if their signed consent is not sought at that time.

An aspect of the introduction that is of special relevance to case-control studies is whether or not the specific disease under study should be mentioned, and whether or not cases and controls should be identified as such in the introduction. While there are no relevant empirical data, it seems likely that a questionnaire will be more salient to cases than controls, and therefore likely to be subject to response bias, if it is specifically identified with the disease from which the cases have recently suffered. It is a common practice, therefore, not to include mention of the disease nor to specifically identify subjects as cases or controls in the introduction. It is advisable, however, to state that the study covers not only those who have had a recent illness but also those who have been well. This statement is intended to overcome the reluctance of some subjects to participate because they have been well and therefore believe themselves to be of no interest to the investigator.

Another item that may be included in the introduction to a questionnaire is some exhortation to the respondent to make an effort to recall the information sought (Cannel 1985). For example, the subject might be told that: 'In this interview we want to get as much information as we can. This includes things which may seem small and unimportant as well as important things. For some of the questions you will need to search your memory thoroughly. We want you to try as hard as you can to give complete and accurate information.'

Figure 6.2 shows a letter designed for a case-control study of Hodgkin's disease to be undertaken by mailed self-administered questionnaire. You will notice that the research organization, study director, research topic, and purpose are disclosed. The research topic and purpose, however, are expressed in terms of the effects of general categories of exposure rather than the aetiology of a particular disease. The estimated time required to complete the questionnaire (which should not be deliberately underestimated) and an assurance of confidentiality are given. Coverage of both 'recently ill' and 'perfectly well' subjects is also stated. This letter was intended for use with both cases and controls.

Instructions

General instructions will usually be necessary only in a self-administered questionnaire. General instructions for interviewers will form part of interviewer training and an interviewer's manual rather than the questionnaire. Instructions relating to specific questions should appear with those questions in the body of the questionnaire, whether it is for self-administration or not. The instructions should include the address for return of the questionnaire; while an addressed return envelope will usually be included, it may easily become separated from the questionnaire. Figure 6.3 gives an example of instructions designed for use with a self-administered questionnaire.

Linking statements

Linking statements break the subject's concentration on a particular topic, provide a brief pause, and establish his or her concentration on a new topic. They may also be used to break the monotony of a long series of questions

The National Health
and Medical Research Council
The University
of Western Australia

**NH&MRC Research Unit in
Epidemiology and Preventive Medic**
University Department of Medicine
The Queen Elizabeth II Medical Centre
Nedlands, Western Australia 6009
Telegrams Uniwest Perth, Telex 92992
Telephone (09)380 1122 ext.

Mr J Doe
13 Plaza Avenue
SMITHTON 6271

Dear Mr Doe

I am writing to ask for your help in a medical research project.

We are studying the relationship between occupations and ways of life and the onset
of certain diseases. Our aim is to improve understanding of the causes of serious
illnesses so that it may be possible to prevent some of them from happening in the
future. To do this we need to get information both from people who are perfectly
well, as well as from those who have had some recent illness.

Would you be willing to help us by completing a brief questionnaire about yourself?

The questionnaire is enclosed. As you can see, it asks questions about your origins,
places where you have lived, jobs you have had, aspects of you and your family's
medical history, and aspects of your way of life. It will take about 30 minutes to one
hour to complete.

I would be most grateful if you could find time to complete this questionnaire. It is
most important to the success of our research that we get information from almost
everyone we contact. The information that you provide will be kept strictly
confidential and used only in the preparation of statistical reports in which you will
not be identified.

If you can help us, please complete the questionnaire as soon as you can and return it
to me in the enclosed envelope. If you cannot help us, please return the questionnaire
anyway with a brief note. I look forward to hearing from you soon.

Thank you for your help.

Yours sincerely

Dr Bruce Armstrong
DIRECTOR

4th April 1985

Figure 6.2   Letter of introduction for a case-control study of Hodgkin's disease
to be conducted by mailed self-administered questionnaire.

THE UNIVERSITY OF WESTERN AUSTRALIA
DEPARTMENT OF MEDICINE

QUESTIONNAIRE ON
OCCUPATION, LIFESTYLE AND HEALTH

INSTRUCTIONS

1. Please read these instructions carefully.

2. Please answer each question unless told to do otherwise.

3. There are two main types of questions:

    (a) Questions to which answers have not been supplied and to which you should write your answer in the space provided.

    (b) Questions to which alternative answers have been supplied. You should select one answer to each, or each part, of these questions and circle the number beside it or under it.

    Example 1

    ARE YOU OVER 16 YEARS OF AGE?
    Circle the number beside you answer.

Yes	①
No	2

    Example 2

    DO YOU EVER NOW TRAVEL TO WORK IN THE KINDS OF VEHICLES LISTED BELOW?
    Circle the number under your answer for each vehicle.

	Yes	No
CAR	①	2
BUS	1	②
BICYCLE	1	②

4. Please ignore any boxes next to the right hand margin, they relate to coding of information for the computer.

5. The information that you provide will be kept strictly confidential and used only in the preparation of statistical reports.

6. Please add any comments that you may wish to make at the end of the questionnaire.

7. Please return the completed questionnaire in the envelope provided to:

    Dr BK Armstrong
    University Department of Medicine
    Queen Elizabeth II Medical Center
    NEDLANDS 6009.

Figure 6.3 Instructions designed for use with a mailed self-administered questionnaire.

on one topic (Dillman 1978). They should not be unnecessarily long, or appear to be demanding, or give unwarranted importance to the succeeding questions. Nor should they contain words or phrases that may bias the succeeding responses. The following are some examples:

- To signify a major change in questioning:

  THE FOOD WE EAT IS AN IMPORTANT PART OF OUR EVERYDAY LIVES. I WOULD NOW LIKE TO ASK SOME QUESTIONS ABOUT THE FOODS THAT YOU USUALLY EAT AND THE AMOUNTS THAT YOU EAT OF THEM.

- To break the monotony of a series of food frequency questions:

  NEXT, I WOULD LIKE TO ASK ABOUT BREAD AND BREAKFAST CEREALS.

- To introduce the demographic questions at the end of the questionnaire:

  FINALLY, I WOULD LIKE TO ASK A FEW QUESTIONS ABOUT YOU FOR STATISTICAL PURPOSES.

Skips or branches

It is commonly necessary to make 'skips' or branch points in a questionnaire where some succeeding questions are not applicable to all respondents. These are points at which both interviewer and respondent error are likely, and succeeding items relevant to the respondent may be missed (Messmer and Seymour 1982).

Probably the most important requirement of skip instructions is that they be placed immediately after the *answer* that leads to the branch point in the questionnaire. Skip instructions should always be worded positively ('Go to question 4') rather than negatively ('Skip question 3').

Complex branching designs are usually only possible in interviewer-administered questionnaires, and can be particularly well handled by computer-assisted telephone interviewing. In self-administered questionnaires, skips are best limited to succeeding parts of the same question as in the following example:

3. OVER THE PAST YEAR, HAVE YOU ENGAGED IN STRENUOUS PHYSICAL EXERCISE AT LEAST ONCE A MONTH—FOR EXAMPLE, JOGGING OR OTHER EXERCISE THAT CAUSES YOU TO SWEAT OR BECOME BREATHLESS?
   Circle the number beside your answer.

──────────────────────────────────── **Yes** 1

(Go to question 4) ← **No** 2

If Yes:

a. HOW OFTEN DID YOU EXERCISE STRENUOUSLY (TO THE
POINT OF SWEATING OR BECOMING BREATHLESS)?
Write the number of times a week or month.

_____ **times a week**

or

_____ **times a month**

b. HOW MANY MINUTES DID THESE SESSIONS USUALLY LAST?

_____ **minutes**

c. WHAT WAS YOUR MAIN FORM OF ACTIVE PHYSICAL
EXERCISE?

_____

A device that may be used to avoid skips in a self-administered questionnaire is the inclusion of a specific 'inapplicable' category among the alternative answers, as in the following example:

HOW OFTEN DO YOU CUT THE FAT OFF MEAT BEFORE YOU COOK OR EAT
IT?
Circle the number beside your answer.

Never	1
Less than half the time	2
More than half the time	3
Always	4
I never eat meat	5

Here use of '**I never eat meat**' as an answer category provided an alternative
answer for everybody and eliminated the need for a skip.

ASKING ABOUT BEHAVIOUR THAT VARIES OVER TIME

Behaviour that varies appreciably over time often presents difficulty in the
design of questionnaires. It will rarely be sufficient to summarize it by way
of a simple question on its 'usual' frequency — both because this summary is
likely to introduce error and because the pattern of variation of the
behaviour with time may be important (see chapter 1). It may be unreasonably burdensome on the respondent to attempt to elicit a usual pattern for
the behaviour (e.g. smoking) for each year of what is considered to be the

aetiologically relevant time period, and division of that period into larger but arbitrarily determined intervals of time (e.g. 0–4 years ago, 5–9 years ago, etc.) introduces the possibility of major changes in behaviour during an interval. Such changes would present problems for both respondents and interviewers, and be likely to increase error in the measurement of exposure.

We recommend an approach to measuring time-variable behaviour that focuses on obtaining details of the behaviour in periods of life in which it has been reasonably stable. Essentially, data are collected in a matrix format, except that reported changes in the subject's pattern of exposure over time determine when a new row is to be completed. This approach has been used in the Lifetime Drinking History described in Skinner and Sheu (1982), in which subjects are first asked about their alcohol consumption in the first year that they drank on a regular basis. Major changes in their drinking patterns are then identified chronologically and, for each pattern, questions are asked about the frequency of drinking, typical and maximum quantity consumed per occasion, types of beverage, style of drinking, and life events related to the next change in drinking pattern.

This approach has also been used to document exposure to the sun in a case-control study of skin cancer conducted following a survey of the prevalence of skin cancer in the town of Geraldton, Western Australia (Kricker *et al.* 1991). Subjects first completed, on their own, a life calendar covering each change of residence, school, occupation, and the number of days they worked each week. At interview, they were asked to identify, on the calendar, years in which major changes in their outdoor activity took place. They were prompted with the suggestion that these changes '. . . could've been due to things like changes in where you lived, changes in the sport you played, changes of school, different jobs, changes in the number of days you worked, and by marriage.' Having identified these years of change and, by inference, periods of comparatively stable outdoor activity, subjects were asked detailed questions about outdoor activity in each period. These questions included the typical numbers of hours outdoors between 9 a.m. and 5 p.m. and 10 a.m. and 2 p.m., on working and non-working days, in both cooler and warmer months of the year, and during summer holidays; frequency of sunbathing; extent of suntan; frequency and severity of sunburn; use of sunscreen preparations; and wearing of a hat.

AIDS TO RECALL

The most commonly used aid to recall is the list of alternative answers supplied as part of a self-administered questionnaire. In an interview, this list may be provided in the form of a card given to the respondent. A list of possible answers may also be given for open-ended questions (e.g. a list of recreational physical activities), but it is essential that it be as comprehensive as possible or it may bias response. Where the list of possible answers to an open-ended question is very long, a list of headings under which all responses might fall can be used instead to stimulate recall. In questions about use of the oral contraceptive pill, it is now common to show the respondent photographs of all present and past formulations to assist her in eliciting the brand actually used. The photographs include the pill itself, the packaging, and the name.

Mitchell *et al.* (1986) reported the effect of three approaches to questioning on use of medications in pregnancy. The first question was open-ended and provided no aids to recall, the second asked about drug use for selected indications, and the third asked about use of specifically named drugs. Among obstetric patients who recalled use of any of five specific drugs, less than a half did so in response to the open-ended question, and 20–40 per cent reported use only when the specific drug was named. Similar results were obtained in a larger study in which 6–40 per cent reported use of 11 drugs only when asked about them by name. It would be reasonable to speculate that recall might have been improved further if photographs of standard formulations of drugs of particular interest had also been used. In this respect, Beresford and Coker (1989) found that 6 out of 14 women who had used postmenopausal hormone replacement therapy for 6 months or more were assisted in their recall of the name and dose by reference to photographs of preparations that had been in use over the preceding 15 years.

A calendar may also be used as an effective aid to recall. Marcus (1982) found that recall of illness and injuries was increased by reference to a wall calendar during questioning. As a means of improving recall of use of birth control methods, Daling (Holt *et al.* 1989; Janet Daling, personal communication) has used a simple month-by-year matrix calendar on which marriages and periods of 'living as married' were first recorded by use of a black marking pen, pregnancies were recorded by use of a blue marker, and then periods of birth control use were recorded, with reference to the other details on the calendar, by use of a red marker. Details for each of the periods of birth control use were then sought and recorded on the main data form. Use of a calendar of residences, schools, and jobs to assist in recall of outdoor activities has been described on page 162.

In each of these examples, calendar time is used to assist recall of and to locate key activities or events which, in turn, are used as stimuli for the recall of some less salient behaviours. This approach is one example of the use of identification of autobiographical sequences to aid recall (Bradburn *et al.* 1987). Autobiographical sequences are groups of events clustered in time, and often organized within some wider framework (e.g. a summer job or an overseas tour) within which memory appears to be organized. Thus any means of entry into an autobiographical sequence, whether, by way of calendar time or through some highly salient event, may assist in recall of events or behaviours of low salience. Thus, for example, asking first about illnesses that may have been indications for the use of particular medications may assist in recall of those medications, and asking about illnesses or injuries may assist in recall of exposure to diagnostic X-rays. These approaches have been used intuitively for years but are now supported by an increasingly strong body of theory and observation (see also Jobe and Mingay 1989).

Recall may also be aided by asking the subject to refer to his or her personal records where they may be relevant. This is more easily done in a mailed questionnaire, where the respondent may refer to the records at leisure, than it is in a personal interview. However, these records may be made available to an interview by notifying the subjects in advance of the proposed lines of questioning and asking that they collect together whatever records they may have.

Care should be exercised in using aided recall procedures for socially desirable behaviours because it may increase over-reporting. It is possible, also, where recall aids are sent by mail in a case-control study, that cases may make greater use of them and therefore increase differential bias in recall.

PREPARING THE QUESTIONNAIRE FOR ADMINISTRATION

Pre-testing

Pre-testing is an essential part of the development of all questionnaires, regardless of whether or not they have been substantially based on previous questionnaires. The objectives of pre-testing are to identify questions that are poorly understood, ambiguous, or evoke hostile or other undesirable responses. Some of the questions that a pre-test should answer are (Dillman 1978):

- Are all the words understood?
- Are the questions interpreted similarly by all respondents?
- Does each closed-ended question have an answer that applies to each respondent?
- Are some questions not answered?
- Do some questions elicit uninterpretable answers?

The steps that should be followed in pre-testing a questionnaire are summarized in Table 6.4.

Obtaining feedback from the respondents is a somewhat neglected aspect of questionnaire pre-testing. Belson (1981) has suggested a formal approach to this process. The questionnaire should be administered in the usual way.

Table 6.4 Steps in the pre-testing and final development of a questionnaire (adapted from Sudman and Bradburn 1983)

1. Obtain peer evaluation of the draft questionnaire.
2. Test the revised questionnaire on a sample of convenience (e.g. yourself, relatives, friends and colleagues).
3. Prepare instructions for use of the revised questionnaire and train interviewers for a pilot test. Problems requiring revision of the questionnaire may be uncovered in this process.
4. Pre-test the questionnaire on a sample (20–50) of respondents representative of the population from which your subjects will be drawn.
5. Obtain comments of interviewers and subjects, preferably in writing.
6. Revise questions that cause difficulty.
7. Pre-test and revise again.
8. Prepare revised instructions and train interviewers for implementation of the study. Revise questionnaire if this process uncovers more problems.
9. Monitor performance of the questionnaire during the early phases of the study and be willing to stop, revise, and pre-test again if necessary.

After completion of administration, each question should be read back with its answer and the respondent asked how he or she arrived at the answer. Probing may be necessary to clarify the answer to this question. A series of questions should then be asked about how each concept in the original question was understood. For example, for the question, 'How many people are there in your household?', the following questions (among others) would be appropriate:

- Did the respondent understand that an exact count was required?
- Did the respondent include himself or herself in the count?
- To what period did the respondent think the question related?
- How did the respondent interpret the term household?

The interview should be taped and listened to by the investigator. This is a demanding form of pre-test, and Belson (1981) suggested that each respondent be asked in detail about only three or four questions. This method, however, has the potential to uncover problems in questions that might otherwise be missed.

Format and layout for printing

Presentation of the questionnaire in printed form is important, especially when it is to be self-administered, both for ease of use and to give it an authoritative appearance that will encourage response. The first page should include the title of the study, the name of the organization conducting it, and the date. In addition, a graphic illustration may make a self-administered questionnaire more attractive to its target population. Pages and questions should be numbered consecutively, and subsections of questions should be indented and identified with letters rather than numbers. As far as possible, questions should not extend over more than one page. Following this rule will generally increase the amount of space between questions, and it is indeed important that the questionnaire not be too congested.

In a self-administered questionnaire the last page should provide space and a specific invitation for any comments that the subject may wish to make. Interviewer-administered questionnaires should provide for the entry of the starting and finishing times and the interviewer's comments.

Ideally, the questionnaire should be printed in booklet form so that it will open flat on a table. This is helpful both to respondents completing a self-administered questionnaire and to interviewers. For interview questionnaires which contain a set of questions that are repeated for the completion of each column of a response matrix (see page 152), it is best if the questions are on a left-hand page and the response matrix on the facing right-hand page. Use may be made of different colours of paper to identify questionnaires or parts of questionnaires to be completed by some respondents but not others.

Translating

The conduct of international, multicentre epidemiological studies often necessitates the translation of a questionnaire into a language other than that in which it was first developed. Translation may also be required when a population contains ethnic minority groups. There is evidence that the intramethod reliability of some questions in a questionnaire is greater when they are administered in the respondent's mother tongue, even when the respondent is multilingual (Becklake *et al.* 1987).

There are four phases in translation of a questionnaire (Del Greco *et al.* 1987):

- preliminary translation
- evaluation of the preliminary translation
- ascertainment of cross-language equivalence
- assessment of validity and reliability.

The preliminary translation aims at producing a translated questionnaire which is as near as possible in meaning to the original. It is best done by someone who understands both the overall objective of the questionnaire and the intent of each question, as well as being expert in both the original language and the language into which the translation is being made. The usual method of evaluating the preliminary translation is to have it translated back into the first language by someone who has not seen the original version. The back-translated version is then compared with the original version, and further work done on questions that have changed their meaning. Some questions may go through the process of re-translation and back-translation several times before they are considered to have been translated correctly. A complementary approach to back-translation in evaluating the preliminary translation is to have bilingual experts evaluate the translation of each question in terms of its content, meaning, clarity of expression, and comparability to the original question.

Cross-language equivalence is determined by administering both the original and the translated versions of the questionnaire to bilingual subjects, and comparing their responses to each. It is usual to give half of the subjects the original questionnaire first and half the translated questionnaire first, to minimize order effects. A high correlation between the responses is taken to indicate cross-language equivalence.

Del Greco *et al.* (1987) noted that the reliability and validity of the questionnaire may not be maintained after translation, and it should be re-evaluated in the translated form. Any change in validity and reliability, however, could be as much due to cultural differences between the two populations as to any problems with the translation.

Where only a few interviews must be conducted in a foreign language, it may be convenient to use a bilingual interviewer who translates from the original questionnaire as he or she interviews. Alternatively, an interpreter may be used. In either of these approaches, it is much more likely than with a carefully translated questionnaire that the questions will not be translated correctly and erroneous responses will be obtained.

SUMMARY

The objectives of questionnaire design are to obtain, with minimum error, measurements of exposure variables essential to the objectives of the study and to create an instrument that is easy for both the interviewer and subject to use, and to process and analyse.

Open-ended questions should be used as far as possible to seek the simple, factual information that is most commonly needed in epidemiological studies. If closed-ended questions are used, the alternative answers offered should be simple, brief, mutually exclusive and as few as possible in number.

The words used in questions should be the usual 'working tools' of the respondents; complex, jargon, vague, and 'loaded' words should be avoided. Questions should:

- be phrased *as* questions
- contain only one concept
- avoid the use of double negatives
- have an unambiguous time reference.

Questions that ask about behaviour or attributes that are socially desirable or undesirable present a particular threat to subjects and require special care in wording.

The way in which questions are set out, the order in which they are presented, the structure of the questionnaire as a whole, and the way it is printed are all important in facilitating use of the questionnaire by interviewers and respondents, in ensuring ease and accuracy of processing data from the questionnaire, and in minimizing error.

Aids may be used to assist subjects in recalling information. They include:

- lists of alternative answers
- photographs of specific agents to which the subject may have been exposed
- a calendar on which key dates are marked
- reference to personal records.

All questionnaires should be pre-tested before being put into routine use. The particular objectives of pre-testing are to see whether the questions are understood and elicit appropriate responses and to ensure that where alternative answers have been provided they cover the full range of relevant answers. Pre-testing should include, at least, initial evaluation by peers and testing on a sample of subjects from the population to be studied.

Translation of a questionnaire into another language should be carried out by a person who is expert in both languages and, ideally, also understands the subject matter. A cycle of translation and back-translation to the original language should be followed until the back-translated questionnaire appears to have the same meaning as the original.

REFERENCES

Aday, L. A. and Andersen, R. (1979). Standard measures of standard variables. In *Health survey research methods*, (ed. L. G. Reeder), pp. 63–66. Washington, US Department of Health Education and Welfare. NCHSR Research Proceedings Series. DHEW Publication No. (PHS) 79-3207.

Becklake, M. R., Freeman, S., Goldsmith, C., Hessel, P. A., Mkhwelo, R., Mokoetle, K., Reid, G., and Sitas, F. (1987). Respiratory questionnaires in occupational studies: their use in multilingual workforces on the Witwatersrand. *International Journal of Epidemiology*, **16**, 606–11.

Belson, W. A. (1981). *The design and understanding of survey questions*. Gower, Aldershot, Hampshire.

Bennett, A. E. and Ritchie, K. (1975). *Questionnaires in medicine*. Oxford University Press, London.

Beresford, S. A. A. and Coker, A. L. (1989). Pictorially assisted recall of past hormone use in case-control studies. *American Journal of Epidemiology*, **130**, 202–5.

Blair, E., Sudman, S., Bradburn, N. M., and Stocking, C. (1977). How to ask questions about drinking and sex: response effects in measuring consumer behavior. *Journal of Marketing Research*, **14**, 316–21.

Bradburn, N. M. and Sudman, S. (1979). *Improving interview method and questionnaire design*. Jossey-Bass, San Francisco, California.

Bradburn, N. M., Rips, L. J., and Shevell, S. K. (1987). Answering autobiographical questions: the impact of memory and inference on surveys. *Science*, **236**, 157–61.

Cannell, C. F. (1985). Experiments in the improvement of response accuracy. In *Survey interviewing—theory and techniques*, (ed. T. W. Beed and R. J. Stimson), pp. 24–62. George Allen and Unwin, Sydney.

Del Greco, L., Walop, W., and Eastridge, L. (1987). Questionnaire development 3. Translation. *Canadian Medical Association Journal*, **136**, 817–8.

Dillman, D. A. (1978). *Mail and telephone surveys*. John Wiley and Sons, New York.

Frey, J. H. (1986). An experiment with a confidentiality reminder in a telephone survey. *Public Opinion Quarterly*, **50**, 267–9.

Helsing, K. J. and Comstock, G. W. (1975). Response variation and location of questions within a questionnaire. *International Journal of Epidemiology*, **5**, 125–30.

Herzog, A. R. and Bachman, J. G. (1981). Effect of questionnaire length on response quality. *Public Opinion Quarterly*, **45**, 549–59.

Hill, A. B. (1953). Observation and experiment. *New England Journal of Medicine*, **248**, 995–1001.

Holman, C. D. J. and Armstrong, B. K. (1983). Hutchinson's melanotic freckle melanoma associated with non-permanent hair dyes. *British Journal of Cancer*, **48**, 599–601.

Holt, V. L., Daling, J. R., Voigt, L. F., McKnight, B. F., Stergachis, A., Chu, J., and Weiss, N. S. (1989). Induced abortion and the risk of subsequent ectopic pregnancy. *American Journal of Public Health*, **79**, 1234–8.

Jobe, J. B. and Mingay, D. J. (1989). Cognitive research improves questionnaires. *American Journal of Public Health*, **79**, 1053–5.

Kricker, A., Armstrong, B. K., English, D. R. and Heenan, P. J. (1991). Pigmentary and cutaneous risk factors for non-melanocytic skin cancer – a case-control study. *International Journal of Cancer*, **48**, 650–662.

Krosnick, J. A. and Alwin, D. F. (1987). An evaluation of a cognitive theory of response-order effects in survey measurement. *Public Opinion Quarterly*, **51**, 201–19.

Leigh, J. H. and Martin, C. R. (1987). 'Don't know' item nonresponse in a telephone survey: effects of question form and respondent characteristics. *Journal of Marketing Research*, **24**, 418–24.

McFarland, S. G. (1981). Effects of question order on survey responses. *Public Opinion Quarterly*, **45**, 208–15.

Marcus, A. (1982). Memory aids in longitudinal health surveys: results from a field experiment. *American Journal of Public Health*, **72**, 567–73.

Messmer, D. J. and Seymour, D. T. (1982). The effect of branching on item non-response. *Public Opinion Quarterly*, **46**, 270–7.

Mitchell, A. A., Cottler, L. B., and Shapiro, S. (1986). Effect of questionnaire design on recall of drug exposure in pregnancy. *American Journal of Epidemiology*, **123**, 670–6.

Poe, G. S., Seeman, I., McLaughlin, J., Mehl, E., and Dietz, M. (1988). 'Don't know' boxes in factual questions in a mail questionnaire. Effects on level and quality of response. *Public Opinion Quarterly*, **52**, 212–22.

Schuman, H., Presser, S., and Ludwig, J. (1981). Content effects on survey questions about abortion. *Public Opinion Quarterly*, **45**, 216–23.

Schwartz, N., Hippler, H. J., Deutsch, B., and Strack, F. (1985). Response scales:

effects of category range on reported behaviour and comparative judgements. *Public Opinion Quarterly*, **49**, 388–95.

Skinner, H. A. and Sheu, W. J. (1982). Reliability of alcohol use indices. The lifetime drinking history and the MAST. *Journal of Studies on Alcohol*, **43**, 1157–70.

Smith, T. W. (1987). That which we call welfare by any other name would smell sweeter. An analysis of the impact of question wording on response patterns. *Public Opinion Quarterly*, **51**, 75–83.

Sobal, J. (1984). The content of survey introductions and the provision of informed consent. *Public Opinion Quarterly*, **48**, 788–93.

Social Science Research Council (1975). *Basic background items for US household surveys*. Social Science Research Council, Washington, DC.

Sudman, S. and Andersen, R. M. (1977). Health survey research instruments. In *Advances in health survey research methods: proceedings of a national invitational conference*, (ed. L. G. Reeder), pp. 7–12. US Department of Health, Education and Welfare, Washington. DHEW Publication No. (HRA) 77–3154.

Sudman, S. and Bradburn, N. M. (1983). *Asking questions: a practical guide to questionnaire design*. Jossey-Bass, San Francisco, California.

7

The personal interview

A series of studies in the early decades of survey research raised the issue of interviewer effects on responses. A classic demonstration was Rice's 1929 study of the causes of destitution. Comparing the results obtained from poverty-stricken respondents by two different interviewers, he discovered that the data collected by one interviewer showed overindulgence in alcohol as the most common cause of destitution while the other interviewer found social and economic conditions the most frequent causes. The case for interviewer bias appeared to be established when it was learned that the first interviewer was a prohibitionist and the second was a socialist. . . . Cannell et al. (1981).

INTRODUCTION

In epidemiology, an *interview* is '. . . a structured procedure with a scientific purpose by means of which the respondent [subject of research], through a series of questions or presented stimuli, is induced to give verbal information.' (Scheuch 1967). The personal interview, whether face-to-face or by telephone, is the commonest method of collecting data on exposure in epidemiological studies.

The objectives of a research interview are the same as those of a research questionnaire: to obtain measurements of exposure variables essential to the objectives of the study and to minimize error in these measurements.

While it is possible to use essentially identical questionnaires to collect data from study subjects by way either of interview or self-administration, the personal interview differs from the self-administered questionnaire in one very important respect: the presence of the interviewer. On the one hand, the interviewer may reduce error by increasing the response rate, motivating the subject to respond well, and probing to obtain complete data when the responses volunteered fall short of what is desired. On the other hand, the interviewer may increase error if by his or her appearance, manner, method of administration of the questionnaire, or method of recording of the responses, he or she exerts a qualitative influence on the subject's responses.

This chapter, then, will deal principally with the role of the interviewer in the research interview and the ways in which the benefits of having an interviewer can be maximized and the potential disadvantages minimized. Other subjects covered include types and styles of interviews, the optimal circumstances for an interview, and aspects of telephone interviewing that differ from face-to-face interviewing.

INTERVIEWER ERROR

There are four general ways in which the performance of interviewers may give rise to error (Hyman *et al.* 1954):

- *asking errors*: omitting questions or changing the wording of questions
- *probing errors*: failing to probe when necessary, biased probing, irrelevant probing, inadequate probing, preventing the respondent from saying all he or she wishes to say
- *recording errors*: recording something not said, not recording something said, incorrectly recording what was said
- *flagrant cheating*: recording a response when a question is not asked or answered.

That these errors do occur has been amply demonstrated in many studies, from which the following examples are drawn.

In a classical study, the American Jewish Committee, in association with the National Opinion Research Center, studied 15 comparatively inexperienced interviewers each of whom administered a 50 question questionnaire to 12 subjects, four of whom were 'planted respondents'. One of the planted respondents played the role of a 'punctilious liberal' — a person incapable of giving an unqualified, categorical response to any question, although friendly to the interviewer — and another played a 'hostile bigot' who required considerable persuasion to answer many of the questions and was 'quite vicious' with the interviewer. On average, each interviewer committed 13 asking errors, 13 probing errors, eight recording errors, and four cheating errors in each interview. All except the cheating errors were highly pervasive, being committed to a similar degree by all interviewers. All interviewers cheated at least once when interviewing the 'hostile bigot'. Four, however, cheated only in a very minor way while another four clearly fabricated large parts of the interview. The interviewers who cheated extensively with the 'hostile bigot' also cheated more than the others when interviewing the 'punctilious liberal', although the overall prevalence of cheating with this respondent was very much less. While the presence of the planted respondents makes these results non-generalizable to the usual interview situation, they do illustrate the extent to which error may arise, especially when the respondent is difficult (Hyman *et al.* 1954).

The extent of interviewer error may also be gauged from studies of interview–reinterview reliability and comparisons between interviewers in the prevalence of characteristics that they record in different random samples from the same population. Studies of interview–reinterview reliability are difficult to interpret because of the contribution of respondent error to disagreement between the two interviews. A number of studies have been carried out, however, in which some subjects have been re-interviewed by the same interviewer and others by a different interviewer. These studies have shown consistent evidence of greater agreement on factual data between two interviews conducted by the same interviewer than between two interviews conducted by different interviewers (Table 7.1).

In an analysis of data collected from 21 counties of Ohio and Michigan in the 1950 US Census, there was significant variation among interviewers in their recording of a number of responses (Hanson and Marks 1958). Variation was present most commonly in 'not applicable' categories of, for example, World War II veteran status, residence in 1949, highest school grade attended, highest school grade completed, now attending school, and wage and salary, self-employed or unearned income. There was also significant variation in some variables that the interviewers may not have liked asking about — for example, highest grade of school not completed and particular occupation and income categories. Similar observations were made with US Health Interview Survey (HIS) interviewers (Koons 1973). In addition, there was substantial variation among HIS interviewers in their recording of chronic conditions.

Table 7.1 Agreement on factual data in interviews and re-interviews obtained by the same or different interviewers (adapted from Hyman *et al.* 1954)

Characteristic	Percentage agreement between interview and re-interview	
	Same interviewer	Different interviewer
Stated age	98	98
Interviewer's estimate of age	90	71
Automobile ownership	96	86
Education		
7 categories	77	67
4 categories	82	79
Church attendance		
4 categories	79	67
2 categories	92	85
Service in World War II	99	98
Which newspaper read	82	82

Another illustration of interviewer error is given by Cannell *et al.* (1977). In the course of studies of the validity of data collected by interview on health service use, they observed that the reporting of contacts with health services fell with increasing experience of the survey by the interviewers. Thus, for example, over 5 weeks of surveying in one study, the proportion of physician office visits that went unreported rose from 18 per cent to 29 per cent. These and other data were taken to indicate that the interviewers lost interest and enthusiasm for the task over time and, in consequence, performed it less well.

Additional relevant data were obtained in a study in which three methods of data collection were compared: the regular HIS interview, the same interview with additional probe questions and a special introductory statement, and collection of data through a self-administered questionnaire left with the respondent. The proportions of hospitalizations not reported with each of these three methods are shown in Table 7.2. The regular interview showed the expected increase in under-reporting with increasing duration of the survey. This increase was absent, however, when the interview included additional probes and introductory material. It appears, therefore, that these additions may have overcome the effects of the interviewers' loss of enthusiasm for the task, as well improving overall reporting. There was no trend towards increased under-reporting with time in the absence of the interviewer.

The above example shows evidence of *interviewer bias* — a tendency for the interviewer, for whatever reason, and by mechanisms which are unclear in this study, to promote under- or over-reporting of particular experiences by the survey subjects. Interviewer error is a matter for concern, whether it is systematic or random. Systematic error (bias), however, is of particular concern when it arises through an interaction between the interviewer and

Table 7.2 Percentage of episodes of hospitalization not reported by week of the survey in a survey of health service use in which data were collected in three different ways (adapted from Cannell *et al.* 1977)

	Method of data collection		
Survey week	Regular HIS[a] interview	His[a] interview with additional probes, etc.	Self-administered questionnaire
1	13.7	8.3	14.4
2	11.0	8.6	16.0
3	16.8	9.2	21.2
4	22.1	8.7	10.5
5	23.7	10.0	16.1

[a] HIS, Health Interview Survey

particular kinds of subjects — for example, cases in a case-control study. The following pages will describe ways of minimizing both systematic and random error.

With specific reference to case-control studies, additional strategies will be necessary to ensure that any residual error is not different between subjects with and without disease. These strategies include each interviewer interviewing the same proportion of cases as of controls, 'blinding' interviewers to the case-control status of subjects, and keeping interviewers in ignorance of the exact objectives of the study.

There is evidence that interviewer error may vary with particular personal characteristics of the interviewer. Some more obvious external attributes of interviewers, such as race, sex, age and social status, are discussed below under 'selection of interviewers'. Other relevant attributes are less obvious, but may underlie subtle effects of the interviewer on the data obtained. For example, in the study described by Blair *et al.* (1977), interviewers who expected the interview to be difficult obtained 4–12 per cent lower reporting of sensitive behaviours than interviewers who did not. Elsewhere, those who expected the behaviours to be under-reported obtained less reports of them than those who did not (Bradburn and Sudman 1979). These observations have implications for both the selection and training of interviewers.

It is the opinion of at least some experts that modern methods of survey interviewing (e.g. the stressing of interviewer neutrality in training, the standardization of questionnaire wording and administration, the development of non-directive probing techniques) have substantially reduced the likelihood that the interviewers' personal attitudes and beliefs will affect the responses obtained (Cannell *et al.* 1981).

TYPES AND STYLES OF INTERVIEWS

Interviews may be structured or unstructured. A *structured interview* is one in which all the interviewer's tasks, and even words, are set down on the interview questionnaire. Structuring may extend not only to the questions to be asked but also to the introductory statement, the prompts to be used in particular circumstances, and even the 'feedback' to be given (if any) in response to answers of particular types.

All the available empirical evidence suggests that highly structured interviews are associated with the lowest rates of error. Such interviews require a highly professional and business-like approach by the interviewer. The emphasis conveyed by the interviewer to the subject is on the task to be done and the need to obtain complete and accurate data.

The objection raised most commonly in regard to highly structured, business-like interviews is that they inhibit the interviewer's development of rapport with the subject. Rapport is presumed to be important to the subject's continuing cooperation and to his or her provision of accurate data.

The use of a 'positively affective and personalized interactive style' of interviewing designed to establish rapport was compared with a more business-like style in a study of a sample of subjects who had had an automobile accident in the preceding four years (Henson *et al.* 1976). There were no significant differences between the two interview methods in the accuracy of reporting of details of the accident. However, the group interviewed in the more business-like manner showed little indication of a fall in accuracy of reporting with time since the accident, whereas a fall was evident in those interviewed with 'rapport'. On the other hand, respondents in the 'rapport' interview gave more information in response to several open-ended questions on health status (for which there was no independent source of data) than those interviewed in a business-like manner. This difference could have been due to the absence of all forms of feedback to the respondent from the business-like interviews. Respondents interviewed with 'rapport' were more likely to report that the interviewer was friendly, but neither group showed any negative reactions to the interview.

Another study has suggested that the development of rapport may have led to biased (under-) ascertainment of symptoms of psychiatric disorder (Dohrenwend *et al.* 1968). In a study of telephone interviews, Rogers (1976) reported that, for interviewers who were perceived as 'warm', respondents were less consistent in reporting education, less willing to report family income, less accurate in reporting their voting behaviour, and more likely to give socially desirable and 'don't know' responses. On the basis of these studies, the Survey Research Center at the University of Michigan abandoned the 'rapport' style in favour of structured interviewing techniques that emphasize the response task.

THE OPTIMAL CIRCUMSTANCES FOR AN INTERVIEW

The optimal circumstances for an interview are determined by *time* and *place*.

Time

Two considerations are relevant (Gorden 1975): the time of the interview in relation to the respondent's usual responsibilities, and the time of the interview with reference to the time when the exposures of interest occurred. For the first, the time should be chosen to minimize, as far as possible, competing demands on the respondent and to find the respondent in the optimal place for the interview (see below). The achievement of these ends for all subjects usually requires that an appointment be made (especially for interviews lasting more than 10–15 minutes) and that the interviewer be able to work both in the evening and on weekends.

Some guide to the times of likely availability of subjects at home, at least for the United States, is given by the results of a 1971 survey (USBC 1973). Table 7.3 lists the probabilities, by hour of the day, that someone 14 years of age or older was home at the interviewer's first call to a house, and compares them with similar data obtained at the 1960 census. As would be expected, people were most often home in the evening. Even then, however, the probability that no one was home was greater than 20 per cent. It is of interest also that the probability of finding someone at home during the day fell by 10 per cent or more between 1960 and 1971; this trend has probably continued. People were hardest to find at home in highly urban areas, and most easily found in farming areas. Except in farming areas, it was twice as hard to find a designated man at home before 4 p.m. as to find a designated woman. Men were more difficult to find at all hours. The easiest group to find at home at any time were those 65 years of age and older.

Day of week is also important in determining whether or not a respondent will be contacted and an interview obtained. In a telephone survey of US Veterans conducted in 1985 and 1986, Weeks *et al.* (1987) found weekday evenings, Saturdays any time, and Sunday afternoons and evenings to be the best time to obtain both an answer to the call and an interview. The evenings gave the highest answer and interview rates. These results applied both for first calls and for repeat calls.

To maximize the accuracy of recall, the interview should take place as near as possible in time to the occurrence of the exposures of interest. The

Table 7.3 Probability of finding someone 14 years of age or older at home at different times of the day in the United States (USBC 1973)

| | Probability | |
Time	1960 Census	1971 Survey
8– 8:59	0.71	0.57
9– 9:59	0.71	0.56
10–10:59	0.69	0.58
11–11:59	0.68	0.59
12–12:59	0.68	0.59
13–13:59	0.69	0.57
14–14:59	0.67	0.57
15–15:59	0.70	0.67
16–16:59	0.72	0.70
17–17:59	0.78	0.74
18–18:59	0.78	0.75
19–19:59	0.80	0.71
20–20:59	0.76	0.78

sensitivity of recall to delay is illustrated by studies of under-reporting of visits to doctors and periods of hospitalization by the time since they occurred (Cannell 1985). Within 10 weeks of discharge, only 3 per cent of hospital admissions went unreported, but this proportion increased to 42 per cent at 51–53 weeks. Similarly, after a delay of 1 week, 15 per cent of physician visits were not reported, while after 2 weeks 30 per cent were missed. This suggests an effect of salince on the persistence of recall, a suggestion that was confirmed by the finding that long periods of hospitalization were recalled better, at all time intervals, than short periods. In practice, in chronic disease epidemiology, and especially in case-control studies, moderate delay in interviewing will add little to the time since the period of aetiologically relevant exposure. For ethical reasons, therefore, and to minimize the effects of illness on responses, it is usual to delay interview until after the subject has recovered from the diagnosis and initial treatment of his or her disease.

Place

The place of interview should be chosen for its convenience to the subject and, as far as possible, to minimize inhibitors of communication (Gorden 1975). In practice, the vast majority of face-to-face interviews are carried out in the subject's home. Within the home, the location for the interview should be chosen so that it is away from distractions that remind subjects of their other obligations in life. This objective may be achieved through time (e.g. when children are at school or after they have gone to bed) as well as through location. The place of interview should be quiet and comfortable. The interviewer should be able to sit facing the respondent (so that the respondent cannot read the questionnaire), ideally at a table so that it is easier for the interviewer to organize his or her papers. Privacy is also important although, like the other ideals, not always attainable. If the respondent may be asked to refer to records during the interview, it will be necessary to interview where the records are kept, or to make arrangements for them to be brought to the interview.

There are some empirical data on the effect of the presence of 'third parties' on responses at interview (Bradburn and Sudman 1979). First, it was noted that a third party was present in a quarter of interviews in spite of instructions to interviewers to the contrary. Thus, where there is a major concern about privacy of the interview, special efforts may have to be made to obtain a private location, or telephone interviewing may be the preferred mode. Second, while the data actually reported appear to be unaffected by the presence of third parties, the presence of a child has been observed to make respondents more uneasy about answering questions about sensitive behaviours, and the presence of an adult may stimulate a higher rate of refusal to answer particular questions. For example, refusal to answer questions on frequency of petting or kissing, sexual intercourse, and masturbation in the past month increased some threefold, from 3–6 per cent to 6–18 per cent, in the presence of a spouse.

THE INTERVIEWER'S TASK

Depending on the nature of the investigation, the interviewer's task may include all or most of sample selection, initial contact with the respondent, elicitation of co-operation, asking questions and obtaining answers, recording of answers, and editing and coding the completed questionnaires.

Sample selection

The interviewer may be required to select subjects for the study if they are identified by random household survey or random digit dialling. Alternatively, if these are the sampling methods (as for selection of controls in a population-based case-control study), a two-step procedure may be adopted in which identification and selection of respondents is done by one field worker and the interviews by another. The choice between these alternatives will be determined by economic and logistic as well as scientific considerations. If interviewers select subjects for the samples, they cannot be blind to their disease status (as is desirable, for example, in a case-control study).

If sample selection is a component of the interviewer's task, details of the sampling scheme and its operation will form part of interviewer training.

Securing the interview

Whether or not the subject has already been contacted by a member of the survey team and an appointment made for the interview, the interviewer must take care to ensure the subject's co-operation. The interviewer should establish his or her identity by showing an official ID card from the institution conducting the research, and make the introductory statement that has been prepared by the investigators (see Chapter 6). It is important that this statement, and any subsequent information that the interviewer gives, should not be too specific regarding the purposes of the study so as not to bias the respondent or increase the salience of the study to a particular class of respondents (e.g. cases in a case-control study or subjects exposed to a particular agent). The interviewer should adopt a positive manner, assuming that the interview will not be refused, and endeavour to enter the house (if that is the location of the interview) as quickly as possible.

The interviewer should be prepared to answer specific questions put by the respondent. Some that commonly arise, and for which prepared answers should be given to the interviewer, are listed in Table 7.4. It is important that

Table 7.4 Questions commonly asked by respondents for which answers should be prepared and given to the interviewer (adapted from SRC 1976)

- How did you happen to pick me?
- Who gave you my name?
- I really don't know anything about this.
- Why don't you talk to my wife, she knows more about this than I do?
- What's all this about anyway?
- What good will this do?
- What's the catch?
- What else am I going to have to do?
- Why do you need my name?
- How can I be sure that you won't tell everyone else what I tell you?
- Why do you want to know that?
- What are you going to do with these answers anyway?

---

the answers given are honest and that they will not bias the interview. It is quite acceptable to give incomplete answers for explicit scientific reasons. For example, in response to 'Who gave you my name?', it would be reasonable to answer: 'The names of some people in the study were given to us by their doctors because they have recently been ill and the doctors want to help find out the causes of disease. The names of others have been selected at random from [*sampling frame*]. I don't know which of these groups you belong to. It is important that I don't know because, to get accurate results from this research, I must ask the questions the same way of everybody. Knowing what group you belong to may affect the way I ask you the questions.' This statement both answers the question and impresses on the respondent the care with which the research is being conducted.

It has also been found to be helpful for the interviewer to have available material that establishes the reputation of the research team (e.g. press clippings that refer to its work, copies of reports of previous work, and other material that demonstrates the value of the work to the community) to assist in establishing his or her bona fides, should that be necessary.

If it appears that the respondent is going to refuse to be interviewed, the positive reasons for participation should be restated (the significance to the community of the research and the reasons why *this* respondent is important) and any implied questions behind the refusal should be answered. As far as possible, a refusal should not be accepted until it is explicit. On occasions, it may be better for the interviewer to withdraw before the refusal has been made explicitly ('I see that I've caught you at a bad time . . .'), and while it may still be possible for a more experienced interviewer to return and obtain the respondent's co-operation.

Asking questions and obtaining answers

Asking

Rules for asking questions in a structured interview are listed in Table 7.5. These rules are largely self-explanatory; their objective is to ensure that a uniform stimulus to response is received by all respondents. The ideal reading speed is about two words a second, rather slower than we would naturally read. Reading the questions slowly not only allows the respondents more time to think about the answers, but has been shown to encourage them to spend more time over the answers and therefore to answer more fully.

Questions should be read with 'correct intonation and emphasis'. Correct intonation and emphasis is rather difficult to define in the general case. It will be achieved by an interviewer if he or she understands fully the intended meaning of the question. This understanding will come as a consequence of careful training. Cannell (1985) observed, after listening to many recordings of interviews, that interviewers were placing the emphasis on different parts of questions and thus giving them different meanings. He found that underlining words that were to be emphasized increased the degree of standardization of question asking.

As noted in Table 7.5, when a respondent mishears or misunderstands a question it should be repeated in full. When the respondent is still unsure of the meaning of a question after repetition, the interviewer should not attempt to explain it but say something neutral like 'Whatever it means to you' (see other permissible probes below). If that does not solve the problem, the question should remain unanswered and the reason for the difficulty noted on the questionnaire.

Table 7.5 Rules for asking questions in highly structured interviews (adapted from SRC 1976 and Brenner 1985)

- Read the questions exactly as they are worded in the questionnaire.
- Read each question slowly.
- Use correct intonation and emphasis.
- Ask the questions in the order that they are presented in the questionnaire.
- Ask every question that applies to the respondent (all inapplicable questions will be identified as such by skip instructions in the questionnaire).
- Use response cards when provided.
- Repeat in full questions that are misheard or misunderstood.
- Use only allowable probes.
- Read all linking or transitional statements exactly as they are printed.
- Do not add apologies or explanations for questions unless they are printed in the questionnaire.

Probing

Probes are additional questions asked or statements made by the interviewer when the answer given by a respondent is incomplete or irrelevant. Probing has two major functions (SRC 1976):

- to motivate the respondent to reply more fully
- to help the respondent focus on the specific content of the question. It must fulfil these functions without biasing the respondent's answers.

The ability to probe an unsatisfactory answer is one of the most important advantages of the personal interview, but it is also a method whereby bias can be easily introduced (e.g. by the interviewer summarizing his or her understanding of the response to the subject when an unclear response has been given, or offering some alternative interpretations of the response from which the respondent can choose). In a highly structured questionnaire, permissible probes for each question and the circumstances under which they can be used may be printed in the questionnaire. Alternatively, a list of acceptable non-directive probes may be given to the interviewers, and their use explained, during the course of training.

The following are non-directive methods of probing:

Repeat the question.   Vague answers may be a consequence of misunderstanding or mishearing of the question, or may arise because the respondent has not had long enough to think about the answer. All that may be required to obtain clarification is to repeat the question after an appropriate introduction like: 'I am not sure that I understand you, let me just ask the question again so that I can be sure to get your answer right. . . .'

The expectant pause.   Waiting expectantly tells the respondent that the interviewer is looking for more information than has been given already.

Repeat the reply.   Repeating the reply aloud while recording it may stimulate the respondent to provide more details.

Neutral questions or comments.   The following are neutral probes that may be used for particular purposes:
   For clarification

- 'What do you mean exactly?'
- 'What do you mean by . . . .?
- 'I don't think that I quite understand. Could you explain that a little?'
- 'In what way?'

For specificity

- 'Would you tell me what you have in mind?'
- 'Could you be more specific about that?'
- 'Can you be any closer about the [date]?'
- 'Can you be more exact?'

For completeness

- 'Anything else?'
- 'What else can you think of?
- 'Can you tell me more about it?'
- 'Are there any other reasons why you feel that way?'

It is usual to probe 'don't know' responses. Often they are given because the respondent did not understand the question, or because he or she needs more time to think about the answer. Thus repetition of the question or an expectant pause may be particularly useful techniques to try. Sometimes some assurance may be necessary like: 'There are no right or wrong answers to these questions, just give whatever answer you think is the right one.'

Feedback

The provision of feedback by the interviewer to the respondent about his or her performance of the response task has been the subject of some research. It was observed that, after asking questions, provision of unprogrammed feedback to respondents formed the highest proportion of interviewer behaviour (Cannell *et al*. 1981). The feedback phrases were almost invariably positive or encouraging to the respondent; they included phrases such as 'uh huh, I see', 'okay', 'that's good', 'all right', 'that's interesting', etc. Moreover, the probability of feedback was greatest in response to poor respondent behaviour, and tended to be most favourable under these circumstances.

As a consequence of these observations, Cannell and his colleagues hypothesized that accuracy and completeness of response could be increased by providing feedback that was contingent on the nature of the subject's responses. Thus, precise and apparently complete responses would be rewarded by feedback like 'Uh, huh, I see, this is the kind of information we want', 'Thanks, you've mentioned . . . things', 'Thanks, we appreciate your frankness' or 'Uh huh, we're interested in details like these', while vague or incomplete responses would be discouraged by phrases like 'You answered that quickly', 'Sometimes its easy to forget . . . Could you think about it again?', or 'That's only . . . things'. Subsequent studies showed that the use of contingent feedback in health-related surveys increased the amount of reporting of most events (e.g. number of doctor visits) and the precision in reporting of some (e.g. dates of medical events). The feedback phrases and the contingencies under which they were to be used were printed in the questionnaire. It was further shown that the combination of contingent feedback with specific instructions regarding the response task and elicitation of a commitment from the respondent to provide accurate and complete information (see Chapter 6) generally provided the most complete data, in comparison with other combinations of these techniques or a control condition in which none was used. It seems likely that the addition of programmed contingent feedback to epidemiological interviews would reduce response error.

Recording responses

The task of recording responses is generally simplified by highly structured interview questionnaires in which the only open questions are those which seek simple factual information. Table 7.6 gives rules for the recording of responses. Their application is generally to the recording of answers to open-ended questions rather than to closed-ended questions, which present few problems.

The emphasis of these instructions for recording responses is on accuracy and completeness. Accuracy means recording exactly what it was that the respondent said. Completeness includes providing all relevant information, including additional things that the respondent may have said that pertain to the objectives of the question; who made the error if an error was made; and whether or not missing information was a consequence of refusal to answer the question, lack of respondent knowledge of the answer, etc.

Table 7.6   Rules for recording responses in interviews (adapted from SRC 1976 and Brenner 1985)

- Make sure that you understand each response.
- Make sure that each response is adequate.
- Do not answer for the respondent (i.e. do not infer a response from an incomplete or inadequate reply).
- Record all response during the interview.
- Begin writing as soon as the respondent begins talking (the respondent's interest may be held by repeating the response aloud as you are writing).
- Use the respondent's own words and record the answers verbatim.
- Include everything that pertains to the question's objectives.
- Note in the questionnaire the nature and place of important probes used.
- Do not erase anything. If a response is wrong, strike it out and enter the correct response and note the source of the error (RE, respondent error; ME, my (interviewer) error).
- Write 'refused' beside any question that the respondent refused to answer.

Editing and coding

The questionnaire should be edited as soon as possible after the interviewer (or respondent) leaves the place of interview and, preferably, before another interview is undertaken. The objectives of editing are to ensure that all entries are legible, any abbreviations used are explained, important probes are noted, interviewer comments are in parentheses (to distinguish them from the respondent's replies), all unclear responses are clarified by parenthetical notes, and reasons are given (again parenthetically) for all missed responses. If editing uncovers missed questions or a missed section of the questionnaire, the interviewer should return to the respondent, with appropriate apologies, and complete them. The cover sheet should be edited to ensure that all identifying data are correctly entered and all other sections (interview start and finish times, call record, etc.) are correctly completed.

Coding may form part of the interviewer's task for closed-ended questions, or for all coded questions in a low-budget study in which the interviewer must also act as the coding clerk. As far as possible, interviewing and coding should be separated. The interviewer should not be required to code responses to open-ended questions during the interview. Coding of answers to closed-ended questions during the interview should be made automatic through the marking of pre-coded response categories (e.g. by circling numbers as in the questionnaire format shown in Chapter 6).

SELECTION, TRAINING, AND SUPERVISION OF INTERVIEWERS

Selection

The typical survey interviewer is a female high-school or college graduate, 30–40 years of age. There is empirical evidence that interview tasks are performed better by women than by men, by college graduates than those with less education, and by persons under 40 years of age (USBC 1972). College students have the reputation of being poor interviewers, although this may be due to lack of training and experience rather than to their young age (Cannell and Fowler 1977). Interviewer productivity increases and technical error rates decrease with increasing experience, to reach a plateau after about 2 years. As noted above, however, experience in a particular interview task may be associated with a fall in the quality of data obtained from respondents (Cannell *et al*. 1977). This observation is an argument for a continuing programme of on-the-job motivation and training, rather than a regular programme of firing experienced interviewers and hiring inexperienced ones. Specific aptitude tests are commonly used in the selection of US Census and Health Interview Survey interviewers, and there is evidence that the results of these tests correlate with subsequent interview performance (USBC 1972; Koons 1973).

Much consideration has been given to matching the interviewer to the respondent on characteristics such as sex, age, race, and socioeconomic status (Sudman and Bradburn 1974). This is probably a more important issue in research into opinions and attitudes than it is for most epidemiological research. Even for opinions and attitudes, matching appears to be important only if the topic of the study is highly related to interviewer or respondent characteristics and the respondent has not arrived at a firm position on it. White respondents, for example, are more likely to express pro-black attitudes if interviewed by a black interviewer than by a white interviewer (even if by telephone; Cotter *et al.* 1982). Antisemitic opinions are less likely to be expressed before an interviewer who appears to be Jewish; and an interviewer's apparent social class was shown to influence reporting of social and political opinions by working-class respondents (Cannell *et al.* 1981). The sex of the interviewer appears to have little effect on attitudes, but is commonly matched in interviews seeking a detailed sexual history. Matching of race may also be beneficial in obtaining co-operation, and logistically convenient if there is significant geographical segregation of races. It is clearly important to employ interviewers who are fluent in the language usually used by the respondents.

It has been common in epidemiological studies to employ nurses or other health professionals to act as interviewers, because of their likely familiarity with the subject matter of the research. They may also be necessary if blood or other biological specimens are to be collected. The employment of health professionals for the US Health Interview survey, however, is discouraged because they 'may tend to diagnose or interpret rather then merely record' (Koons 1973). No empirical data were offered to support this position.

Training

The training of interviewers has been shown empirically to improve their performance, particularly in reducing under-reporting of information and item non-response (Billiet and Loosveldt 1988). A carefully planned and structured programme of training of interviewers is essential to the success of epidemiological studies.

A general approach to the training of field workers has been outlined in Chapter 5. The specific training of US Health Interview Survey interviewers has been outlined by Koons (1973). Briefly, new interviewers are first given a package of self-study materials which includes administrative materials, a copy of the questionnaire, an interviewer's manual, and copies of letters sent to respondents. Interviewers then receive 5 days of classroom instruction which covers the interviewer's manual, the questionnaire and related forms, and interviewing techniques. The teaching techniques used in the classroom include lectures, reading of portions of the interviewer's manual, answering questions, group discussion, written exercises, and the conduct of mock interviews covering situations that the interviewer may face. The interviewer also participates in practice field interviews accompanied by an observer who coaches as required and completes an observation report. The interviewer is assessed on whether questions were asked correctly, whether probes were used correctly, whether the responses were recorded accurately,

Table 7.7   Contents of a typical interviewers' manual (adapted from SRC 1976)

- The sample survey:
  When is a survey made?
  What kinds of questions are asked?
  How is survey information used?
  Types of surveys
  Conducting a survey.

- The role of the interviewer.

- Introduction to the interview:
  Initial contact
  Securing the interview.

- Using the questionnaire:
  Introduction to the format of questionnaires
  Asking the questions
  Skip patterns
  Complex questions.

- Probing and other interviewing techniques:
  Probing
  The use of feedback.

- Recording answers and editing the questionnaire.

- Call and call-back strategy:
  Making contact
  Making an interview appointment
  Dealing with reluctant respondents.

- Telephone interviewing.

- Sampling principles and procedures:
  Sampling methods
  Selecting the respondent's household
  Selecting the respondent.

- Administrative procedures and office forms and records.

- Ethical principles for interviewers and the maintenance of confidentiality.

and whether other behaviours were appropriate.

The interviewer is accompanied by a supervisor for the first two days of the first interviewing assignment. All interview questionnaires completed during the first 8 weeks of interviewing are edited by the supervisor, errors identified, and a report on the errors given to the interviewer. In the supervised interviews, the supervisor acts as an observer only. The supervisor discusses his or her notes with the interviewer immediately on leaving the place of interview and, in addition, edits the questionnaire and prepares a written report. Thereafter, interviewers receive continued training through additional home study assignments and staff meetings.

The interviewers' manual

Each study that requires the collection of data by personal interview should have an interviewers' manual. An interviewer's manual is a specific form of the general procedures manual outlined in Chapter 5. It contains material general to all interviews and also material specific to the particular study for which it has been prepared. Table 7.7 outlines the topics applicable to interviewing in epidemiological research which are covered in a general manual prepared by the Survey Research Center of the University of Michigan (SRC 1976).

It is often useful to include a copy of the questionnaire in the manual, interleaved with pages of question-by-question explanation and instructions for the interviewer. An example of this approach is shown in Figure 7.1.

Supervision

The general principles of quality control during the course of collection of epidemiological data in the field have been outlined in Chapter 5. With respect to interviewing, they include:

- prompt editing by a supervisor or another experienced editor of the work completed by each interviewer
- timely performance of range and logic checks by computer
- periodic observation of the work of each interviewer
- re-interview of a proportion of subjects by a supervisor or other experienced interviewer
- comparison of the distribution of variables among interviewers
- analysis of trends in the variables over time.

The importance of observation or re-interview is underscored by the fact that only 12 per cent of interviewer errors could be identified by a careful examination of the completed questionnaires (Cannell *et al.* 1975). Tape

H7.   HOW MANY BROTHERS AND SISTERS DO YOU HAVE, EITHER LIVING OR DEAD?
       PLEASE INCLUDE ONLY BROTHERS AND SISTERS RELATED BY BLOOD.

       `Related by blood' includes half brothers and half sisters.

H8.   WHAT RACE DO YOU CONSIDER YOURSELF?

White	=> 1
Black	=> 2
Native American/Eskimo	=> 3
Asian	=> 4
Hispanic	=> 5
REFUSED	=> 7
OTHER _____	=> 8
UNKNOWN	=> 9

       For responses that do not fit into any categories, write down the response on the line to the right of
       `OTHER'.

H9.   WHAT IS THE HIGHEST LEVEL YOU ATTENDED IN SCHOOL?

Elementary school		=> 1
Middle or Junior High School		=> 2
High School		=> 3
Technical or Trade School		=> 4
College		=> 5
Graduate School		=> 6
REFUSED	(go to H11)	=> 7
OTHER _____		=> 8
UNKNOWN	(go to H11)	=> 9

       Examples of technical or trade schools are beautician school, computer training school, auto repair
       school, etc. Professional schools (medical school, law school, business school, etc.) are
       encompassed within the general term `graduate school'.

       Note that this question refers only to levels of attendance, rather than the level at which a subject
       graduated and completed. Thus if a respondent attended college but did not graduate, the code for
       her response would still be `5' (college).

       If the response is not listed among the choices given below the question, write down the response
       on the line beside `OTHER'. If the subject responds that she doesn't know or refuses to give an
       answer, enter the corresponding code and skip to question H11.

H10.   HOW MANY YEARS DID YOU COMPLETE AT THAT LEVEL?

       The answer to this question refers to the number of years of the highest level of education.

Figure 7.1 Example of question-by-question instructions to interviewers
adapted from an interviewers' manual used in a multicentre collaborative
case-control study of uterine sarcoma and cervical adenocarcinoma (Schwartz
et al. 1991).

recording of interviews is an acceptable alternative to supervisor observation of interviewers (Cannell *et al.* 1975). An example of its use in epidemiology can be found in Maclennan *et al.* (1977).

If a tape recorder is used, it is essential that the interviewer is familiar with its use and makes sure that it is working correctly and ready for operation before he or she enters the house. A simple request to the respondent, 'The University has asked me to tape these interviews if that's agreeable to you', is usually sufficient to obtain his or her consent to the recording. The recorder should be placed on the table between the interviewer and the respondent and thereafter forgotten, as far as possible.

It is important that these quality control procedures are carried out in a timely fashion and that there is prompt feedback to interviewers, either by way of direct supervisory communication or through staff meetings. Where problems have been identified and corrected, continuing surveillance should be maintained to ensure that the correction has been successful. It may be necessary to terminate the services of an interviewer who persistently presents work that fails the quality control checks.

A more detailed account of the supervision of interviewers is given in Koons (1973).

SPECIAL ASPECTS OF TELEPHONE INTERVIEWING

Differences between telephone and face-to-face interviewing

It is generally held that the principles outlined above apply to telephone interviewing even although they have been derived almost solely from research into and experience of face-to-face interviewing. The evidence that this is true is very limited. Telephone interviewing is probably not 'simply the transfer of face-to-face techniques to the telephone' (Miller and Cannell 1982). Use of visual cues, such as 'show cards', is impossible on the telephone, and must be compensated for in questionnaire design. There is evidence that this compensation may lead to response differences (Groves and Kahn 1979). In addition, other non-verbal communication, both from interviewer to respondent and from respondent to interviewer, is absent. The 'expectant pause', for example, cannot be used as a probe for additional information on the telephone. It is also more difficult for the interviewer to establish the legitimacy of the interview on the telephone. The pace of the interview may be faster (because of the need to keep talking), leading to hurried and, perhaps, less throughtful responses. On the positive side, the telephone should eliminate non-verbal biasing activity by the interviewer, and the greater 'distance' between the interviewer and the respondent may encourage more honest reporting of sensitive behaviours. Empirical data, however, have not shown consistent evidence of these effects (Colombotos 1969; Groves and Kahn 1979).

Miller and Cannell (1982) found that use of a commitment procedure, explanation of the response task, and programmed feedback had similar but less strong effects in telephone interviews to those that had been observed in face-to-face interviews. In particular, it appeared that contingent feedback was comparatively ineffective when added to the other two techniques. They hypothesized that this lack of effect may have been due to the need to include a good deal of 'back channel' feedback in the interview to ensure the respondent that the interviewer was still on the line and listening. This non-contingent feedback may have reduced the power of the contingent feedback.

Possible enthusiasm for telephone interviewing should be tempered by two additional considerations.

(a) There may be differences between cultures in the performance of this interviewing method. Most of the data that we have on it come from the United States, where telephone ownership is high and individual's use of the telephone is high. This familiarity with the telephone may make it a more acceptable medium for interviewing in that country than in some other countries. Siemiatycki *et al.* (1984) in Canada and O'Toole *et al.* (1986) in Australia found evidence that the quality of data collected by telephone interview in those countries was as high as that collected by face-to-face interview or by mail.

(b) Communications research identifies two kinds of telephone user: the 'business caller' and the 'social caller' (Cutler and Sharp 1985). While there are a number of differences between these two polar types of telephone user, in essence, the former uses the telephone mainly as a tool, resents calls, and avoids answering as far as possible, while the latter sees the telephone as a friend and welcomes calls. The existence of the former type, particularly, could give rise to important effects on data quality in certain circumstances.

Supervision of telephone interviews

Telephone interviewing offers considerable advantages in its ease of supervision. The interviewers may all be working together in the same building as the supervisor, and it is a comparatively simple matter for the supervisor to listen to and code interviewer behaviour in selected interviews without influencing either interviewer or respondent behaviour (subject, of course, to any legal or ethical constraints on such procedures).

Computer-assisted telephone interviewing

Computers have the potential to facilitate the interviewer's task and increase the accuracy of asking questions, giving programmed probes and feedback, and recording responses. In addition, computer-assisted telephone interviewing (CATI) may reduce the time taken to prepare questionnaires and to process the data (Taylor 1981). The availability to the supervisor of the computer screen currently visible to the interviewer also greatly facilitates observation of interviews (Groves 1981). The capabilities of present computer-assisted telephone interviewing systems have been summarized by Nicholls (1988). They include:

- administrative management of the survey sample
- on-line call scheduling and selection of cases to be called as each interviewer becomes free
- on-line interviewing including
  - screen display of instructions and questions
  - capacity to change screen displays in response to prior answers
  - display of permissible responses to closed questions
  - on-line editing of responses leading to acceptance or rejection, or generation of a probe or additional question
  - acceptance by extended text answers to open-ended questions
  - automatic branching or skipping
  - capacity to interrupt and resume interviews in mid course and to change and add information as necessary
- on-line monitoring of interviews by a supervisor
- automatic record keeping with respect to calls, response rates, interviewer productivity, etc.
- preparation of data sets ready for the next stage of processing.

Present evidence on the realization of the potential value of CATI is somewhat mixed. Harlow *et al.* (1985) conducted a study of data obtained by telephone from proxy respondents for cases and controls in a case-control study of colorectal cancer based on death certificates. They found no differences in the proportions of unresolved 'don't knows' and the quality of the interview, as assessed by the interviewer, between CATI and 'hard-copy' telephone interviews. The CATI interviews, however, took longer and were associated with less recording of comments and use of probes by the interviewers. The mean differences between CATI and hard-copy interviews on these variables, however, were much less than the differences between means for individual interviewers. The finding that CATI interviews are, on average, longer appears to be a consistent one (Groves and Mathiowetz 1984; Catlin and Ingram 1988). Groves and Mathiowetz (1984) found only small differences in response rates, reactions of interviewers and respondents, and the values of the health statistics sought between CATI and hard copy interviewing. Interviewer variability was less with CATI, and there were fewer skip errors. It seems likely that the advantages of CATI in terms of questionnaire design and data processing, and the evidence of some reduction in error associated with it, will eventually outweigh any disadvantages that it may have.

Some software for computer-assisted interviewing is now available for personal and lap-top computers (Birkett 1988; Smucker *et al*. 1989). Use of this software may extend some of the potential benefits of computer-assisted interviewing to face-to-face interviewing, or to projects that do not have easy access to bigger systems.

SUMMARY

The personal interview is the commonest method of collecting data on exposure in epidemiological studies. It differs principally from other methods by the presence of the interviewer; a presence that can have both positive and negative effects on the quality of the data obtained.

The interviewer's tasks may include sample selection and establishment of initial contact with the subject as well as asking questions and obtaining answers, recording responses, and initial editing and coding of the questionnaire. Whatever the initial approach to subjects, the interviewer must be skilled in obtaining the cooperation of the subjects. Interviewers should be provided with an appropriate introductory statement and model answers to questions that subjects are likely to ask.

Interviews may be structured or unstructured. Available evidence suggests that the former, in which the interviewer's tasks and words are all set out in detail on the questionnaire, are associated with the least error.

When asking questions, interviewers should read them slowly, with correct intonation and emphasis and exactly as they are worded in the questionnaire. Questions should be asked in the order that they are presented in the questionnaire; all questions relevant to each subject should be asked; and all linking and transitional statements should be read exactly as written. Probing should be non-directive and aimed at obtaining more complete and more relevant responses. Provision of question-by-question feedback which is contingent on the quality of the response can be used to improve the quality of responses.

The emphasis in recording responses should be on accuracy in recording exactly what it was that the respondent said, and completeness in providing all relevant information. The questionnaire should be edited as soon as possible after the interview so that any problems can be corrected while the interviewer's memory of the interview is still fresh and the subject still potentially available.

The best interviewers are generally female college graduates under 40 years of age. Interviewer productivity increases and technical error rates decrease with increasing experience of the interviewer. Training improves the performance of interviewers, and should be carried out in accordance with a carefully planned programme of instruction which includes practice in the field. As part of their training and for ongoing maintenance of standards, interviewers should be provided with a specific study manual. A programme of continuing training and supervision is advisable.

The principles that apply to interviewing face-to-face generally apply also to interviewing by telephone. Telephone interviewing offers considerable advantages in its ease of supervision. Computer-assisted telephone interviewing can also make the interviewer's task easier and reduce the time taken to prepare questionnaires and process the data. Lap-top computers may bring some of the advantages of computer-assisted telephone interviewing to face-to-face interviewing.

REFERENCES

Billiet, J. and Loosveldt, G. (1988). Improvements of the quality of responses to factual survey questions by interviewer training. *Public Opinion Quarterly*, **52**, 190–211.

Birkett, N. J. (1988). Computer-aided personal interviewing. A new technique for data collection in epidemiologic surveys. *American Journal of Epidemiology*, **127**, 684–90.

Blair, E., Sudman, S., Bradburn, N. M., and Stocking, C. (1977). How to ask questions about drinking and sex: Response effects in measuring consumer behavior. *Journal of Marketing Research*, **14**, 316–21.

Bradburn, N. M. and Sudman, S. (1979). *Improving interview method and questionnaire design*. Jossey-Bass, San Francisco, California.

Brenner, M. (1985). Survey interviewing. In *The research interview: uses and approaches*, (ed. M. Brenner, J. Brown, and D. Canter), pp. 9–36. Academic Press, London.

Cannell, C. F. (1985). Overview: response bias and interviewer variability in surveys. In *Survey interviewing, theory and techniques*, (ed. T. W. Beed and R. J. Stimson), pp. 1–23. George Allen and Unwin, Sydney.

Cannell, C. F. and Fowler, F. J. (1977). Interviewers and interviewing techniques. In *Advances in health survey research methods: proceedings of a national invitational conference*, (ed. L. G. Reeder), pp. 13–23. US Department of Health Education and Welfare, Washington. NCHSR Research Proceedings Series. DHEW Publication No. (HRA) 77-3154.

Cannell, C. F., Lawson, S. A., and Hausser, D. L. (1975). *A technique for evaluating interviewer performance*. Institute of Social Research, University of Michigan, Ann Arbor, Michigan.

Cannell, C. F., Marquis, K. H., and Laurent, A. (1977). A summary of studies of interviewing methodology. *Vital and health statistics*, Series 2, No. 69. DHEW Publication No. (HRA) 77-1343.

Cannell, C. F., Miller, P. V., and Oksenberg, L. (1981). Research on interviewing techniques. In *Sociological methodology 1981*, (ed. S. Leinhardt), pp. 389–437. Jossey-Bass, San Francisco, California.

Catlin, G. and Ingram, S. (1988). The effects of CATI on costs and data quality: a comparison of CATI and paper methods in centralized interviewing. In *Telephone survey methodology*, (ed. R. M. Groves, P. P. Biemer, L. E. Lyberg, J. T. Massey, W. L. Nicholls and J. Waksberg), pp. 437–450. John Wiley and Sons, New York.

Colombotos, J. (1969). Personal versus telephone interviews: effect on responses. *Public Health Reports*, **84**, 773–82.

Cotter, P. R., Cohen, J., and Coulter, P. B. (1982). Race-of-interviewer effects in telephone surveys. *Public Opinion Quarterly*, **46**, 278–84.

Cutler, T. A. and Sharp, K. F. (1985). Telephone interviewing: the meaning of the medium. In *Survey interviewing, theory and techniques, (ed. T. W. Beed and R. J. Stimson), pp. 136-157.* George Allen and Unwin, Sydney.

Dohrenwend, B. S., Colombotos, J., and Dohrenwend, B. P. (1968). Social distance and interviewer effect. *Public Opinion Quarterly*, **32**, 410-22.

Gorden, R. L. (1975). *Interviewing: strategy, techniques and tactics.* Dorsey, Homewood, Illinois.

Groves, R. M. (1981). A researcher's view of the SRC computer-based interviewing system: measurement of some sources of error in telephone survey data. In *Health survey research methods, third biennial conference*, (Ed. S. Sudman), pp. 88-98. US Department of Health and Human Services, Washington. DHHS Publication No. (PHS) 81-3268.

Groves, R. M. and Kahn, R. L. (1979). *Surveys by telephone. A national comparison with personal interviews.* Academic Press, New York.

Groves, R. M. and Mathiowetz, N. A. (1984). Computer assisted telephone interviewing: effects on interviewers and respondents. *Public Opinion Quarterly*, **48**, 356-69.

Hanson, R. H. and Marks, E. S. (1958). Influence of the interviewer on the accuracy of survey results. *Journal of the American Statistical Association*, **53**, 635-55.

Harlow, B. L., Rosenthal, J. F., and Ziegler, R. G. (1985). A comparison of computer-assisted and hard copy telephone interviewing. *American Journal of Epidemiology*, **122**, 335-40.

Henson, R., Cannell, C. F., and Lawson, S. (1976). Effects of interviewer style on quality of reporting in a survey interview. *Journal of Psychology*, **93**, 221-7.

Hyman, H., Cobb, W. J., Feldman, J. J., Hart, C. W., and Stember, C. H. (1954). *Interviewing in social research.* University of Chicago Press, Chicago.

Koons, D. A. (1973). Quality control and measurement of nonsampling error in the Health Interview Survey. *Vital and health statistics*, Series 2, No. 54. DHEW Publication No. (HSM) 73-1328.

Maclennan, R., Da Costa, J., Day, N. E., Law, C. H., Ng, Y. K., and Shanmugaratnam, K. (1977). Risk factors for lung cancer in Singapore Chinese, a population with high female incidence rates. *International Journal Cancer*, **20**, 854-60.

Miller, P. V. and Cannell, C. F. (1982). A study of experimental techniques for telephone interviewing. *Public Opinion Quarterly*, **46**, 250-69.

Nicholls, W. L. (1988). Computer-assisted telephone interviewing: A general introduction. In *Telephone survey methodology*, (ed. R. M. Groves, P. P. Biemer, L. E. Lyberg, J. T. Massey, W. L. Nicholls and J. Waksberg), pp. 377-85. Wiley, New York.

O'Toole, B. I., Battistutta, D., Long, A., and Crouch, M. K. (1986). A comparison of costs and data quality of three health survey methods: Mail, telephone and personal home interview. *American Journal of Epidemiology*, **124**, 317-28.

Rogers, T. F. (1976). Interviews by telephone and in person: quality of responses and field performance. *Public Opinion Quarterly*, **40**, 51-65.

Scheuch, E. K. (1967). Das interview in der sozialforschung. In *Handbuch der epirischen sozialforschung, Vol. 1*, (ed. R. König), p. 138. F. Enke, Stuttgart.

Schwartz, S., Welss N. S., Daling, J. R., Newcomb, P. A., Liff, J. M., Gammon, M. D., Thompson, W. D., Watt, J. D., Armstrong, B. K., Weyer, P., Isaacson, P. and Ek, M. (1991). Incidence of histologic types of uterine sarcoma in relation to menstrual and reproductive history. *International Journal of Cancer*, **49**, 362–7.

Siemiatycki, J., Campbell, S., Richardson, L., and Aubert, D. (1984). Quality of response in different population groups in mail and telephone surveys. *American Journal of Epidemiology*, **120**, 302–14.

Smucker, R., Block, G., Coyle, L., Harvin, A., and Kessler, L. (1989). A dietary and risk factor questionnaire and analysis system for personal computers. *American Journal of Epidemiology*, **129**, 445–9.

Sudman, S. and Bradburn, N.M. (1974). *Response effects in surveys. A review and synthesis.* National Opinion Research Center Monographs in Social Research, Aldine, Chicago.

SRC (Survey Research Center) (1976). *Interviewers' manual* (revised edition). Institute of Social Research, University of Michigan, Ann Arbor, Michigan.

Taylor, D.G. (1981). Observations on the behaviour of automated telephone interviewing. In *Health survey research methods, third biennial conference*, (ed. S. Sudman), pp. 99–100. US Department of Health and Human Services, Washington. DHHS Publication No. (PHS) 81–3268.

USBC (US Bureau of the Census) (1972). *Investigation of census bureau interviewer characteristics, performance and attitudes: a summary.* Working Paper No. 34, US Government Printing Office, Washington.

USBC (US Bureau of the Census) (1973). *Who's home when?* Working Paper No. 37, US Government Printing Office, Washington.

Weeks, M.F., Kulka, R.A., and Pierson, S.A. (1987). Optimal call scheduling for a telephone survey. *Public Opinion Quarterly*, **51**, 540–9.

8

Use of records, diaries, and proxy respondents

> *Anyone who has ever worked with medical records knows that they are an imperfect source of scientific data. The records contain all the idiosyncrasies and errors that can occur in the communication of human observations. . . . The recorded data often consist of anecdotal generalities rather than precise specifications; the statements often represent opinions or interpretations rather than descriptions of observed evidence; important information may sometimes be absent or unobtainable; and the remarks made by one doctor may sometimes contradict those made by another.* (Feinstein et al. 1969a)

INTRODUCTION

In this chapter we consider the use of records, diaries, and proxy respondents, all of which are important methods of measurement of exposure in epidemiology.

USE OF RECORDS

Scope of records

The term *record* will be used here to describe data recorded for a purpose other than the epidemiological study of interest. Records useful for epidemiological research include medical (inpatient and outpatient), pharmacy, disease registry, birth certificate, death certificate, and environmental records. Records may be paper records, such as most medical records, or computerized records such as death certificate files.

A common element in the use of records is that part or all of the data collection has already been carried out. To gain insight into the accuracy of the information, the researcher should become familiar with the process of data recording that has already occurred.

For example, in the United States, the information on birth certificates is recorded at each hospital, usually by the medical records staff or the obstetric nursing staff. The National Center for Health Statistics has published a procedure manual (NCHS 1987a), but generally, there is no uniform training of recorders. The personal information (mother's age, education) is recorded on the birth certificate from a questionnaire developed by each hospital, which is administered during the mother's hospital stay, and placed in the mother's hospital chart. The medical information (method of delivery, months of prenatal care, complications) is abstracted from the mother's and infant's inpatient records and the prenatal records if they are available. The attending physician verifies the accuracy of the medical information and signs the form, and the state or local vital registration office checks for completeness and queries incomplete or inconsistent certificates.

The medical information on death certificates in most countries is recorded by a physician or coroner. However, the doctor signing the form may not be the decedent's primary physician, and may be unfamiliar with the decedent's past medical history or the circumstances surrounding the death. In many countries, the funeral director is responsible for recording personal items concerning the decedent (age, marital status, usual occupation, type of business or industry) through an informant. The informant, usually a relative, is named on the certificate. In the United States, the National Center for Health Statistics provides procedure manuals (NCHS 1987*b*, *c*) for physicians and funeral directors, which may be modified by states to meet their needs. Formal training in completion of death certificates is provided by some medical schools and by some state or local vital record offices. State or local record departments review the records, and provide informal training to physicians and funeral directors during call-backs to clarify information.

The information in hospital records may include an admission form completed by a clerk; handwritten notes by physicians, nurses, and other health workers; results of diagnostic tests (X-rays, laboratory tests); reports from consultations with sub-specialists; operation reports or reports of other therapeutic procedures; and a typewritten discharge summary, usually dictated by a physician. The notes by the health care providers include information volunteered by or solicited from the patient, information from the physical examination of the patient, medical diagnoses, and prescribed medicines or other therapeutic procedures.

These examples highlight some of the limitations of the use of records compared with data collection by structured interview. When a structured interview is used, the researcher attempts to collect the same information in the same manner for all subjects. In contrast, when records are used, the researcher has little control over how questions are phrased, the definition of terms, what items are recorded, and the order in which they are recorded. Moreover, records are often produced by a large number of recorders with little uniform training. Records are also subject to many of the same sources of error as interviews, including erroneous reports by the subject (e.g. self-report of alcohol use), or errors in the entry of information into the record. Further, treatment information in outpatient records may indicate only the intended treatment; a record of a drug prescription, for example, does not necessarily mean that the medication was taken.

Advantages to the use of records

There are several advantages to the use of records over other methods of data collection. The study costs are usually low, and the study time is reduced because some or all of the data collection has been carried out by others.

More importantly, despite the limitations of records, the accuracy of selected data items can be better than that obtained by personal interview. The primary advantage of records is that they can provide prospectively recorded information, collected on exposures in the past. The prospective nature of records minimizes errors due to poor recall of the exposure, or due to lack of knowledge of the exposure by the subject. For example, use of pharmacy records in a case-control study of prescription drug use could overcome lack of recall or knowledge by subjects of the names of drugs taken.

Medical records are generally assumed to be more accurate than subject interview for medical conditions, diagnostic X-ray procedures, and prescription drug use. Indirect support for the superiority of records comes from the poor to moderate agreement between questionnaire data and medical records. The concordance between medical diagnoses in records and reports by subjects varies widely across conditions and between studies (Harlow and Linet 1989). In a study of older women, the reported κ coefficients for agreement between personal interview and medical records were 0.63 for benign breast disease, 0.70 for diabetes, and 0.78 for hypertension (Paganini-Hill and Ross 1982). Subject reports of X-ray procedures appear to be particularly poor. Tilley *et al.* (1985) found κ of 0.37 for agreement between physician records and mothers' recall after more than 10 years, of trunk X-ray during pregnancy Graham *et al.* (1963) found that only 19 per cent of diagnostic radiography and 59–71 per cent of fluoroscopic examinations were accurately recalled. Studies of drug use have focused on oral contraceptive use and postmenopausal oestrogen use (Harlow and Linet 1989), and suggest moderate agreement. For agreement between personal interview and physician records of use of exogenous oestrogen (ever vs. never), κ ranged from 0.51 to 0.71 across three studies (Horwitz *et al.* 1980; Spengler *et al.* 1981; Paganini-Hill and Ross 1982) with a reported correlation of 0.63 for total duration of use (Paganini-Hill and Ross 1982).

Records may be less vulnerable than retrospective interviews to certain sources of error. Telescoping of exposures from the past into a more recent time period may affect records less than interviews. Walter *et al.* (1988) found that women report more Pap smears over the previous 5 years than their medical records suggest, and report their last smear as more recent than indicated in their outpatient records. Records may be less influenced by social desirability bias as well; in one study, psychiatric diagnoses were reported twice as often in medical records as in interviews (NCHS 1973). In addition, differential exposure measurement error between those with and without disease is less likely to affect prospectively recorded records than retrospective interviews, providing the exposure information used is limited to that recorded before the onset of disease (or other outcome) or symptoms of the disease.

A final advantage in the use of records is the potential for a high response rate. The use of birth records affords a complete sample of births within an entire state. Computerized pharmacy records of a health maintenance organization (Stergachis 1989) may offer near-complete data on a well-defined population. Response rates can be particularly high if subject contact is not required to permit use of the record. In such studies, information can be obtained even when the subject is dead or his or her current address unknown. Approval from human subject review committees for such studies can often be obtained if confidentiality can be assured; for instance, if personal identifying information such as name and address are not abstracted from the records and abstractors sign a commitment to confidentiality.

Unfortunately, not all studies that make use of medical records achieve a high response. In some studies, subjects or next-of-kin must recall the names of health care providers before medical records can be obtained. Permission or a written response from the provider or hospital is often required. Response rates from physicians can be low (Stolley *et al.* 1978; Tilley *et al.* 1985) and, in one study, 31 per cent of hospitals refused access to their records (Savitz and Grace 1985). Finally, records can be lost or no longer available, for example when the physician has died.

Reliability and validity of record information

Studies of the agreement between medical records and questionnaire data, such as those cited above, provide only indirect information on the validity of records, because they were interpreted under the assumption that discrepancies between the two methods were due to errors in the interview data. Of course medical record data are subject to error as well, but few direct studies of the reliability and validity of record information have been conducted.

It is necessary, first of all, to ask how reliable are the types of measurements that are documented in medical records. A comprehensive study of the reliability of physical examination information was conducted among Vietnam veterans (CDC 1989). Subjects had a second examination by a different physician on the same day as their first examination. The inter-physician κ for agreement on common conditions (conditions affecting at least 5 per cent of subjects) ranged from a high of 0.47 for ear canal abnormalities and 0.45 for abnormal heart sounds (murmurs, systolic clicks, or gallop sounds) to a low of −0.05 for prostate abnormalities (enlargement or tenderness). The correlation between blood pressure readings was 0.54–0.73 for systolic and 0.45–0.73 for diastolic blood pressure. Biochemical analyses of blood from repeated blood samples (analysed in the same batch) were highly reproducible; correlations ranged from 0.87 for albumin to 0.99 for cholesterol.

Further information on the validity of medical records comes from studies in which records were compared to a more accurate source of data. Two such studies suggest that medical records are only a moderately accurate source of information on prescription drug use. In a Veterans Hospital study, only 74 per cent of prescriptions listed in hospital pharmacy records were recorded in the medical chart (Monson and Bond 1978). Moreover, only 38 per cent were correctly recorded in terms of drug name, strength, dosage, and directions. In a study by Gerbert *et al.* (1988), four methods of measuring the use of several drugs among patients with chronic obstructive pulmonary disease were compared (based on a single physician visit): chart review, patient interview, physician interview, and videorecording of the consultation between patient and physician. By simultaneously considering the four methods, it appeared that chart review of the drugs tended to be highly specific (specificity estimates of 0.95–1.0). But the proportion of drugs prescribed that were noted (the sensitivity) ranged from 0.60–0.82.

Certain exposures in records, such as alcohol use, smoking, and occupation, originate from self-report by the subject. For these exposures, comparison of records to interviews provides some information about the validity of the records, because the interview may be the more valid source. Brownson *et al.* (1989) compared information in hospital medical records (abstracted for a cancer registry) to that obtained by a telephone interview with the subject. In comparison to the interview, hospital medical records could be used to correctly classify 57 per cent of alcohol drinkers (sensitivity) and correctly classify 96 per cent of the non-drinkers (specificity). A similar comparison for smoking led to a sensitivity of 0.80, a specificity of 0.91, and a Spearman rank correlation coefficient of 0.93 across four levels of packs smoked per day. Exact agreement of US Census three-digit occupational codes was achieved for 70 per cent of occupations and 72 per cent of industries. These statistics may be somewhat misleading, however, as they were based only on records with information that could be coded. They do not reflect the problem of missing data, which is discussed below.

The occupation reported on death certificates has a further source of error: the information is provided by a proxy respondent. The accuracy of this variable is discussed in the section on proxy respondents below.

Sources of error and quality control procedures for record abstraction

Records should be selected as the method of exposure measurement only after consideration has been given to the quality of the data collection process that has already been carried out. Then, quality control procedures should be applied to the remaining steps of data collection. When computerized records are used, range and logical checks on the data items should be performed as a minimum requirement. For paper records, the challenge is to reduce an unstructured text into a well-defined set of coded variables. Explicit criteria are needed to minimize the need for judgement and interpretation by the abstractor.

When data are to be abstracted from records, most of the general quality control procedures outlined in Table 5.3 can be applied to the abstraction process. These include the design of a clear, easy-to-use abstraction form, development of a detailed protocol for abstraction of the information, thorough training of abstractors, and pre-testing of the protocol. Figure 8.1 gives an example of a data abstraction form and Figure 8.2 an example of the protocol for coding a few data items from an abstractor's manual.

Quality control during data collection should include re-abstraction of some percentage of the work done by each abstractor to identify items that are unreliably abstracted. Regular staff meetings should be held to discuss abstracting and coding issues and to maintain staff commitment to the project. All forms should be edited by an editor, by computer, or both. The development of small portable microcomputers has also made it useful for record abstractors to enter data direct from records to computer, with performance of logic and range checks in the process to permit immediate correction of errors. This removes at least one error-prone step in data collection.

In addition to these general procedures for reducing error, attention needs to be paid to sources of error particular to information ascertained from records (Feinstein *et al.* 1969*a*, *b*; Horwitz and Yu 1984; Hilsenbeck *et al.* 1985). These include:

- lack of complete coverage by records of the time period of interest
- missing information on the exposure or covariates of interest
- lack of uniform order of information in the record
- ambiguous or inconsistent information within and between records.

These sources of error are described in more detail below, along with quality control procedures that may reduce them.

The emphasis of the following sections is on abstracting data from written medical records. However, many of the sources of error and quality control

CANCER SURVEILLANCE SYSTEM CONFIDENTIAL REPORT OF NEOPLASM   RESUBMIT

NOTE: _____ CHT # _____

(CSS USE ONLY) Inst
Deletion: ☐ AHI ☐ File Seq #   K=   * CR#   CkD   File #   Inst Seq #

Coder   Editor   ☐ X-FILE ☐ OS   ☐ POTENTIAL CORRECTION ☐ CORRECTION (Circle all corrections in red)   ☐ INSTITUTION SEQUENCE #1 (Code all data items)   ☐ INSTITUTION SEQUENCE #2-6 (Code blue shaded data items)

PATIENT NAME   LAST   FIRST   MIDDLE

ADDRESS   STREET   CITY   STATE   SEX   MARITAL STATUS   RACE   SPANISH ORIGIN/ MAIDEN NAME

AGE   SPOUSE/PARENT/SPONSOR NAME: SS #   BIRTHPLACE   RESIDENCE AT DX (CITY/STATE)
☐ Address confirmed: Admit date >6 mos from dx date

USUAL OCCUPATION   INDUSTRY   INSURANCE   TOBACCO HX

WAS DX MADE ELSEWHERE? ☐ YES, DATE   ☐ CLINICAL DX ONLY   (CSS USE ONLY) ☐ CSS by NAME ☐ ATR   ITEMS IN BOLD TYPE TO BE COMPLETED AT HOSPITAL
CHECKED: ☐ CSS by SS #   DATE:

IF YES: INSTITUTION/CITY/STATE   INSTITUTION #

ORIG. SLIDE #:   CHART #   ADDRESS VERIFIED IN PHONE BOOK: ☐ Patient's ☐ Post Office   ACCESSION #   19____

SEQUENCE   PREVIOUS PRIMARIES: SITE/DX DATE/PLACE OF DX   OS MALIG CODE

TYPE OF CHART (Check One):   ☐ OUTPT ONLY   ☐ INPT ADMIT ONLY   ☐ CHEMORX ONLY   CONSULT ONLY INST #   SS #
☐ OUTPT FOLLOWED BY INPT ADMIT WITHIN 2 MO. ☐ RADIATION ONLY ☐ PATHOLOGY ONLY

PRIMARY SITE   SITE CODE (CSS USE)   ZIP CODE

PATHOLOGY (INCLUDE MO./DAY/YR; SLIDE #; SPECIMEN; FINAL PATH DX) GROSS/MICRO; EOD INFO INCLUDING TUMOR SIZE; # OF REGIONAL LN'S; # AND SIZE OF ⊕LN'S)   BIRTHDATE

CHART #
CLASS   DATE ADMIT

Reporting Source   Primary Sequence
DXDATE
Primary Site
Histology
DXCONF   DXPROC

MO/DAY/YR PHYSICAL EXAM (INCLUDE CHIEF COMPLAINT)   MO/DAY/YR ENDOSCOPIES/SURGERIES (INCLUDE NAME OF PROCEDURE AND FINDINGS)   GROUP HEALTH INSURANCE ☐ YES ☐ NO

CENSUS TRACT

MO/DAY/YR X-RAY/SCANS

MO/DAY/YR STAGE   T ___ N ___ M ___ OTHER: T N M
SOURCE   TNM

MO/DAY/YR ERA/PRA   ERA (DX DATE ≥ 1988)
☐ Report in chart; specify lab:
MO/DAY/YR LAB (SERUM/URINE PROTEIN ELECTROPHORESIS; ACID PHOS)   ☐ Results in chart   PRA VALUE (DX DATE ≥ 1988)
☐ Ordered; results unknown
MO/DAY/YR DISCHARGE DX (SIGN-OUT DX)   ☐ Unknown; no info   ERA VALUE (DX DATE ≥ 1990)
☐ ERA POS   ☐ PRA POS
☐ ERA NEG   ☐ PRA NEG   PRA VALUE (DX DATE ≥ 1990)
Value: Value:
☐ fmol/mg ☐ ICC ☐ Other: 1 4 7 10

FIRST COURSE DEFINITIVE THERAPY (INCLUDE MO/DAY/YR; DOCUMENT ALL PLANNED RX; RX GIVEN, OR ANY REASON RX NOT GIVEN)   EOD
STAGE   LAT   DATE 1st RX
RADIATION   SSS   (DX DATE ≥ 1988) REASON FOR NO SSS   S C R B N U H O D O O C H M O R D G
(DX DATE ≥ 1988)LUNG & LEUKEMIA: RAD TO CNS   RX

STATUS AT ☐ ALIVE ☐ DEAD DATE   (CSS) FU: STATUS: VITAL STATUS   DATE LAST FOLLOWED/FU SUBM
LAST CONTACT ☐ CLINICALLY FREE OF CA ☐ WITH CA ☐ UNKNOWN   ☐ CASE OPENED   ☐ CODER ENTERED FU
AUTOPSY? ☐ YES ☐ NO ☐ UNKNOWN (EXPIRED OUTSIDE THIS INSTITUTION) ☐ CLOSE TO FU   ABSTRACTOR   DATE ABST

PHYSICIANS: ENTER ADDRESS/PHONE # OF NEW PHYSICIAN ON BACK   1. FU PHYSICIAN/INSTITUTION   2. ALTERNATE FU PHYSICIAN   3. SURGERY   4. RADIATION THERAPY   5. CHEMOTHERAPY

FU INSTITUTION INDICATOR

ORIG/AHI ENTERED: CORR ENTERED: X-FILE ENTERED: ☐ OS ONLY/NO CORR
Reorder from Lancer Ltd 509-922-0260 Dial Toll Free 1-800-541-2232 20/3-9

Figure 8.1 Example of a record abstraction form: cancer registry abstraction form (Cancer Surveillance System, Fred Hutchinson Cancer Research Center, David B. Thomas, MD, DPH, with permission).

FOR BREAST CASES (Site 174.0-174.6, 174.8-174.9, 175.9)

Field 45   Estrogen Receptor Protein Status (for cases diagnosed 1/88 or later)

          0   Estrogen receptor assay not done
          1   Estrogen receptor: Positive
          2   Estrogen receptor: Negative
          3   Estrogen receptor: Borderline
          4   Ordered but results not on chart
          9   Unknown; no information

Field 47   ERA Value (for cases diagnosed 1/90 or later)

NOTES:
   1.   Leave ERA fields 45 and 47 blank for cases that do not meet the above site/dx date restrictions.

   2.   DEATH CERTIFICATE ONLY AND AUTOPSY ONLY CASES MUST BE CODED "9" IN FIELD 45.

   3.   If abstract clearly indicates per clinician/pathologist "No ERA" or "ERA not done" code 0 in field 45. If there is no indication this is a physician's statement code 9 in field 45.

   4.   Code the value given if stated in femtomoles/mg (if value is stated to be < 5, code value as 4, if stated to be ≤ 5, code value as 5).

   5.   If ERA is done using immunofluorescent or immunocytochemistry (ICC) technique the ERA value will not be coded in fields 47, however, the value should be noted on the abstract.

Figure 8.2   Example from a record abstraction protocol: coding of oestrogen receptor assay (Cancer Surveillance System, Fred Hutchinson Cancer Research Center, David B. Thomas, MD, DPH, with permission).

procedures described apply to other types of records as well, and some also apply to computerized records.

Incomplete coverage of the time period of interest

Records should only be selected as the method of exposure measurement if the data required are expected to be available for a large proportion of subjects; additionally, the completeness of coverage within the records themselves should also be considered.

   The time period covered by the record may not be the complete time period of interest. Outpatient medical records cover only the time period a subject has been with the provider or clinic. Medical conditions or personal information such as occupation relevant to earlier time periods may be only variably recorded. A related problem is the use of multiple providers during a given time period. For example, a subject may have seen several physicians or used multiple pharmacies, and the researcher may not have access to all providers. In one study, the agreement on use of oral oestrogens was substantially higher for interview compared to medical records than interview compared to pharmacy records ($\kappa = 0.51$ and $\kappa = 0.21$ respectively; Paganini-

Hill and Ross 1982). The authors attribute this to subjects' use of pharmacies other than the community medical centre pharmacy that was surveyed.

One concern with incomplete coverage is that differential misclassification can be introduced if the time periods of coverage are systematically different between cases and controls. Suppose a case-control study were to be conducted of myocardial infarction in relation to certain medications within a health maintenance organization. If cases had been enrolled for an average of 10 years and randomly selected controls had been enrolled for an average of 5 years, this selection of controls would almost certainly have led to differential measurement error in medication history. To minimize this bias, cases and controls (or those exposed and unexposed in a cohort study) should be matched or stratified on the date of commencement of their records and on length of time with the provider.

Finally, records or certain volumes of records may be lost, no longer in storage, or otherwise unavailable (Horwitz and Yu 1984). A system of recording the volume numbers should be used to ensure that all volumes of a subject's medical record are obtained.

Missing information in records

Information of interest to the researcher is often missing in records. As noted earlier, even patient care information such as drug prescriptions is sometimes not recorded in medical records (Gerbert *et al.* 1988; Monson and Bond 1978). Symptoms, risk factors, or personal information may be even less consistently noted in medical records. In an experimental study, medical students recorded on average 63 per cent of the 'pertinent' items from a mock patient interview when they took notes during the interview, and only 43 per cent when they recorded the notes after the interview (May and Miller 1977). Moreover, there is a tendency to omit negative findings rather than positive ones. For example, no information in a record on smoking could either mean that the question was not asked, or that it was asked and a negative answer was obtained but not recorded.

A particular problem with the use of records is that records may have been selected for the availability of information on the primary exposure, but information on potential confounders may not be recorded for many subjects, or may be recorded in insufficient detail. For example, Brownson *et al.* (1989) found that among records of cancer patients, 15 per cent had missing information on smoking, 25 per cent on alcohol consumption, and 36 per cent on occupation. These deficiencies would lead to an inability to control fully for the effects of confounding variables.

An additional problem is that missing information may be related to the disease or exposure under study. For example, the physician may be more likely to ask a question on family history of breast cancer among women with benign breast disease, which would lead to more reports of a positive history even in the absence of any true association. The selection of an appropriate reference date may lessen the problem of differential recording of exposures between those with and without the disease. A reference date for each case before the onset of symptoms of the disease could be selected, and a similar date assigned to each control. Information in a record recorded after that date would not be abstracted. This procedure could also help to blind data abstractors to the disease status of subjects.

Supplemental data collection is one solution to missing data. Certain exposures may be measured by record review and others by interviews conducted with the subject, the physician, or the next-of-kin. For example, if the primary exposure in a study were use of a particular class of drugs, pharmacy records might be used, but information on smoking, occupation, etc., would be ascertained by personal interview. Alternatively, interviews could be conducted only for those subjects with missing items in the record. However, this approach should be used cautiously; any difference in the proportion of missing data between cases and controls would lead to a difference in exposure measurement methods between groups, which could produce differential measurement error.

The coding of missing information in records can present problems. For each item of data, the researcher must decide whether no mention of the item in the record implies that the exposure is absent or should be treated as missing data. At times when a data item is missing in a medical record, it can be assumed with reasonable confidence that the condition is absent. For example, if a woman's obstetric and delivery record has no mention of placenta praevia, it is unlikely to have occurred. Items such as this could be coded on the abstraction form simply as 'yes' or 'no', with no mention of the condition in the record coded as 'no'. On the other hand, if there is any doubt about the meaning of missing information, such as missing information on smoking, it should be coded as 'missing' so that its further treatment can be considered at the time of analysis. Additional detail about missing information might be useful: for example, a 'missing' laboratory test result might be coded as 'not done', 'ordered but results not in chart', or 'no information'. The protocol in Figure 8.2 gives an example of the detailed coding of missing information for oestrogen receptor status.

Unfortunately, differentiating 'missing information' from 'condition absent' may be difficult for abstractors. In two studies of coding errors made by well-trained data abstractors, miscoding of 'missing' as 'no' was a common mistake (Herrmann et al. 1980; Horwitz and Yu 1984)

Lack of uniform order of information in records

Another common source of error in record abstraction is that information recorded in the chart is sometimes missed by abstractors (Horwitz and Yu 1984). In a study of medical intervention surrounding delivery (Caesarean section delivery, electronic fetal monitoring, amniotomy, etc.), abstractors coded as absent 10 per cent of the events that were recorded in the chart (Hewson and Bennett 1987). Errors in the opposite direction were rare: almost no absent events were coded as present.

These errors stem from the lack of uniform order of information in the medical record. Information on certain items may appear in different places in records of different subjects, and may be missed by the abstractor. The usual approach is for the abstractor to review the entire medical record or to read major sources of information such as the hospital admission form, the history and physical, the discharge summary, and laboratory reports (in some specified order), and to record the information on the data collection form as it is found. This is in contrast to a personal interview, where the interviewer can collect information in the order that the items appear on the questionnaire.

The design of the data collection form and the training of abstractors need to take into consideration this unique aspect of medical record abstracting (Hilsenbeck *et al.* 1985; Horwitz and Yu 1984). If possible, the data collection form should be one page only, so that abstractors do not need to flip pages forward and back to record information as it is found. Use of two columns of items on the page and use of abbreviations for item descriptions can help to limit the form to one page. Instructions and lists of responses usually found on an interview form can be omitted from the abstraction form and included in the abstractor's manual instead. Figure 8.1 gives an example of a one-page abstraction form.

The data abstraction form should be structured in a way that is logically related to the structure of the record. Items that are likely to be grouped together in the record should be in the same section of the form. For example, the subject's age and sex would first appear on the hospital admissions form, and these items might form the first section of the abstraction form. Abstractors should be familiar with the organization of medical records, and have the ability to scan large amounts of information. In addition, the training of abstractors and the data collection manual should specify in which parts of the record each item is likely to be found.

Use of check lists for items of interest leads to fewer missed items than if open-ended questions are used. In the state of Washington, when birth certificates were formatted with an open-ended question on birth complications, only 33 per cent of Caesarean section deliveries and 52 per cent of breech presentations were recorded in comparison with hospital reports of these conditions (Frost *et al.* 1984). When a format was introduced that listed each complication of interest, over 90 per cent of Caesarean sections and breech presentations were recorded.

After abstraction is complete but before returning the record, abstractors should completely review the data form to search for data items that were missed. Use of a coloured pen on a black and white form helps in detecting missed items.

Uncertainties and inconsistencies in records

A final problem in record abstraction is the handling of uncertainties and inconsistencies in the records. Records often include information recorded with an indication of uncertainty. For example, 'possible asthma' may be recorded in a chart, based on the patient's report of history of attacks in the absence of signs at the time of the visit, with no subsequent follow-up information. How should qualifiers such as 'possible', 'probable', or 'consistent with' affect the coding of the condition? Or, how should a test value of '< 20' be recorded? Decisions such as these should be made by the researcher and specified in the abstractor's manual rather than be left to the abstractor's judgement. The existence of such difficulties, if not anticipated, should be uncovered during pre-testing of the abstraction form.

Inconsistencies occur when conflicting information is recorded within a subject's record, or when technical terms are used differently between records. One source of inconsistencies within and between records is the large number of data recorders. Information in hospital records in particular is likely to be recorded by multiple providers — the primary physician, residents, specialists, and nurses — and the multiple recorders can lead to conflicting information on the same item (Horwitz and Yu 1984; Hermann et al. 1980). Even standardized tests such as the Apgar score of infant condition at birth can be applied differently by different health care providers. In a study of uncomplicated births at five hospitals, the proportion of infants who scored a perfect 10 on the five-minute Apgar test ranged from 58 per cent at one hospital to none at another (Hewson and Bennett 1987).

Medical terms are interpreted differently not only between providers, but also between abstractors. Herrmann et al. (1980) found that inter-abstractor agreement was poorest for items that required judgement on the part of the abstractors. In particular, among six pre-existing conditions abstracted from hospital records of trauma patients, the inter-rater agreement was lowest for obesity ($\kappa = 0.41$).

To minimize inconsistencies, the aim of the abstractor's manual and the emphasis of the training of abstractors should be on the standardized extraction of information from records. Abstractors should be familiar with medical terminology, and more importantly, well trained in the definitions of terms used in the study. Boyd et al. (1979) found that when physician-abstractors were provided with explicit definitions of terms, the inter-rater κ values for measures of several symptoms of Hodgkin's disease were higher (0.75–0.93) than when physicians worked without the use of explicit criteria (0.29–0.59).

Feinstein et al. (1969a) suggest separating abstracting from coding, to promote the uniform application of coding rules. Abstractors first record all items requiring coding as words and abbreviations, and then coders code the items numerically. This allows one or a few staff members to specialize as coders, and enables coding to be checked without re-accessing the records. On the other hand, this two-step process could increase study costs, has not been demonstrated to reduce error, and could conceivably introduce error through misunderstanding of the abstract by the coder. It may, therefore, be appropriate only for variables with complex coding rules. The form in Figure 8.1 was designed for this two-step procedure.

Feinstein *et al.* (1969*a*) also suggest ranking the sources of information in priority order to resolve conflicts within records. For example, data from the primary source (e.g. laboratory slips) should be abstracted in preference to secondary sources (e.g. laboratory values in the medical notes). Conflicting information in a record can also reflect true change over time in a patient (even over a very short time, such as in a trauma patient). The record abstraction instructions should make clear the preferred time to which the observation should relate, in relationship to the start of the record, the disease diagnosis, or the reference date.

A final source of inconsistency within or between records is that laboratory tests often differ between hospitals or over time in analytical method, units of measurement, and upper and lower limits of detection or reporting. Consideration needs to be given to handling differing units of measure (e.g. birth weight may be recorded in pounds in some records, kilograms in others) and various laboratory analytical techniques. Abstractors should not perform conversions. Instead, for example, an abstraction form might include two items for birthweight — one if it is recorded in pounds, another if it is recorded in kilograms.

Summary

The prospective nature of records makes them an attractive source of information that may be less subject to the biases of retrospective interview. Their use in exposure measurement, however, has limitations. In particular, the researcher has little control over the availability of records for each subject for the time period of interest, the items recorded, the definition of terms used, and the order of information in the records. Careful design of the record abstraction form, precise definition of terms, and abstractor training can reduce some of these sources of error. Additional quality control procedures include matching cases and controls with respect to length of time with the health care provider, use of a reference date, making preferential selections when conflicting information appears in a record, and coding missing items as 'missing information' rather than 'condition absent' when appropriate.

USE OF DIARIES

Scope of diaries

Diaries refer here to detailed prospective records of exposure kept by the subject. This method has been used to measure physical activity (La

Porte *et al.* 1979), sexual activity (Kunin and Ames 1981; Hornsby and Wilcox 1989), alcohol consumption (Hilton 1989), and other frequent exposures. Diaries are also used to measure dietary intake; these are usually termed *food records* (Marr 1971; Freudenheim *et al.* 1986; Witschi 1990). *Health diaries* are used to measure symptoms, minor illnesses, medication use, and medical care (Roghmann and Haggerty 1972; Verbrugge 1980, 1984).

Diaries are generally open-ended, and take the form of a booklet in which the subject records each occurrence of a particular behaviour in the level of detail requested by the research worker. Open-ended diaries usually take the form of a journal with one entry per line, with columns indicating the details needed. Figure 8.3 gives an example of a diet diary. This form is designed for a new page to be started each day and one food to be recorded per line, with columns for recording the time of food consumption, the food description, and the amount eaten. One column is for future coding by the study staff. The diary also incorporates detailed instructions for recording the information required (see Figure 8.4).

Diaries can also take other forms. They can be closed-ended or partly closed-ended. For example, types of physical activities may be printed on the form, with columns for the subject to prospectively record his daily frequencies of the listed activities. Open-ended diaries allow more accurate specification of the type of exposure, but closed-ended diaries reduce the amount of coding required. Diaries in which few or no entries are expected for most days, such as a diary of doctor visits, can take the form of a monthly

CIRCLE DAY: SU   M   T   W   Date: _____

	Time	Place Code	Food/Beverage Description	Amount	Coder Use
1					
2					
3					
4					
5					

Figure 8.3   Example of a diary form: diet diary (© Nutrition Coordinating Unit, Women's Health Trial, Tufts University Nutrient Data Center; Margo N. Woods, ScD, Sherwood L. Gorbach, MD, with permission).

GUIDELINES FOR KEEPING A FOOD RECORD

1. <u>4-Day Food Record</u>: Start your food record at midnight Saturday (12:01 a.m. Sunday morning) and keep it until Wednesday night at 12:00 p.m. (midnight).

2. <u>Record foods and beverages</u> immediately after eating or drinking:
   - use pen
   - do not include water or medications
   - do not change present eating habits during collection of food record
   - include all meals, snacks and beverages actually consumed anytime of the day or night
   - include vitamin and mineral supplements
   - if "diet" or other special product, copy nutrition information from label
   - include type and amount of added fat
   - use brand name wherever possible

3. <u>Start a new page for each day</u>.

4. <u>List only one food per line</u>. Skip a line between each item.

5. <u>Time</u>: Record the time to the nearest hour and whether meal was consumed in A.M. or P.M.

6. <u>Place</u>: Put down the letter where food was eaten: Home=H; Away=A.

7. <u>Describing Amounts</u>:
   - Weigh all solid food using the scale provided, and record how much you ate in ounces. (Example: cheese, cheddar 1 oz.)
   - Weigh food after cooking and after removing parts that you do not plan to eat, such as bones or skin.
   - Measure all liquids using the clear measuring cup provided and record in cups. (Example: milk, 2% 3/4 C.)
   - If scales are not available, measure the portion consumed using tablespoons (TB), teaspoons (tsp), cups (C), inches (in), or list the number of small items (Example: 15 raisins).

      .
      .
      .

8. <u>Describing foods, beverages and supplements</u>:
   - PROTEIN FOODS:
     - <u>Meat, Fish, and Poultry</u>:
       - cooked or raw weights
       - trimmed, partially trimmed or untrimmed
       - with or without bone/shell
       - method of preparation
       - type, cut or part, grade or % fat
       - light or dark poultry
       - poultry with or without skin
       - oil or water packed fish

   - MILK PRODUCTS:
     - type or percent fat
     - dairy or non-dairy
     - liquid or powder

   - FRUIT AND MIXTURES:
     - fresh, frozen, canned or dried
     - cooked or raw weight
     - sweetened or unsweetened

      .
      .
      .
      .

9. <u>Recipes</u>:
   - For each recipe used, complete a recipe form at the back of this booklet.
     - Record no more than one ingredient per line.
     - In the food record, refer to the letter of the recipe used.
     - If the recipe is consumed again, indicate the new serving size in the same measurements as before.
     - No cooking directions are required.
     - Record total yield of recipe and amount eaten in the same measurement, or record proportion of total recipe eaten.

10. <u>After completing your four day food record</u>, go back to the guidelines and check (✓) each item listed and make sure you have followed all the instructions.

Figure 8.4 Example of diary recording instructions for subjects: diet diary (© Nutrition Coordinating Unit, Women's Health Trial, Tufts University Nutrient Data Center; Margo N. Woods, ScD, Sherwood L. Gorbach, MD, with permission).

calendar. When disparate behaviours are being recorded, e.g. both symptoms and doctor visits, diaries can have a ledger format, with separate sections for the different types of entries (Verbrugge 1980).

A method related to diaries is *short-term recall of exposure*, i.e. telephone or face-to-face interviews covering the behaviour in question over defined, usually short, periods of time. For example, subjects may be telephoned, once or several times, and asked to report all foods eaten in the last 24 hours (Witschi 1990). This method is a hybrid between the face-to-face interview and the self-completed diary, and shares some of the advantages and limitations of each method.

Advantages and limitations of diaries

Diaries are assumed to be highly accurate in measuring current behaviour because they do not rely on memory. In particular, the use of prospective recording eliminates telescoping, and facilitates the collection of information on events of low salience that are quickly forgotten, such as foods eaten. Diaries also allow the collection of greater detail about the exposure than is possible by questionnaire. For example, foods can be weighed or measured by the subject before consumption, or recreational physical activities can be timed.

A further advantage is that diaries do not require the subject to summarize his pattern of behaviour, while questionnaires often ask about 'usual' behaviour. For example, the pattern of alcohol drinking can vary greatly from day to day or from week to week (Alanko 1984). A diary kept for a sufficient time period can capture this kind of variation. Another example comes from a comparison between a diary estimate of frequency of sexual intercourse and a question on usual frequency (Hornsby and Wilcox 1989). The reported usual frequency was overestimated by almost 50 per cent compared to the diary. The authors attributed this to a tendency to consider 'usual' frequency as being that in the absence of menses, travel, illness, or other transient factors.

The primary limitation of the use of diaries is that only current exposure can be measured. Diaries are a measure of past exposure only if current and past behaviour are highly correlated.

In addition, diaries generally demand more time and skills from subjects than do other methods. Subjects need basic measurement and recording capabilities. The training of subjects in the skills needed to keep an accurate diary can be time consuming for both the subjects and study staff. Moreover, subjects need the motivation to maintain the diary over the required time period.

These limitations may make it difficult to recruit a representative sample of the population of interest and to obtain a high response rate. A review of response rates across studies of health diaries found a range of 50–96 per cent

(Verbrugge 1980). Participation rates and rates of full completion of diaries among participants have been found to be lower for those with less than a high-school education, those of lower social class, those who are over age 65, and those who have experienced recent stressful life events (Marr 1971; Gersovitz *et al.* 1978; Verbrugge 1984).

Another disadvantage of diaries is the complexity of processing the information. For diet diaries, for example, each food item recorded must be numerically coded, food portions must be standardized, and a computer program and associated database are needed to convert the wide range of foods to nutrients. Some systems have as many as 9000 food codes (Willett 1990, pp. 31–32).

The training and monitoring of subjects and the lengthy coding procedures tend to make the use of diaries expensive. Roghmann and Haggerty (1972) estimated that 7 hours of interviewers' and coders' time were spent per family for an initial interview plus a 28-day health diary, including an average of 2.6 personal visits and 2.5 telephone calls.

These disadvantages have led to limited use of diaries in epidemiology. They have been used primarily as a comparison method for validation studies of questionnaires or other methods. However, diaries could be an appropriate method for exposure measurement in prospective cohort or cross-sectional studies. The advantage of increased accuracy needs to be weighed against the disadvantages of subject burden and study cost. Hilton (1989) has argued that a retrospective interview on alcohol use is nearly as accurate as a diary and is easier to administer. Among a sample of moderate to heavy drinkers he found a correlation of 0.89 between the two methods, with minimal under-reporting in the interview (59 drinks/month on average on the interview compared with 61 on the diary). Willett *et al.* (1985) reported that the validity of nutrients computed from a 1-week diet diary is greater than that of a retrospective food frequency questionnaire, using as the standard three other 1-week diaries completed over a 1-year period. The correlation of calorie-adjusted fat intake from the 1-week diary with the standard was 0.64, while the correlation of fat intake from the questionnaire with the standard was 0.52. He suggested, however, that the expense of diet diaries should be considered in choosing between the two methods (Willett 1990, p. 108). Allen *et al.* (1954) found that a health diary was clearly superior to interview. Twice as many minor illnesses were reported in the diary as by interview.

Sources of error and quality control procedures for diaries

Although diaries are generally more accurate than questionnaires, they are still subject to a range of errors. Most of the quality control procedures outlined in Table 5.3 can be applied to diary studies to improve the validity of the exposure measurement. The development of a detailed study procedure manual, pre-testing of the procedures, and monitoring of data collection are important in any data collection effort. In addition, several sources of error specific to diaries need to be considered (Marr 1971; Roghmann and Haggerty 1972; Gersovitz *et al*. 1978; Verbrugge 1980; Sempos *et al*. 1985; Gibson 1987; Witschi 1990). These include:

- the time period covered may not be sufficient to reflect the subject's 'true exposure'
- the act of keeping the diary may affect the behaviours being recorded
- errors may be introduced because the subjects serve as the primary data collectors
- the coding of diaries may be more complex than for other methods.

These issues and suggested quality control procedures are discussed below.

Selection of diary recording period

Although diaries can only directly measure a few days or weeks of exposure, they are usually intended to reflect the subject's exposure over some longer period of time. Thus, while a one-day diary might be perfectly accurate as a measure of exposure during that day, the validity of that measure depends on how well it captures the true variable of interest, for example, exposure over the preceding year. The diary should include a sufficient number of days and a sufficient spread of days over time to account for day-to-day, weekday-to-weekend, month-to-month, or season-to-season variation in exposure. For example, nutrient intake has been shown to differ on weekends from weekdays and to vary by season (Marr 1971).

The formulas in Chapter 5 (pages 118–19) offer guidance as to the number of randomly selected days each subject should keep a diary. Formulas are given for determining the number of parallel measures needed per subject to achieve a specified validity or to minimize study costs. Related formulas are given by Liu *et al*. (1978), Beaton *et al*. (1979), and Sempos *et al*. (1985).

For example, suppose calcium intake is to be studied prospectively in relationship to bone loss. Calcium intake will be measured by a diet diary, and the number of diary days needs to be determined. Assume that a pilot study demonstrated that for calcium intake measured on two random diary days (X_1 and X_2), the reliability coefficient, $\rho_{X_1 X_2}$, was 0.41. Then under the assumption that X_1 and X_2 are parallel measures, the validity coefficient for a one-day diary, ρ_{TX_1}, would be estimated as $\sqrt{0.41} = 0.64$. Equation 5.5 could then be used to determine the number of days, k, needed to achieve a validity coefficient, ρ_{TA}, of say 0.8 for the diary measure A, calcium intake averaged over k days:

$$k = \frac{0.8^2(1 - 0.41)}{0.41(1 - 0.8^2)} = 2.6.$$

This result indicates that three random days of diary per subject would be needed. Using similar computations, 2 days would be needed to achieve a validity coefficient of 0.7, and 7 days for a validity of 0.9. These results are similar to those of an empirical study which assessed validity against a standard of 64 days of food records per subject on average (Freudenheim *et al.* 1987).

Selecting the time period for a diary involves practical as well as stastistical considerations. Randomly selecting days over the entire time period of interest is statistically the most efficient approach to capturing variation in exposure over time. However, for convenience, diary days are usually consecutive for some time period (2 days to 1 month) and then repeated one or more times if necessary to capture month-to-month variation. For example, to measure recreational physical activity, two or more 1 week diaries spread over a year may be needed. Distribution over a whole year is important for measurement of behaviours that vary seasonally.

The assumptions of equal and uncorrelated errors in the equations that yield number of diary days (see Chapter 5) are unlikely to hold when X_1 and X_2 represent measured exposure on two consecutive days. In this situation, the errors may be correlated, either positively or negatively. For example, if there were seasonal variation in dietary intake, the errors in X_1 and X_2 might be positively correlated since both reflect the same season. Conversely, higher than average recreational physical activity one day may tend to be followed by no activity on the next day, i.e. the errors may be negatively correlated.

One approach to selecting the number of consecutive days of recording is similar to the approach for selecting the number of random day diaries. The equations in Chapter 5 can be used, but with X_1 and X_2 representing two multiple-day diaries. A reliability study could be conducted in which subjects complete, for example, two 7-day diaries, with the two 7-day periods randomly selected throughout a year. Then variables X_1 and X_2 can be created so that they represent two 1-day diaries from random times in the year, or two 2-day diaries, etc. The researcher can then estimate how many 1-day, 2-day, 3-day, . . ., records spread over a year would be needed to achieve a certain level of validity. This might indicate, for example, that three 1-day records or two 2-day records were equally good, and the two 2-day diaries might be selected by the researcher as more convenient to administer.

Reactivity

Diaries are intended to measure the subject's usual behaviour over some time period. One concern with diaries is that the act of keeping a diary may lead to a change in behaviour (Verbrugge 1980; Sempos *et al.* 1985). This is an example of *reactivity*, that is, that 'the process of measuring may change that which is being measured,' (Campbell and Stanley 1963). Record keeping may sensitive subjects to their actions or feelings, and may lead them to change towards more socially desirable or health-conscious behaviours. For example, recording recreational exercise might lead to an increase in physical activity during the diary period, or recording symptoms may sensitize a subject to recognize minor symptoms that might otherwise go unnoticed. In addition, subjects might change behaviours to simplify record keeping. Subjects may avoid preparing lengthy recipes on diary days, to avoid recording the many ingredients. Reactivity has not been empirically documented when diaries are used, but been demonstrated to affect behaviour during direct observation by the researcher (Baum *et al.* 1979).

Discussion of the problem of reactivity during training of subjects might reduce this source of error. Subjects could be told that for scientific reasons it is important to assess their usual behaviour. For example, part of the written instructions for a diet diary could inlcude:

Don't change what you usually eat.

- Eat as you normally do
- Give a complete, true record
- No one is judging what you eat

Reactivity decreases over time in direct observation studies, as the subject becomes habituated to the observer (Baum *et al.* 1979). However, long diary periods cannot be recommended because they are unduly burdensome for the subjects.

Inaccuracies due to study subjects as data collectors

When diaries are used to measure exposure, the study subjects themselves are the primary data collectors. Subjects may record information inaccurately due to deception (e.g. under-reporting socially undesirable behaviours), lack of understanding of the recording techniques, or lack of motivation. Many of the quality control procedures previously outlined to minimize errors by data collectors can and should be adapted to the situation where the subjects are the data collectors.

In particular, study subjects should be trained, preferably in person, in the diary recording techniques. An overview of the diary recording methods is presented, followed by detailed specific examples. Examples of topics that would be covered in a training session on keeping a diet diary are given in Table 8.1. The trainers and those who develop the written instructions must be familiar with the coding scheme, so that the level of detail needed for accurate coding of items is recorded by the subjects. For example, if the database for coding food records has different codes for fresh, canned, and frozen vegetables, then subjects must record this information. Subjects should also be taught how to handle any unusual situations, such as illness, or food eaten outside the home which cannot be weighed. The training

Table 8.1 Example of topics covered in training subjects to complete a diet diary

---

Importance of accurate records (to motivate subjects not to change behaviour).

Scope of records:
 General instructions to record the type of food, brand name, method of storage (fresh, frozen, canned), method of preparation, and amount eaten.

 How and when to record (e.g. record immediately after eating or drinking, list only one food per line).

Recording foods:
 Examples of recording milk products, meats, desserts, packaged foods, supplements.

 How to weigh or measure foods.

 Recording recipes.

Recording in unusual situations—illness, travel, restaurant foods that can't be weighed or measured.

Reviewing records for accuracy and completeness.

Importance of subject to study (to motivate subjects to keep accurate diary).

Logistics:
 When to start and stop recording.
 Who to call with problems.

Review of sample completed diary form.

Practice in completing form.

---

session would also include review of examples of completed forms, and practice in completing the diary. To reduce the staff time needed to train each subject, part of the instruction could be presented on videotape.

Detailed written instructions should also be given to each subject (see Figure 8.4). In addition to the material covered in the training session, the instructions should include the date to start the diary, the date to end the diary, and the name and telephone number of the person to call with any questions.

Subjects should also be instructed in how frequently to record information. Frequent recording reduces errors due to poor memory (Kunin and Ames 1981), but increases the subject burden. Diaries requiring periodic entries during the day should take the form of a small booklet that can be carried in a handbag or pocket.

Beyond understanding the data recording procedures, subjects need to be motivated to spend the time and effort to record information accurately. Enthusiastic trainers who can explain the importance of each subject's involvement can help motivate subjects.

After initial training, the data collection needs to be monitored. The quality control principles of continued training and motivation of the data collectors also apply to diaries. Phone calls often need to be made to remind subjects of the day to begin, and then again to ask about any problems within the first few days of keeping the diary. Subjects should be asked to review their records for accuracy and completeness each day. After the diaries are returned, they should be reviewed immediately by a study editor for unclear entries or missing data. Long diaries should be reviewed periodically. The editor should review with the subject any specific problems, and should also discuss any general recording problems the subject appears to be having if future diaries are to be collected.

There is some evidence that accuracy decreases over time because of fatigue with the study. Gersovitz *et al*. (1978) found a decline in accuracy of diet records over a 7-day period. Verbrugge (1980) noted that reported health events such as illnesses and physician visits tended to drop over time independently of any seasonal effects. This may be due to reactivity early in the study leading to an increase in reported health events, followed by fatigue leading to under-reporting. Several well-spaced shorter time periods rather than long recording periods might minimize subject fatigue as well as capturing month-to-month variation.

Errors in coding

As noted above, open-ended diaries can yield a large amount of information that requires detailed coding. Open-ended food diaries, for example, require code numbers for thousands of types of foods, which relate to a database of nutrients in foods. Because coding of diaries can be a complex task, quality control procedures specific to this step need to be developed (Dennis *et al*. 1980). Coders should be selected who are familiar with the exposure (e.g. nutritionists for food diaries) and are meticulous in dealing with details. As in any type of study, there is a need for training of coders and practice sessions, and for monitoring of coders' work by periodic re-coding by another coder. In large-scale studies, coders may be given an examination to become 'certified' in the coding procedures; this improves accuracy and standardization across coders. Coders should refer uncertain situations to the lead coder or editor for resolution, and staff meetings should include exercises and discussion of items that have led to coding problems. The codebook containing the codes and detailed coding procedures should be updated by the lead coder whenever changes are made.

An alternative to manual numeric coding of all diary entries is direct key entry of the text (or appropriate key words). Sophisticated computer programs can then automate the coding and analysis. Willett (1990, p. 32) lists resources for both manual and automated coding of diet diaries.

Reliability studies of coding have identified several sources of error (Youland and Engle 1976; Henry *et al.* 1987):

- incomplete description of items which require coder judgement
- hand conversions by coders (e.g. cups to weight)
- transposed numbers.

Incomplete description of items can be avoided by appropriate training of subjects and by call-backs to subjects. To avoid errors in hand calculation, all calculations should be performed by computer. For example, a program to convert a diet diary to nutrients should have the capability to convert cups to weight or food dimensions to weight when necessary. A check digit can be included in each code, so that transposition errors can be identified by the data entry program (Gibson 1987). Computer range and logic checks on the raw data (e.g. quantity of each food) and the computed variables (e.g. kilocalories per day intake) can also identify some coding errors. In one study of coding 4-day diet diaries, continued improvement of documentation, automated conversions, computerized edit checks, and increased experience of coders resulted in an improvement of inter-coder reliability of dietary fat intake from 0.92 to 0.98 (Henry *et al.* 1987).

Summary

The use of diaries may be a highly accurate method of measuring present common behaviours. The limitations of diaries, in comparison with interview methods, are the greater burden on subjects, which may lead to a poorer response rate, and the greater cost for subject training and for coding of the data. The accuracy of diary information can be enhanced by use of multiple diary days spread over a sufficient time period, and by careful training of subjects and coders.

USE OF PROXY RESPONDENTS

Proxy or surrogate respondents are people who provide information on exposure in place of the subjects themselves (index subjects). They are used in epidemiology when the subjects of study are for some reason (e.g. death, dementia, youth, lack of knowledge of their exposure) unable to provide the data required. Their use may allow an increase in the number of subjects available and provide a more representative group for study (Nelson *et al.* 1990). The potential importance of the latter point has been demonstrated empirically by Greenberg *et al.* (1986) who found, in a case-control study of oral cancer, that the consumption of cigarettes and hard liquor was more commonly reported in cases for whom information was collected from proxies than it was in subjects interviewed directly. Exclusion from the analysis of cases for whom proxy respondents were interviewed led to a weakening of the associations between oral cancer and alcohol and tobacco.

In this section, we review evidence on the quality of information provided by proxy respondents and offer some practical guidance as to their use in epidemiological studies.

Reliability of data provided by proxy respondents for living subjects

The reliability of data provided by spouses or other kin as proxies for living subjects has been documented in a number of studies (Table 8.2). While the data from these studies are of variable quality, some conclusions can be drawn.

The extent of agreement between subjects and proxies was highly variable from one exposure variable to another. There was good agreement on height, weight, and educational level, and moderate agreement on smoking history. Agreement on components of diet, however, was only fair; values of κ were in the range 0.28–0.53. Agreement was particularly poor on an index of vitamin A consumption, with values of κ varying between 0.11 and 0.37.

There was evidence, for some variables, of bias in the responses given by proxies relative to that in responses given by index subjects. Proxies reported fewer jobs on average than did the index subjects (Blot *et al.* 1978; Rocca *et al.* 1986). This tendency to under-report occupations may extend to the reporting of specific occupational exposures, as Blot and McLaughlin (1985) noted that proxy respondents in a case-control study of lung cancer were less likely to report occupational exposure to asbestos than subjects who responded for themselves. In one study spouses (mainly wives) reported higher mean daily cigarette and coffee consumptions than did the subjects (Kolonel *et al.* 1977). Proxies appeared to underestimate intensity of exposure to passive smoking at home (Cummings *et al.* 1989). In one study, husbands reported that their wives ate smaller portions of food than the wives reported themselves (Humble *et al.* 1984). This apparent underestimation of food intake was not evident for frequency of intake, and was not present in wives' estimates of their husbands' intakes.

The question arises whether the extent of disagreement between proxy respondents and index subjects is greater than would be expected in a comparison of the responses of single subjects at two different points in time. In this regard, in a study of recall of medical history and diet, Herrmann (1985*a*, *b*) found little evidence to suggest that the agreement of subjects with themselves over an interval of 3 months or more, but with reference to the same time period, was any better than the agreement of subjects with proxies. Thus, for at least some variables, exposure data obtained by interview

Table 8.2 Summary of results of studies[a] in which data obtained by personal interview from living subjects were compared with data collected independently from proxy respondents for these subjects

Measurement	Number of studies	Relative bias[b]	Agreement (%)	κ or r[c]
Height (estimated)	2	No (1)[d]	92–93[e]	0.93 (1)[d]
Weight (estimated)	3	No (1)	64–79[f]	0.95 (1)
Highest grade of education	2	NR[g]	80–82	0.96 (1)
Last or present job	2	NR	86–97	NR
Number of jobs	1	Yes	63	0.49
Life events	1	NR	91	NR
Presence of a number of medical conditions	2	No (1)	60–100	0.69 (1)
Present use of oral contraceptives	1	No	94	0.54
Presence of a number of medical conditions in family	1	NR	86–100	NR
Smoking habits	3	NR	83–99	NR
Cigarettes or packs per day	6	Yes/No (2)[h]	53–69[i]	0.30–0.80 (4)
Age started smoking	2	No (1)	70[j]	0.57 (1)
Age stopped smoking	1	NR	NR	0.87
Any smokers at home in childhood	1	NR	91	0.76
Number of smokers at home in childhood	1	Yes	NR	0.79
Any smoker at home as an adult	1	NR	76	0.51
Number of smokers at home as an adult	1	Yes	NR	0.67
Passively exposed to tobacco smoke in immediate work area	1	NR	78	0.50

Table 8.2   *cont.*

Measurement	Number of studies	Relative bias[b]	Agreement (%)	κ or r^c
Hours of passive exposure to tobacco smoke at work each week	1	Yes	NR	0.46
Drinking habits	2	NR	92–100	NR
Frequency or amount of alcohol drinking	4	No (3)	56–83	0.40–0.92 (3)
Age began drinking	1	No	68[j]	NR
Coffee intake	1	Yes[k]	76[l]	NR
Tea intake	1	No	94[l]	NR
Present or recent past intake of various foods	5	No (4)	36–75	0.31–0.53 (4)
Usual serving size of foods	1	No/Yes[m]	63–64	0.28–0.32
Dietary vitamin A index	2	No/Yes (2)[n]	27–52[o]	0.11–0.37 (2)
Dietary vitamin C index	1	No	28–36	0.34–0.62

[a] Kolonel *et al.* (1977); Blot *et al.* (1978); Krueger *et al.* (1980); Marshall *et al.* (1980); Humble *et al.* (1984); Herrmann (1985a); Rocca *et al.* (1986); Cummings *et al.* (1989); Metzner *et al.* (1989).

[b] Refers to presence of difference between mean values for proxies and subjects.

[c] Pearson, Spearman or intraclass correlation coefficient.

[d] Numbers in brackets refer to numbers of studies on which assessment of bias or estimate of κ or r were based.

[e] Agreement to within 1 inch or 1 per cent.

[f] Agreement to within 5 lb or 5 per cent.

[g] NR = not reported.

[h] In one study, spouses over-estimated consumption by 14 per cent. One other study reported no bias.

[i] Agreement to within 5 cigarettes a day.

[j] Agreement to within 2 years.

[k] Spouses overestimated consumption by 22 per cent.

[l] Agreement to within 1 cup per day.

[m] Husbands underestimated wives' serving sizes by average of 10 per cent. No bias in wives' estimates of husbands' serving sizes.

[n] Inclusion of serving size in the index produced a 24 per cent underestimate of wives' intake by the husbands in one study. In another, wives overestimated husbands' intakes.

[o] Agreement within tertiles or quintiles of distribution of index.

Table 8.3 Summary of results of studies[a] in which data obtained from living index subjects were compared with data collected from proxy respondents after the index subjects had died

Measurement	Number of studies	Relative bias[b]	Agreement (%)	κ or r^c
Height (estimated)	1	Yes	64[d]	0.52
Weight (estimated)	1	Yes	64[d]	0.48
Year of birth	1	NR[e]	92	–
State of birth	1	NR	98	–
Urbanization of birthplace	1	Yes	85[g]	0.76
Age at migration	1	No	90	0.86
Highest grade of education	1	No	72	–
Last or usual job	2	No (1)[f]	70–78[h]	0.61 (1)[f]
Total number of jobs held	1	Yes	–	–
Exposure to specific occupational hazards	1	No	50–86	0.07–0.62
Smoking habits	4	No (3)	92	–
Cigarettes per day	3	No/Yes (3)[i]	51[g]	0.25–0.44 (2)
Age started smoking	2	No/Yes (1)[i]	–	0.48 (1)
Years of smoking	2	No (2)	–	0.91 (1)
Recent intake of various foods	1	No	41–52[k]	0.14–0.24

[a] Lerchen and Samet (1986); McLaughlin *et al.* (1987); Rogot and Reid (1975); Todd (1966).
[b] Refers to presence of difference between mean values for proxies and subjects.
[c] Pearson correlation coefficient.
[d] Agreement over four categories.
[e] NR = not reported.
[f] Numbers in brackets refer to numbers of studies on which assessment of bias or estimates of κ or r were based.
[g] Agreement over three categories.
[h] Included agreement at up to four-digit level of occupational classification.
[i] Rogot and Reid (1975) found that proxies reported a higher average level of consumption than did index subjects, whereas Todd (1966) and Lerchen and Samet (1986) did not.
[j] In the study by McLaughlin *et al.* (1987), proxies reported a higher average age at starting smoking in males only.
[k] Agreement over five categories of food frequency for six food items.

of proxy respondents may be no more likely to be in error than data obtained from the index subjects themselves.

Reliability of exposure data provided by proxies for dead subjects

Several studies have addressed the quality of data provided by proxy respondents after the subject of the study has died (Table 8.3). These studies have shown generally good agreement between proxies and index subjects over simple demographic variables, such as year of birth, state of birth, urbanization of birthplace, age at migration (the population studied by Rogot and Reid was a population of British and Norwegian migrants to the United States), and whether or not the index subject had been a smoker. Moderate levels of agreement were observed with respect to estimated height and weight, highest grade of education, and the last or usual job. Agreement was poor on number of cigarettes smoked per day, age at starting smoking, frequency of intake of several foods, and exposure to specific occupational hazards (see Lerchen and Samet 1986). These levels of agreement appeared not to be as good as those observed between proxies and index subjects who were living at the time the proxy was interviewed (Table 8.2); this difference may be explicable, in part at least, by the usually longer recall period when the subject is dead.

With respect to relative bias, there was a tendency for proxies to overestimate height and underestimate weight (Rogot and Reid 1975), provide higher estimates of the degree of urbanization of the subject's birthplace (Rogot and Reid 1975), underestimate the number of jobs that index subjects had had (Lerchen and Samet 1986; see also Pickle *et al.* 1983), overestimate cigarette consumption (one of three studies; Rogot and Reid 1975), and perhaps to overestimate age at commencement of smoking (McLaughlin *et al.* 1987). Among these variables, there was evidence also of underestimation of number of jobs and overestimation of cigarette consumption in studies involving living index subjects (Table 8.2).

That the bias, for dead subjects at least, may sometimes be differential and have an appreciable effect on study results was shown by Greenberg *et al.* (1985). An original proportional mortality study of nuclear shipyard workers, based on reports by next-of-kin of whether the decedent had worn a radiation detector and engaged in 'nuclear work', had shown an increased mortality from cancer in workers exposed to radiation, while a subsequent cohort study based on work records had not. In a re-analysis of the proportional mortality study, use of exposure classifications from records rather than the next-of-kin reduced the ratio of the adjusted proportional cancer mortality rate in nuclear workers from 1.96 to 1.53, the same as that in nonnuclear workers. The authors found that while the next-of-kin of men who died from cancer recalled their occupations without net bias, the kin of men who had died from other causes substantially underestimated the prevalence of work with radiation in the decedents.

Reliability of exposure data on death certificates

A number of studies have compared data derived from death certificates (provided most often by the next-of-kin) with data provided by the decedent during life. The most often quoted study is that of Heasman *et al.* (1958) which compared the occupations on death certificates of current and former coal miners with their actual job in the mines. They observed a tendency, at least partly due to coding practices, to promote men with lower-status jobs into the higher status category of 'faceworkers' (hewers and getters), and a much smaller tendency to promote ordinary miners to supervisors. These tendencies appeared to be greater among retired than currently employed mineworkers. Similar results were obtained across all occupations by comparison of earlier census records with death certificates of men, 45–64 years of age, who died in the United States in 1950 (Kaplan *et al.* 1961). Actual agreement as to occupation, in 10 groups, varied between 52 per cent for labourers and 84 per cent for farm workers (overall 71 per cent). Agreement between census records and birth certificates with respect to the occupation of the father was better (overall 77 per cent) and there was no evidence of 'promotion' of the father.

The levels of agreement between occupation on death certificates and some *pre mortem* source of this information appear to have changed little over the years. For example, Steenland and Beaumont (1984) found agreement with respect to 3-digit occupation codes in 51 per cent of cases for usual occupation and 70 per cent of cases for last occupation. Agreement was less for women and non-whites than it was for white males. Using 5-digit codes, Shumacher (1986) found that occupation agreed in 67 per cent of individuals and industry agreed in 68 per cent.

Educational level, an alternative to occupation as a measure of socioeconomic status, has likewise shown evidence of *post mortem* promotion. In a study of death certificates in New York State and Utah, Shai and Rosenwaike (1989) found a high degree of error in recording of educational status in subjects who had either not started or not completed high school, in almost all instances in favour of a higher level of education.

Accuracy of recording of other sociodemographic variables on death certificates has also been documented (Hambright 1969*a,b*). In US census records and death certificates for 1960, there was 69 per cent agreement on single year of age with up to 93 per cent agreement on 10-year age group depending on sex, age, and race. For marital status, agreement was good in single, married, and widowed categories, but poor in the divorced. There was very good overall agreement, 99.6 per cent, on skin colour (white, negro, other non-white); other non-white were the least well identified. There was poorer agreement on a detailed description of race. Nativity was well reported (whether US or foreign born, 98 per cent agreement). Again, agreement on detail — actual country of birth — was less (93 per cent in those shown as foreign born on both records); there was least agreement on countries that had undergone substantial changes in political geography since World War I (e.g. Yugoslavia and Austria).

Missing data in reports by proxies

Missing data are potentially a greater problem in information provided by proxies, because the proxies may never have known the facts sought, or be more prone to forget them than the index subject because of the lower salience of the information for them.

Several studies have reported the prevalence of missing data (item non-response) in information provided by proxy respondents. Rogot and Reid (1975) found that the prevalence of non-response by proxy respondents varied from 17 per cent (for smoking) to 24 per cent (for age at migration) across seven variables. Rocca *et al.* (1986) obtained an appreciable proportion of 'don't know' responses from proxies only for history of general anaesthesia (27 per cent), history of blood transfusion (10 per cent), history of antacid drug use (21 per cent), dementia in second-degree relatives (12 per cent), and age of mother and father at the subject's birth (27 per cent) among a wide range of variables covering socio-demographic characteristics, personal and family medical history, life habits, and animal contacts. McLaughlin *et al.* (1987) found that 35 per cent of proxies could not provide information on the age when the index subject began smoking, compared with 1 per cent of the subjects themselves.

Pickle *et al.* (1983) examined the performance of particular types of proxies in providing complete information. While the prevalence of non-response was appreciably higher in the spouse than the subject for questions regarding smoking, occupational exposure to asbestos, and history of cancer in the parents and grandparents, the prevalence of non-response was generally lower in the spouse than in other proxy respondents. Siblings, however, provided more complete data for country of birth and history of cancer in the parents and grandparents. The average percentages of missing data for each respondent over the 10 variables reported by Pickle *et al.* (1983) were:

- subject 10.1 per cent

- spouse 19.5 per cent
- siblings 17.7 per cent
- offspring 21.0 per cent
- other proxies 31.2 per cent.

With respect to age at uptake of smoking, McLaughlin *et al.* (1987), found that siblings and other proxies had the highest prevalence of non-response and parents of male subjects and spouses of female subjects the lowest. This sex difference may relate to the ages at which smoking was taken up in people who are now old—teenage and early adult life in men and middle life in women.

Issues in the use of proxy respondents

Design of studies making use of proxy respondents
The design of studies which include proxy respondents should include proxies for non-diseased subjects (controls) as well as for diseased subjects (cases) (Nelson *et al.* 1990). Ideally, where proxy respondents must be used for some subjects in a study, they should be used for all subjects of the study in addition to obtaining data direct from the index subjects who are able to provide it. This approach allows evaluation of the extent of error due to the use of proxy respondents in both cases and controls (by comparison of responses obtained from proxies and index subjects when both provide data) and the potential for applying a correction for this error in the analysis (see Chapter 5).

Cost is probably the only disadvantage of obtaining proxy respondents for all subjects in a study in which they must be used for any. A suitable alternative approach, particularly in large studies, would be to obtain both proxy and subject data in samples of subjects sufficiently large to estimate the reliability of the proxy responses with reasonable precision (see Chapter 4).

Dead controls for dead cases?
Because the quality of response given by a proxy respondent may be different when the index subject has died, it is tempting to suggest that dead controls should be used for dead cases. This approach would also match proxy respondents for cases to proxy respondents for controls. Gordis (1982) pointed out, however, that since death may have resulted from diseases caused by the exposure under study, the selection of dead controls may lead to biased estimates of the prevalence of the exposure in the source population and thus biased estimates of its effect. This phenomenon has been demonstrated empirically by McLaughlin *et al.* (1985a) with respect to smoking, drinking, and the use of medications.

The potential bias outlined above may be dealt with either by selecting living controls and obtaining proxy responses for them, or by endeavouring to exclude from among the dead controls those who have died from diseases thought to be caused by any of the exposures of interest (McLaughlin *et al.* 1985*b*). We prefer the former approach, adequately supported by a comparison of the responses obtained from proxies and living subjects, because of the very highly selected nature of a control series made up of dead people and the uncertainty about whether deaths related to the exposures of interest can ever be adequately excluded. The evidence of McLaughlin *et al.* (1985*b*) is that they cannot, at least for smoking.

Selection of proxy respondents

Selection of the proxy respondents to be used should be based on consideration of which person within the subject's family would be most likely to know the facts required. Evidence reviewed above (Pickle *et al.* 1983) indicates that close relatives — spouse, sibling, parent, or child — usually provide more complete data than other proxy respondents. The spouse or child will generally know more about the subject's adult life, while a parent or sibling will generally know more about his or her childhood and young adult life. Consideration should be given to obtaining the consensus view of more than one proxy respondent on the exposures of interest, especially when the whole of life is of interest.

Because the choice of the proxy respondent is inevitably restricted by the availability of particular classes of relatives, there may be advantage in matching on proxy type or, at least, endeavouring to balance the distribution of proxy types among cases and controls so that this variable can be taken into consideration in the analysis.

Sample size

Use of proxy respondents will generally necessitate an increase in the sample size of a study over what would otherwise have been considered necessary. This is because of the likely greater degree of error in proxy responses, leading to attenuation of the observable measure of effect, and the likely higher prevalence of item non-response (Nelson *et al.* 1990). Allowance for the effects of measurement error in sample size estimation is dealt with in Chapter 3. Assumptions about the likely prevalence of item non-response and the resulting reduction in effective sample size for each variable would be necessary to take this factor into account in estimating the required sample size.

Questionnaire design

Evidence reviewed above indicates that proxy respondents are more likely to be unable to reply or to be in error than index subjects themselves when detailed data are sought (e.g. age at starting smoking, and details of occupational history in someone who has had many jobs). It may be desirable, therefore, in the interests of reducing the burden on respondents, to seek rather simpler data from proxy respondents than from index subjects, or to simplify the questionnaire for both.

Pickle *et al.* (1983) have suggested that a question should be asked of proxy respondents regarding the closeness of their knowledge of the index subject. This variable may be used later in the evaluation of the reliability of proxy data and as a stratification variable in the analysis.

Analysis

The analysis of studies that make use of proxy respondents is beyond the scope of this book. It has been reviewed by Walker *et al.* (1988) and Nelson *et al.* (1990). It is enough to say here that where data are collected from both index subjects and proxy respondents among both cases and controls, as we have advocated above, the broadest range of analytical options is available. It should be noted, in addition, that when this is done rules should be set down in advance of the analysis as to which data will be used in each class of subjects for analyses involving each variable (Nelson *et al.* 1990). These rules will have regard to:

- prior perceptions as to the validity of each data source
- the likelihood of differential measurement error between cases and controls
- the likely consequences of a case series biased by the loss of dead subjects
- the effects of the reduction in sample size that would result from the exclusion of the dead.

Summary

There is substantial error in data provided by proxy respondents. This error is more likely to be present in measurements of variable and low-impact characteristics, and where detail is required, than in measurements of fixed and high-impact characteristics, and where the data required are comparatively simple. There are indications that random error in the responses of proxy respondents, for diet and smoking at least, may be no greater than in the responses from the subjects themselves. However, responses obtained from proxies, for some variables at least, may be biased relative to those obtained from the index subjects. In particular, proxy respondents may under-enumerate occupations and occupational exposures and report the subject as having a higher-status job than he or she really had. Quantitative variables related to smoking may also be reported with bias.

Item non-response is more common in data provided by proxy respondents than by the index subjects. Close relations generally provide more complete data than proxy respondents who are more distantly related, or not related at all.

In undertaking studies making use of proxy respondents, the following are recommended:

(a) The study design should include proxies for non-diseased subjects as well as diseased subjects, but dead controls should not be sought, preferentially, for dead cases.

(b) The sample size should be increased to allow for the greater error and prevalence of missing data that are likely.

(c) The proxy respondents selected should generally be close relatives and, as far as possible, those most likely to know the facts sought.

(d) Questionnaire design should make allowance for the reduced detail that may be available from proxy respondents so that respondent burden is not excessive.

REFERENCES

Alanko, T. (1984). An overview of techniques and problems in the measurement of alcohol consumption. In *Research advances in alcohol and drug problems*, Vol. 8, (ed. R. G. Smart, F. B. Glaser, Y. Israel *et al.*), pp. 209–26. Plenum Press, New York.

Allen, G. I., Breslow, L., Weissman, A., and Nisselson, H. (1954). Interviewing versus diary keeping in eliciting information in a morbidity survey. *American Journal of Public Health*, **44**, 919–27.

Baum, C. G., Forehand, R., and Zegiob, L. E. (1979). A review of observer reactivity in adult–child interactions. *Journal of Behavioral Assessment*, **1**, 167–78.

Beaton, G. H., Milner, J., Corey, P., McGuire, V., Cousins, M., Stewart, E., deRamos, M., Hewitt, D., Grambsch, P. V., Kassim, N., and Little, J. A. (1979). Sources of variance in 24-hour dietary recall data: implications for nutrition study design and interpretation. *American Journal of Clinical Nutrition*, **32**, 2456–9.

Blot, W. J. and McLaughlin, J. K. (1985). Practical issues in the design and conduct of case-control studies: Use of next of kin interviews. In *Statistical methods in cancer research*, (ed. W. J. Blot, T. Hirayama, and D. G. Hoel), pp. 49–62. Radiation Effects Research Foundation, Hiroshima.

Blot, W. J., Harrington, J. M., Toledo, A., Hoover, R., Heath, C. W., and Fraumeni, J. F. (1978). Lung cancer after employment in shipyards during World War II. *New England Journal of Medicine*, **299**, 620–4.

Boyd, N. F., Pater, J. L., Ginsburg, A. D., and Myers, R. E. (1979). Observer variation in the classification of information from medical records. *Journal of Chronic Diseases*, **32**, 327–32.

Brownson, R. C., Davis, J. R., Chang, J. C., DiLorenzo, T. M., Keefe, T. J., and Bagby, J. R. Jr (1989). A study of the accuracy of cancer risk factor information reported to a central registry compared to that obtained by interview. *American Journal of Epidemiology*, **129**, 616–24.

Campbell, D. T. and Stanley, J. C. (1963). *Experimental and quasi-experimental designs for research*. Rand McNally, Chicago.

CDC (Centers for Disease Control) (1989). *Health status of Vietnam veterans. Supplement B: medical and psychological data quality*. US Department of Health and Human Services, Atlanta, Georgia.

Cummings, K. M., Markello, S. J., Mahoney, M. C., and Marshall, J. R. (1989).

Measurement of lifetime exposure to passive smoke. *American Journal of Epidemiology*, **130**, 122–32.

Dennis, B., Ernst, N., Hjurtland, M., Tillotson, J., and Grambsch, V. (1980). The NHLBI nutrition system. *Journal of the American Dietetic Association*, **77**, 641–7.

Feinstein, A. R., Pritchett, J. A., and Schimpff, C. R. (1969a). The epidemiology of cancer therapy III. The management of imperfect data. *Archives of Internal Medicine*, **123**, 448–61.

Feinstein, A. R., Pritchett, J. A., and Schimpff, C. R. (1969b). The epidemiology of cancer therapy IV. The extraction of data from medical records. *Archives of Internal Medicine*, **123**, 571–90.

Freudenheim, J. L., Johnson, N. E., and Smith, E. L. (1986). Relationships between usual nutrient intake and bone-mineral content of women 35–65 years of age: longitudinal and cross-sectional analysis. *American Journal of Clinical Nutrition*, **44**, 863–76.

Freudenheim, J. L., Johnson, N. E., and Wardrop, R. L. (1987). Misclassification of nutrient intake of individuals and groups using one-, two-, three-, and seven-day food records. *American Journal of Epidemiology*, **126**, 703–13.

Frost, F., Starzyk, P., George, S., and McLaughlin, J. F. (1984). Birth complication reporting: the effect of birth certificate design. *American Journal of Public Health*, **74**, 505–6.

Gerbert, B., Stone, G., Stulbarg, M., Gullion, D. S., and Greenfield, S. (1988). Agreement among physician assessment methods: searching for the truth among fallible methods. *Medical Care*, **26**, 519–35.

Gersovitz, M., Madden, J. P., and Smiciklas-Wright, H. (1978). Validity of the 24-hr dietary recall and seven-day record for group comparisons. *Journal of the American Dietetic Association*, **73**, 48–55.

Gibson, R. S. (1987). Sources of error and variability in dietary assessment methods: a review. *Journal of the Canadian Dietetic Association*, **48**, 150–5.

Gordis, L. (1982). Should dead cases be matched to dead controls? *American Journal of Epidemiology*, **115**, 1–5.

Graham, S., Levin, M. L., Lilienfeld, A. M., Dowd, J. E., Schuman, L. E., Gibson, R., Hempelmann, L. H., and Gerhardt, P. (1963). Methodological problems and design of the Tristate Leukemia Survey. *Annals New York Academy of Science*, **107**, 557–69.

Greenberg, E. R., Rosner, B., Hennekens, C., Rinsky, R., and Colton, T. (1985). An investigation of bias in a study of nuclear shipyard workers. *American Journal of Epidemiology*, **121**, 301–8.

Greenberg, R. S., Liff, J. M., Gregory, H. M., and Brockman, E. (1986). The use of interviews of surrogate respondents in a case-control study of oral cancer. *The Yale Journal of Biology and Medicine*, **59**, 497–504.

Hambright, T. Z. (1969a). Age on the death certificate and matching census record. United States—May–August 1960. *Vital and Health Statistics Series 2*, Vol. 29. US Department of Health, Education and Welfare, Washington. (US DHEW PHS Pub. No. 1000, Series 2, No. 29.)

Hambright, T. Z. (1969b). Comparability of marital status, race, nativity, and country of origin on the death certificate and matching census record. United States—May–August 1960. *Vital and health statistics series 2*, Vol. 34. US Department of

Health, Education and Welfare, Washington. (US DHEW PHS Pub. No. 1000, Series 2, No. 34.)

Harlow, S.D. and Linet, M.S. (1989). Agreement between questionnaire data and medical records: the evidence for accuracy of recall. *American Journal of Epidemiology*, **129**, 233–47.

Heasman, M.A., Liddell, F.D.K., and Reid, D.D. (1958). The accuracy of occupational vital statistics. *British Journal of Industrial Medicine*, **15**, 141–6.

Henry, H.J., Shepard, E.A., Woods, M., and Blethen, E. (1987). Quality control procedures to monitor the effects of coding four-day food records in the Women's Health Trial (Abstract). American Dietetic Association Meeting Abstracts, Atlanta, Georgia.

Herrmann, N. (1985*a*). Retrospective information from questionnaires I. Comparability of primary respondents and their next-of-kin. *American Journal of Epidemiology*, **121**, 937–47.

Herrmann, N. (1985*b*). Retrospective information from questionnaires II. Intra-rater reliability and comparison of questionnaire types. *American Journal of Epidemiology*, **121**, 948–53.

Herrmann, N., Cayten, C.G., Senior, J., Staroscik, R., Walsh, S., and Woll, M. (1980). Interobserver and intraobserver reliability in the collection of emergency medical services data. *Health Services Research*, **15**, 127–43.

Hewson, D. and Bennett, A. (1987). Childbirth research data: medical records or women's reports? *American Journal of Epidemiology*, **125**, 484–91.

Hilsenbeck, S.G., Glaefke, G.S., Feigl, P., Lane, W.W., Golenzer, H., Ames, C., and Dickson, C. (1985). *Quality control for cancer registries*. US Department of Health and Human Services, Washington.

Hilton, M.E. (1989). A comparison of a prospective diary and two summary recall techniques for recording alcohol consumption. *British Journal of Addiction*, **84**, 1085–92.

Hornsby, P.P. and Wilcox, A.J. (1989). Validity of questionnaire information on frequency of coitus. *American Journal of Epidemiology*, **130**, 94–9.

Horwitz, R.I. and Yu, E.C. (1984). Assessing the reliability of epidemiologic data obtained from medical records. *Journal of Chronic Diseases*, **37**, 825–31.

Horwitz, R.I., Feinstein, A.R., and Stremlau, J.R. (1980). Alternative data sources and discrepant results in case-control studies of estrogens and endometrial cancer. *American Journal of Epidemiology*, **111**, 389–94.

Humble, C.G., Samet, J.M., and Skipper, B.E. (1984). Comparison of self- and surrogate-reported dietary information. *American Journal of Epidemiology*, **119**, 86–98.

Kaplan, D.L., Parkhurst, E., and Whelpton, P.K. (1961). *The comparability of reports on occupation from vital records and the 1950 census*. Vital Statistics Special Reports, Vol. 53, No. 1. US Public Health Service, Washington.

Kolonel, L.N., Hirohata, T., and Nomura, A.M.Y. (1977). Adequacy of survey data collected from substitute respondents. *American Journal of Epidemiology*, **106**, 476–84.

Krueger, D.E., Ellenberg, S.S., Bloom, S., Calkins, B.M., Maliza, C., Nolan, D.C., Phillips, R., Rios, J.C., Rosin, I., Shekelle, R.B., Spector, K.M., Stadel, B.V., Stolley, P.D., and Terris, M. (1980). Fatal myocardial infarction and the role of oral contraceptives. *American Journal of Epidemiology*, **111**, 655–74.

Kunin, C.M. and Ames, R.E. (1981). Methods for determining the frequency of sexual intercourse and activities of daily living in young women. *American Journal of Epidemiology*, **113**, 55–61.

La Porte, R.E., Kuller, E.H., Kupfer, D.J., McPartland, R.J., Matthews, G., and Caspersen, C. (1979). An objective measure of physical activity for epidemiologic research. *American Journal of Epidemiology*, **109**, 158–68.

Lerchen, M.L. and Samet, J.M. (1986). An assessment of the validity of questionnaire responses provided by a surviving spouse. *American Journal of Epidemiology*, **123**, 481–9.

Liu, K., Stamler, J., Dyer, A., McKeever, J., and McKeever, P. (1978). Statistical methods to assess and minimize the role of intraindividual variability in obscuring the relationship between dietary lipids and serum cholesterol. *Journal of Chronic Diseases*, **31**, 399–418.

McLaughlin, J.K., Blot, W.J., Mehl, E.S., and Mandel, J.S. (1985a). Problems in the use of dead controls in case-control studies I. General results. *American Journal of Epidemiology*, **121**, 131–9.

McLaughlin, J.K., Blot, W.J., Mehl, E.S., and Mandel, J.S. (1985b). Problems in the use of dead controls in case-control studies II. Effect of excluding certain causes of death. *American Journal of Epidemiology*, **122**, 485–94.

McLaughlin, J.K., Dietz, M.S., Mehl, E.S., and Blot, W.J. (1987). Reliability of surrogate information on cigarette smoking by type of informant. *American Journal of Epidemiology*, **126**, 144–6.

Marr, J.W. (1971). Individual dietary surveys: Purposes and methods. *World Review of Nutrition and Dietetics*, **13**, 105–64.

Marshall, J., Priore, R., Haughey, B., Rzepka, T., and Graham, S. (1980). Spouse-subject interviews and the reliability of diet studies. *American Journal of Epidemiology*, **112**, 675–83.

May, J.R. and Miller, P.R. (1977). Note-taking and information recall: an empirical study. *Journal of Medical Education*, **52**, 524–5.

Metzner, H.L., Lamphiear, D.E., Thompson, F.E., Oh, M.S., and Hawthorne, V.M. (1989). Comparison of surrogate and subject reports of dietary practices, smoking habits and weight among married couples in the Tecumseh diet methodology study. *Journal of Clinical Epidemiology*, **42**, 367–75.

Monson, R.A. and Bond, C.A. (1978). The accuracy of the medical record as an index of outpatient drug therapy. *Journal of the American Medical Association*, **240**, 2182–4.

NCHS (National Center for Health Statistics) (1973). Net differences in interview data on chronic conditions and information derived from medical records. *Vital and health statistics*, series 2, Vol. 57, 1–58. (DHEW Publ. No. (HSM) 73–1331.)

NCHS (National Center for Health Statistics) (1987a). *Hospitals' and physicians' handbook on birth registration and fetal death reporting*. US Department of Health and Human Services, Hyattsville, Maryland.

NCHS (National Center for Health Statistics) (1987b). *Physicians' handbook on medical certification of death*. Department of Health and Human Services, Hyattsville, Maryland.

NCHS (National Center for Health Statistics) (1987c). *Funeral directors' handbook on death registration and fetal death reporting*. US Department of Health and Human Services, Hyattsville, Maryland.

Nelson, L. M., Longstreth, W. T. Jr, Koepsell, T. D., and van Belle, G. (1990). Proxy respondents in epidemiologic research. *Epidemiologic Reviews*, 12, 71–86.

Paganini-Hill, A. and Ross, R. K. (1982). Reliability of recall of drug usage and other health-related information. *American Journal of Epidemiology*, 116, 114–22.

Pickle, L. W., Brown, L. M., and Blot, W. J. (1983). Information available from surrogate respondents in case-control interview studies. *American Journal of Epidemiology*, 118, 99–108.

Rocca, W. A., Fratiglioni, L., Bracco, L., Pedone, D., Groppi, C., and Schoenberg, B. S. (1986). The use of surrogate respondents to obtain questionnaire data in case-control studies of neurologic disease. *Journal of Chronic Diseases*, 39, 907–12.

Roghmann, K. J. and Haggerty, R. J. (1972). The diary as a research instrument in the study of health and illness behavior. *Medical Care*, 10, 143–63.

Rogot, E. and Reid, D. D. (1975). The validity of data from next-of-kin in studies of mortality among migrants. *International Journal of Epidemiology*, 4, 51–4.

Savitz, D. A. and Grace, C. (1985). Determinants of medical record access for an epidemiologic study. *American Journal of Public Health*, 75, 1425–6.

Sempos, C. T., Johnson, N. E., Smith, E. L., and Gilligan, C. (1985). Effects of intraindividual and interindividual variation in repeated dietary records. *American Journal of Epidemiology*, 121, 120–30.

Shai, D. and Rosenwaike, I. (1989). Errors in reporting education on the death certificate: some findings for older male decedents from New York State and Utah. *American Journal of Epidemiology*, 130, 188–92.

Shumacher, M. C. (1986). Comparison of occupation and industry information from death certificates and interviews. *American Journal of Public Health*, 76, 635–7.

Spengler, R. F., Clarke, E. A., Woolever, C. A., Newman, A. M., and Osborn, R. W. (1981). Exogenous estrogens and endometrial cancer: a case-control study and assessment of potential biases. *American Journal of Epidemiology*, 114, 497–506.

Steenland, K. and Beaumont, J. (1984). The accuracy of occupation and industry data on death certificates. *Journal of Occupational Medicine*, 26, 288–96.

Stergachis, A. (1989). Group Health Cooperative. In *Pharmacoepidemiology*, (ed. B. L. Strom), pp. 149–160. Churchill Livingstone, Edinburgh.

Stolley, P. D., Tonascia, J. A., Sartwell, P. E., Tockman, M. S., Tonascia, S., Rutledge, A., and Schinnar, R. (1978). Agreement rates between oral contraceptive users and prescribers in relation to drug histories. *American Journal of Epidemiology*, 107, 226–35.

Tilley, B. C., Barnes, A. B., Bergstralh, E., Labarthe, D., Noller, K. L., Colton, T., and Adam, E. (1985). A comparison of pregnancy history recall and medical records: implications for retrospective studies. *American Journal of Epidemiology*, 121, 269–81.

Todd, G. F. (1966). *Reliability of statements about smoking. Supplementary Report*, Research Paper 2A, pp. 25–7. Tobacco Research Council, London.

Verbrugge, L. M. (1980). Health diaries. *Medical Care*, 18, 73–95.

Verbrugge, L. M. (1984). Health diaries – problems and solutions in study design. In *Health survey research methods*, (ed. C. F. Cannell and R. M. Groves), pp. 171–92. Research Proceedings Series. National Center for Health Services Research, Rockville, Maryland. (DHHS Pub. No. PHS 84-3346.)

Walker, A. M., Velema, J. P., and Robins, J. M. (1988). Analysis of case-control data derived in part from proxy respondents. *American Journal of Epidemiology*, **127**, 905–14.

Walter, S.D., Clarke, E.A., Hatcher, J., and Stitt, L.W. (1988). A comparison of physician and patient reports of pap smear histories. *Journal of Clinical Epidemiology*, **41**, 401–10.

Willett, W. (1990). *Nutritional epidemiology*. Oxford University Press, New York.

Willett, W.C., Sampson, L., Stampfer, M.J., Rosner, B., Bain, C., Witshci, J., Hennekens, C.H., and Speizer, F.E. (1985). Reproducibility and validity of a semiquantitative food frequency questionnaire. *American Journal of Epidemiology*, **122**, 51–65.

Witschi, J.C. (1990). Short-term dietary recall and recording methods. In *Nutritional epidemiology*, (ed. W. Willett), pp. 52–68. Oxford University Press, New York.

Youland, D.M. and Engle, A. (1976). Practices and problems in HANES. *Journal of the American Dietetic Association*, **68**, 22–5.

9

Measurements in the human body or its products

Ideally in an epidemiological study [subjects] should be classified into exposure groups according to their concentration of bioactive chemical at the biological receptor. (Droz *et al.* 1991)

INTRODUCTION

An exposure always leaves a trace, either transient or permanent, in the exposed subject. As a result, the exposure can sometimes be measured directly in the subject's internal environment: in cells, body fluids, or body products. These measurements are commonly described as 'biological measurements' or measurements of 'biological markers', although the measurement procedures, in most cases, do not make use of biological properties but are, rather, chemical or physical in nature.

Three types of biological measurements can be used to measure exposure:

(a) The concentration of the substance of interest itself in various biological media, such as blood, urine, expired air, hair, adipose tissue, saliva, etc.

(b) The concentration of products of biotransformation of the substance in the same media.

(c) The biological effects that result from contact of the agent with the human body.

The substances measured are, in some instances, *endobiotic*, that is, body constituents that are normally present and necessary, at some concentration, for healthy bodily function (e.g. hormones). In others, they are *xenobiotic*: agents that are foreign to the human body such as drugs, cosmetics, and environmental contaminants absorbed through the skin, lungs, or gastrointestinal tract.

The biological effects of these substances may be harmless or harmful, reversible or irreversible after cessation of exposure, and may appear early or late after exposure begins. Logically, those effects measured to evaluate exposure should not be the disease under study itself, or any of its direct effects. The inhibition of serum pseudocholinesterase by exposure to organophosphorus pesticides (Lauwerys 1985) is an example of a reversible and substantially harmless effect, at least at low levels of exposure. On the other hand, effects such as chloracne after exposure to chlorinated organic compounds, skin erythema after irradiation, and the very early radiological manifestations of pneumoconioses are indicators of harmful exposure, although some may be reversible.

In general, biological effects are measured when there is no possibility of measuring the agent or its biotransformation products in the body; this is the case for physical agents like sound or electromagnetic waves. Thus, for example, changes in the skin due to degeneration of dermal collagen have been used as indicators of total accumulated exposure to sunlight (Holman and Armstrong 1984). In addition, biological effects, when they can be measured accurately, may sometimes provide a more error-free measure of the actual exposure of interest (e.g. total accumulated exposure to the sun) than an alternative subjective measurement (e.g. a personal interview).

The epidemiological application of measurements of exposure in the human body and its products, together with increasingly refined measurements of biological effects for exposure, individual susceptibility, and outcome determination, characterize what has come to be called molecular epidemiology. This is a field rich in potential (Hulka *et al*. 1990) and increasingly in results.

The detailed rationale, development, application, and technical interpretation of biological measurements belong largely to experts in disciplines other than epidemiology. This chapter deals particularly with those aspects of these measurements which demand most directly attention or personal action from the epidemiologist during the course of a study, like sampling, storage of biological specimens, and quality control procedures. Following a general account of the characteristics, value, and limitations of biological measurements, particular aspects of the measurement of exposure to xenobiotic and endobiotic compounds will be considered separately and exemplified, respectively, with reference to measurement of exposure to carcinogens and measurement of diet. Quality control and the establishment of 'banks' of biological specimens will be given special attention.

THE VALUE AND LIMITATIONS OF MEASUREMENTS IN THE HUMAN ORGANISM

In principle, measuring an exposure directly in the human body or its products can make an exposure assessment:

- *objective*, that is, independent of the observed persons' perceptions and substantially independent of the observer if instrumental or laboratory methods are used
- *individualized*, that is, exactly targeted on each subject at times relevant to causation of the disease under study

• quantitatively *specific* and *sensitive* to the exposure of interest.

Here 'specificity' denotes the ability of a method to respond only to the agent of interest without or with minimal response to other agents, and 'sensitivity' denotes the ability to respond in a quantitative way to the agent down to a very low limit of detection. For practical purposes, 'very low' means a level well below the minimum concentration likely to induce a detectable biological effect.

Because of these favourable characteristics, biological measurements of exposure may be regarded in principle as the optimal ones, at least for present exposure.

In practice, biological measurements are *objective* to the extent that they are automated and that the technicians in charge of the procedure are ignorant of the status (exposed or not exposed, case or control) of the subjects. Subjectivity on the part of the subjects of the study is introduced when they must participate cooperatively in the collection of specimens (e.g. when the collection of urine specimens is required; a complete 24-hour collection may be difficult to achieve). Similarly, subjectivity may affect instrumental measurements when, for example, the subject must exhale air into instruments that detect and measure volatile compounds (e.g. carbon monoxide and alcohol).

Individualization of the measurements is absolute with biological measurements, apart from errors of identification of specimens and readings. Individualization of the measurement is a prime strength of biological measurements. Still, if the wrong compartment within a person's body is sampled, or samples are taken at the wrong time, an exposure may be missed completely when it might have been correctly identified by a cruder measurement in the environment, or by answers to a questionnaire.

The possibility of achieving a high degree of *specificity* for single substances or biologically relevant fractions (e.g. the active site of a hormonally active molecule) represents the other major strength of biological measurements.

Recent developments, particularly in the area of immunoassays using monoclonal antibodies, have provided some highly specific methods of measurement of both endobiotic and xenobiotic substances. However, many methods still fall short of optimal specificity. For example, in radioimmunoassays of cotinine, non-specific cross-reactivity with other substances in the urine may reduce specificity if volumes of urine larger than 20 μl are used. These cross-reacting substances prevent the use of large volumes of urine to increase the sensitivity of the assay when the concentration of cotinine is low, and call for a more complex process of prior extraction and concentration (Van Vunakis *et al.* 1987).

A common problem affecting specificity, particularly in biological measurements of metals, is incomplete 'speciation'. Measurements of metals in biological specimens are still based mainly on tests for the elementary metal, while biological properties such as kinetics and toxicity are usually specific to a particular chemical form of the metal. For example, trivalent chromium salts are less water soluble than hexavalent chromium salts, are less capable of crossing biological membranes, and have different tissue and organ affinities; they also exhibit different toxicities. Occupational exposure to hexavalent chromate causes lung cancer in man, and hexavalent chromic acid is capable of producing skin ulcers and perforation of the nasal septum (IARC 1990). These effects have not been observed with trivalent chromium compounds.

Biological measurements have the potential to be more specific for relevant exposure than measurements in the environment (see Chapter 10). Measurements in the environment estimate the *available* dose of an agent or, at best, the *administered* or external dose (intake), while biological measurements estimate the *absorbed* or internal dose (uptake) (see Figure 1.2). Thus, for example, biological measurements of exposure to an airborne agent occurring in the workplace, unlike measurements of its concentration in the air, will reflect individual variations in factors such as the use of respirators, personal hygiene, and metabolism. They will also usually measure the presence of an agent in the body whatever its external sources and route of entry. Depending on the object of the investigation, this may be an advantage or a disadvantage. For example, as noted on page 10, in an investigation of the possible role of aluminium in the aetiology of Alzheimer's disease, all sources of intake and not just, say, that from antacid drugs, would need to be taken into account. In this case, a biological measurement reflecting the total body uptake of aluminium would be appropriate. On the other hand, in a study of the relationship between pollution from car engine exhaust gases and myocardial infarction, the use of blood carboxyhaemoglobin concentration, an accurate measure of recent exposure to carbon monoxide, would be inappropriate, at least by itself, because it measures exposure to carbon monoxide from all sources, including tobacco smoke. In this case, a measurement in the environment or by way of interview might be more pertinent.

Biological measurements may also, in some circumstances, permit estimation of the *active* or biologically effective dose, namely the dose at the level of the structures (organs, cells, subcellular and molecular constituents) which are targets of the action of the agent.

Specificity, combined with absolute individualization and objectivity, allow the possibility that biological measurements will be able to measure 'the right thing in the right person in the right way'. These characteristics are even more important for epidemiological purposes than high *sensitivity*, an asset that biological methods of measurement also posses, often to a high degree. Pursuit of sensitivity has often been spectacularly successful. For example, the most sensitive technique for detecting adducts of carcinogens with DNA (^{32}P post-labelling) needs as little as 10 mg of tissue, a quantity orders of magnitude smaller than that required by other analytical methods (Randerath *et al*. 1988).

Whether or not biological measurements also allow measurement 'at the right time', that is at a time relevant aetiologically to the disease under study, depends on the natural history of the disease, the characteristics of the biological marker, and the study design. In case-control studies biological measurements are suitable only if there is evidence that they can measure exposure at the relevant times in the past and that they are not altered by the occurrence of disease. These limitations do not apply to measurements in prospective cohort studies, although in these studies measurements at a single point or even several points in time may not be able to capture the long-term pattern of exposure.

Problems in the timing of biological measurement, added to error in the assay procedure and short-term physiological variability, may produce appreciable misclassification of subjects with respect to the relevant exposure and reduce or eliminate the gains in accuracy of exposure measurement that might otherwise have been anticipated. These possibilities underline the need for validity and/or reliability studies comparing alternative methods of biological measurements of exposures, and comparing biological with other kinds of measurements (e.g. interview-based measurements or measurements in the environment), before biological measurements can be confidently adopted for widespread use in epidemiological studies.

In addition to the above considerations, the practical usefulness of biological measurements depends on their feasibility and cost. Both will be influenced by the nature of the specimens required, the logistic difficulties in collecting them, and the technology required to make the actual measurements. Feasibility will also be influenced by the adverse effects that inclusion of some biological measurements may have on the willingness of subjects to participate. Costs may be substantially reduced in prospective studies by storage of specimens and analysis only of those from subjects who develop disease and a sample of those who do not. Issues related to storage ('banking') of specimens for later use are discussed in the last section of this chapter.

MEASUREMENT OF XENOBIOTIC COMPOUNDS

Principles of sampling

The principal matters to be specified in a sampling scheme are the body sites (tissues and products) from which the samples will be taken, and the times and numbers of the samples. They are determined substantially by the kinetics of absorption, distribution, storage, metabolism, and elimination of the xenobiotic substances in question.

Knowledge of the distribution of a substance and of the products of its biotransformation or its early effects within the body, and the time course of these processes, is essential for correct sampling. Plasma or, more exactly, plasma water is most often the central compartment in which an agent becomes distributed after absorption. From this compartment it may be transferred into a number of other compartments (e.g. blood cells, liver, fat, cerebrospinal fluid, and urine). Some of these compartments are of particular importance because they may lend themselves to easy sampling (e.g. urine, saliva, and hair). In general, the distribution of a substance involves more than a single compartment, with some organs or tissues concentrating it, either because they are targets of the action or because they act as storage sites.

Biological measurements on the substance itself, on metabolites, or on markers of effect can be made either during exposure or after exposure has ended. When past exposure is being measured, the time since exposure began and/or ended must be taken into consideration. In the simplest case, the substance itself is measured in plasma in the post-exposure period with the body behaving as a single, homogeneous compartment and with the disapperance of the substance from plasma governed by first-order (single exponential) kinetics. In this case a constant proportion R of the substance

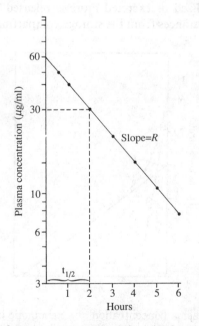

Figure 9.1 Fall in plasma concentration of a xenobiotic compound for which the body behaves as a single, homogeneous compartment obeying first-order kinetics (reproduced with permission from Klaassen 1980).

present at a time t is lost in the subsequent very small time interval Δt. If the plasma concentration values are plotted on the natural logarithmic ordinate of a graph with time on the arithmetic abscissa, the value of the fractional constant of elimination R is given by the slope of the straight line going through the points (Figure 9.1). The biological half-life ($t_{1/2}$), namely the time for the concentration of the substance to be reduced by half, can also be read directly from the graph as the time interval between any two concentrations, the second of which is half of the first. Alternatively, it can be obtained as $t_{1/2} = \ln 0.5/R = 0.693/R$ a relationship from which R can be derived reciprocally once the value of $t_{1/2}$ has been obtained graphically.

If the body behaves as a system of several compartments, exchanging reversibly or irreversibly at different rates with the central plasma compartment, the curve of the concentration of the substance in plasma will be composed of as many single exponentials as there are compartments. A two-compartment model is represented in Figure 9.2 in which lines A and B represent the two single exponentials. The exponential with the shallower slope (B) on this semilogarithmic plot corresponds to the compartment from which the elimination of the substance is the slowest. This may often be a storage site like plasma proteins (e.g. albumin for many xenobiotics), liver and kidney, fat (for all lipophilic substances), bone, etc. The substance in these storage sites is always in equilibrium with the free substance, and as the free substance is metabolized or excreted more is released from storage. The disappearance of substances from the storage compartment(s), as expressed

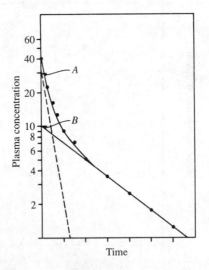

Figure 9.2   Fall in plasma concentration of a xenobiotic compound for which there are two compartments of distribution in the body, each obeying first-order kinetics, as represented by lines A and B (reproduced with permission from Klaassen 1980).

by the rate of elimination, may be very slow, in the order of years (e.g. lead from bone).

Very often measurements will be taken during continuous or intermittent exposure rather than in the post-exposure phase. The former can be regarded as a particular case of the latter, with very short pulse exposures separated by very short intervals. Figure 9.3 shows the concentration curve of nicotine in the plasma of a smoker; each cigarette produces a pulse exposure. After about five cigarettes a plateau level of nicotine is reached which fluctuates with and between each cigarette smoked subsequently (Teeuwen 1988). The plateau is reached asymptotically at $t = \infty$, but 90–95 per cent of the plateau level is reached in a time equal to 3–4 half-lives, whatever the frequency of the repeated exposure. However, the level of the plateau depends, for a given half-life, on the frequency of the repeated exposure (Rowland and Tozer 1980). The plateau occurs when the concentration lost in the interval T between two exposures exactly equals the rise in concentration given by a new absorbed dose.

Samples can be taken directly from secondary compartments rather than from the central one, plasma water. If this is done the relevant items of information become the concentration versus time curve in the secondary compartment sampled and its relationship to the absorbed dose and the amount of the exposure. Secondary compartments in which elimination occurs, such as urine and expired air, may simply reflect, *moment by moment* and in

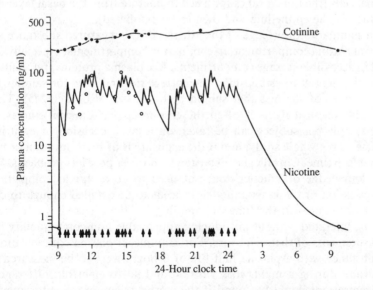

Figure 9.3 Concentration curves of nicotine and cotinine in the plasma of a smoker where each arrow (↑) represents the smoking of one cigarette delivering 1.1 mg of nicotine (reproduced with permission from Teeuwen 1988).

accordance with fixed proportionality factors, the concentration curve of the substance in plasma water. They may be, therefore, not only particularly convenient and easy to sample but also capable of providing as much information as would be derived from the analysis of plasma. Other secondary compartments may accumulate and store substances circulating in plasma. For example, fat accumulates lipophilic substances such as PCBs (used industrially for example as insulators in electrical capacitors and found both in workplace and general environments) and the insecticide DDT. The concentration of a substance in such storage compartments, when measured at a particular time, will reflect the cumulative exposure to it up to that time.

For secondary compartments containing metabolites of the parent substance (and even more so for markers of biological effect), the relationship of the concentration vs. time curve to absorbed dose and to exposure is less direct. It may indeed be quite complex, requiring both extensive empirical data and complex formal modelling for an exact description. For example, a few empirical data exist on the times of appearance and disappearance, in relation to exposure, of the micronucleus marker (a non-specific indicator of exposure to DNA-damaging agents) in erythrocytes, lymphocytes, and exfoliated buccal mucosa cells (Vine 1990). In these cases, the micronucleus marker appears almost immediately following exposure in circulating lymphocytes, after about 3–4 days in red cells (the time from exposure to the appearance of new red cells in the blood) and after about 5–7 days in epithelial cells (the time it takes for a cell to migrate from the basal layer to the surface of the epithelium and then to be exfoliated).

In summary, knowledge of the kinetics of the measured substance in the central plasma compartment, in elimination compartments, especially urine, and in accessible storage compartments, like plasma proteins, fat, nails, and hair, is essential to establishing the correct *site* and *time* for sampling and the number of samples that should be taken (see also page 245). Time is especially critical if, as is often the case in epidemiological studies, only one sample per subject can be taken on a given occasion or even in the course of the whole study, and if the exposure is of brief duration or highly variable in time. Chronic, near constant exposures pose less problems. While this knowledge of kinetics does not need to go as far as complete characterization of the kinetic model, it needs to be detailed enough to define what differences in the time of sampling for the different study subjects can be tolerated without introducing appreciable non-comparability in the measurements of their exposure. For example, if plasma concentrations of a substance with a plasma half-life of 3 hours were to be measured after exposure during a night-work shift, four fold to eightfold differences in concentrations could be found if the workers were examined sequentially throughout the day, without there being any appreciable differences in exposure.

Two other matters arising from knowledge of the kinetics of xenobiotic compounds should be noted.

(a) This knowledge does not only allow the establishment of the conditions for valid measurements. It may also permit back-calculation of the initial absorbed dose from the observed concentration in the body, and knowledge of the time since exposure.

(b) Kinetic parameters are not narrowly fixed biological constants, but vary as a function of age, previous exposure to the same substance, or concurrent exposures to other substances which may modify rates of metabolism — for example, by way of enzyme induction or inhibition. There is widespread exposure to substances, such as alcohol and tobacco, capable of inducing P-450-dependent microsomal monoxygenases which metabolize many lipid-soluble xenobiotics (Berlin *et al.* 1984; Bartsch *et al.* 1988). The potential for the introduction of further variability in biological measurements of exposure (Saracci 1984) as a result of other exposures must therefore be carefully considered in the light of available knowledge on the metabolism of the xenobiotic under study. Where this potential exists, collection of information on these other exposures is essential to a correct interpretation of the study.

Assays for xenobiotic compounds

Analytical procedures for biological measurement of xenobiotic compounds to suit the medium- to large-scale needs of epidemiological research have only recently become available. These procedures are also suitable for routine 'biological monitoring' of working or general populations, which shares with epidemiology a number of practical requirements.

A 1979 report stated that 20 compounds, of which seven were metals, could be analysed in humans with reasonably valid methods and without undue disturbance of the subjects (Berlin *et al.* 1979). Six years later a review put at 53 the number of compounds which could be validly measured in specimens of blood, plasma or serum, urine, breast milk, placenta, hair and nails, expired air, and faeces. Included in the 53 were 12 metals (elements and inorganic or organic compounds of them), five organochlorine pesticides, four polyhalogenated hydrocarbons of low volatility, six volatile halogenated hydrocarbons, five aromatic and aliphatic hydrocarbons, 19 other organic compounds, and three internal asphyxiants (Zielhuis 1985).

To be usefully applied, analytical methods need to be complemented, as outlined above, by information on the distribution and kinetics in the body of the substance to be measured. For example, carbon monoxide can be measured either to assess exposure to this compound itself or to methylene chloride, a volatile solvent widely used as an aerosol propellant, paint stripper, degreasing agent, and fat extractant. The measurements can be made either in blood, measuring carboxyhaemoglobin, or on carbon monoxide levels in expired air, the half-life of carbon monoxide being the same in both compartments. However, if the measurement is to assess external exposure to carbon monoxide, the half-life is 5 hours, while if the agent present in the environment is methylene chloride, the half-life is some 10 hours. In this case carbon monoxide derives from the biological transformation of methylene chloride, which continues after exposure has ceased (Zielhuis 1985).

Similarly, as shown in Figure 9.3 (Teeuwen 1988), the plasma concentration of nicotine after daytime exposure to tobacco smoke, which has a half-life of only about 2 hours, rapidly reverts to a low baseline level when smoking is stopped overnight. Its main metabolite, cotinine, however, has a longer half-life of 24 hours. As a consequence, not only are its fluctuations around the plateau concentration smaller, but its concentration remains high so that it can still be assayed even in the post-exposure phase, say, next day.

Some metals and asbestos have very long half-lives. Lead, for example, remains in the blood for several weeks, cadmium for years. In some circumstances, measurement of their concentrations at one point in time may reflect reasonably accurately cumulative exposure to that point. Care, however, must be exercised. Figure 9.4 shows a considerable difference between tremolite (a variety of amphibole asbestos) and chrysotile asbestos, when cumulative exposure (measured here in millions of particles per cubic foot years), assessed by work history and environmental measurement, is plotted against the concentration of fibres in the lungs of deceased miners (Sébastien *et al.* 1986). The amphibole concentration in the lung increases linearly with cumulative exposure; but the chrysotile concentration levels off, indicating an equilibrium between rates of deposition and clearance. While the reasons for

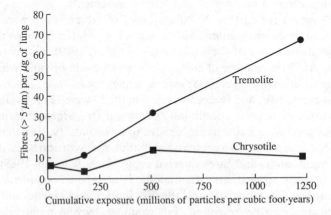

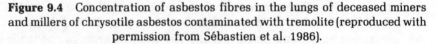

Figure 9.4 Concentration of asbestos fibres in the lungs of deceased miners and millers of chrysotile asbestos contaminated with tremolite (reproduced with permission from Sébastien et al. 1986).

this difference are poorly understood (the data available on the deposition and clearance of the two types of asbestos are not so different as to explain the observed effect), the difference highlights the danger of simply taking, without qualification, fibre concentration in the lungs at a single point in time as reflecting cumulative exposure.

Assays for carcinogens

There has been a great expansion in methods of biological measurement of xenobiotic carcinogens over the last decade. Carcinogens aptly illustrate the whole spectrum of possible biological measurements of exposure. For convenience they will be grouped, in this discussion, into measurements of carcinogens and other metabolites and measurements of the biological effects of carcinogens.

Measurements of carcinogens and their metabolites

Measurements of carcinogens and their metabolites may be specific or non-specific. Mutagenic activity in urine reflecting exposure to mutagens or pro-mutagens, and urinary thioethers reflecting exposure to electrophilic substances, are the most popular non-specific markers of exposure to carcinogens. Because of their non-specificity they are, for example, appreciably influenced by substances in tobacco smoke. However, they may be of use in directing attention to unsuspected exposure to mutagens or electrophilic substances during the last 1–3 days, rather than for the quantitative assay of a single substance. More specific measurements of exposure to carcinogens include measurement of free carcinogens and their metabolites, and of chemical adducts of carcinogens with macromolecules in cells and body fluids.

Adducts are 'addition products' resulting from covalent binding of the reactive form of a carcinogen to macromolecules like nucleic acids and proteins. Measurement of adducts to DNA extracted from cells is the most direct measurement available of exposure at the level of the cellular target of carcinogen action, and constitutes, in principle, an internal dosimeter unequalled among existing biological markers. Measurements have been made in human subjects of DNA adducts with several polycyclic hydrocarbons, nitrosamines, aflatoxins, and aromatic amines.

These and other examples, as well as measurement methods and problems, have been reviewed in two recent volumes (Bartsch *et al.* 1988; Hulka *et al.* 1990). The quantity of DNA required for immunoassays is of the order of 100 μg, and the sensitivity of the order of 1 adduct per 10^6–10^8 nucleotides. The techniques are relatively uncomplicated, and can thus be used on the numbers of subjects that might be required for epidemiological studies. Even smaller, of the order of 10 μg, is the quantity of DNA required for the ^{32}P post-labelling assay (Randerath *et al.* 1981), which has the advantage of not requiring advance knowledge of which adducts to look for, as it can detect the presence of any adduct with a high sensitivity of 1–2 adducts per 10^{10} nucleotides. The method is, however, technically elaborate, particularly if identification of the specific chemical producing the adduct is to be pursued.

The usefulness of DNA adducts as measures of exposure to carcinogens and mutagens is limited by a number of as yet poorly elucidated factors which affect the measured concentrations. These factors include:

- production of several different adducts by a single compound
- rates of removal of adducts that depend on DNA repair and cell turnover, and vary according to adduct, organ, and tissue
- inter-individual variation in formation of adducts
- background presence of certain adducts
- stability in storage
- intra-laboratory and inter-laboratory variability in assay.

A critical issue for the application of measurements of adducts in epidemiology is their persistence in target tissues including blood cells and tissues like intestinal or respiratory mucosa which, under certain conditions, can be sampled through biopsy or surgery. Lymphocytes are widely used for the measurement of adducts. They can themselves be possible target cells, although non-proliferating lymphocytes contain low concentrations of activating enzymes and are less capable of adduct formation than other cells (Lucier and Thompson 1987), or they can take up reactive carcinogens from the variety of tissues with which they come into contact. As the lifespan of different lymphocyte subpopulations may vary from a few days to several years, and this and the size of these populations can be influenced by a variety of immunological stimuli, the persistence of DNA adducts in lymphocytes and the period of time over which they measure exposure cannot be estimated in general. Some human data indicate the possibility of persistence for several weeks (Haugen *et al.* 1986).

Since some adducts are removed from cellular DNA and RNA by repair enzymes and excreted in urine, measurement of nucleic acid adducts in urine can be used to reflect recent exposure. Its accuracy for this purpose, however, is influenced by variability in the capability for repair of DNA.

Protein adducts may also be useful in measuring exposure to carcinogens, although they have no role in the carcinogenic process. The most investigated up to now have been adducts with haemoglobin. Their use is analogous to the use of glycosylated haemoglobin to monitor exposure of diabetic patients to blood glucose which provide a picture of exposure to excess glucose integrated over time. Carcinogens of diverse structure have been shown to bind to haemoglobin *in vivo*, either directly, as with alkylating agents, or after metabolic activation. Adducts of haemoglobin with ethylene and propylene oxides, 4-aminobiphenyl, benzo(*a*)pyrene, and some *N*-nitroso compounds, have been measured in human samples. These adducts appear to be stable over the lifespan of the average erythrocyte (120 days) and therefore offer a measure of cumulative exposure over a period of several months.

More recently, adducts of albumin (with aflatoxin, for example) have been investigated and may also prove useful as markers of recent exposure, given that most xenobiotics are metabolized in the liver, where albumin is synthesized, and that the half-life of albumin is not too short (20 days).

Measurement of the biological effect of carcinogens

Several indicators of early biological effects of carcinogens are measurable in somatic cells or germ line cells. They include gene mutations, chromosomal aberrations, sister chromatid exchanges, micronuclei, and unscheduled DNA synthesis. Some of these early markers have been measured in groups exposed to ionizing radiation or chemical agents. Indicators arising later in the process of carcinogenesis, such as measurement of tumour markers or of abnormalities in exfoliative cytology, may not measure exposure in any direct way but simply indicate the presence of malignant cells.

As measurements of exposure to carcinogens, all measurements of biological effects are non-specific. This restricts their usefulness for exposure measurement, particularly as quantitative measures, except in certain cases. One such exception is the quantitative indication of cumulative exposure to ionizing radiation given by structural chromosomal aberrations in lymphocytes. This exception occurs because ionizing radiation can induce aberrations in all stages of the cell cycle. Structural chromosomal aberrations in lymphocytes are not useful, however, for measuring exposure to most chemical carcinogens. This is because these carcinogens usually require metabolic activation and the cell must be in the S-phase (i.e. during the period of DNA synthesis) when exposure occurs, or pass an S-phase between exposure and observation, if aberrations are to be observed. Most circulating lymphocytes are in the resting phase (Bloom 1981) and can only go into the S-phase after mitogen stimulation in *vitro*, by which time a substantial and variable proportion of aberrations will have been eliminated by repair processes.

MEASUREMENT OF ENDOBIOTIC COMPOUNDS

Introduction

Endobiotic compounds include not only substances that are produced endogenously but also exogenous compounds that are of importance to normal body function, for example nutrients. It may be possible to infer nutrient intake from biological measurements of nutrients or their effects. These measurements are being undertaken increasingly, both because analytical methods have improved and because the error associated with other methods of measuring nutrient intake is often substantial. Measurement of other endobiotic compounds has been used more to elucidate the pathogenesis of and role of host factors in disease, rather than to measure exposure to external causes of disease. Where such measurements are known to be influenced by external agents, however, they may assist in drawing inferences about exposure to these agents.

Principles of sampling

Sampling to measure physiological compounds demands knowledge of their distribution in tissues and in time which, unlike that of xenobiotic compounds, is substantially influenced by homeostatic mechanisms. The concentrations of endobiotic compounds depend on time in various systematic ways. They vary with age — as instanced by the falling plasma concentration of calcitonin and the rising concentration of parathormone with increasing age — and in response to external stimuli, like the response of gastrointestinal and pancreatic hormones to food intake. Major hormonal variations take place during the menstrual cycle. Diurnal variation of as much as 30 per cent to 50 per cent is found, for example, in the plasma concentrations of corticosteroids, catecholamines, and oestriol. The concentrations of nutrients are also subject to diurnal variation in relation to eating and homeostatic mechanisms, and to sizable fluctuations from day to day caused by variations in diet.

These within-person variations have an important effect on the use of endobiotic compounds as markers of exposure to external agents. For example, when plasma total cholesterol concentration, a non-specific marker of lipid intake, was measured twice at an interval of 2 years, it showed a ratio of within-person to between-person variance of 0.54 (Shekelle *et al.* 1981) equivalent to an intraclass correlation coefficient (R) of 0.65. As explained in Chapter 3, this implies that if one random measurement of plasma total cholesterol concentration is taken for a number of subjects, a true relative risk of, say, 2.00 between two classes of subjects with different average values of plasma cholesterol would be attenuated, because of the intra-individual variability over time, to an observable relative risk of 1.57. For β-carotene concentration a ratio of within-person to between-person variances of 0.62 ($R = 0.62$) has been reported for a 4-week interval between measurements (Tangney *et al.* 1987). This implies that a single measurement would reduce a true relative risk from 2.00 to an observed relative risk of 1.53. For 24-hour urinary sodium, a marker of sodium intake, a ratio of within-person to between-person variances as high as 3.20 has been reported ($R = 0.24$), which would imply a reduction of a true relative risk from 2.00 to an observed relative risk of 1.18 (Liu *et al.* 1979). When practical, the use of the average of multiple measures per subject over the appropriate time period improves the precision of the exposure measurement and lessens the attenuation of the relative risk (see Chapter 5).

Biological measurements of diet

Second to the direct measurement of body size or fatness, measurements of nutrient concentrations in body fluids were the most frequent direct measurements made on human subjects in the 564 papers from the *American Journal of Epidemiology* reviewed in Chapter 1 (see Table 1.1.). The use of these measurements, and of measurements of nutrient effects, is increasing and so it is considered important to give some specific attention here to biological measurements of diet. They are treated in much more detail in Willett (1990).

A biological measurement suitable for an epidemiological investigation of diet should be specific and sensitive for the dietary component (nutrient, group of related nutrients, or food item) of which the uptake is to be measured. Unfortunately, even the best available biological measurements do not represent purely the effect of dietary uptake, and the boundary between measurements of exposure and measurements of biological effect—that is, nutritional status—is not well defined. Specificity can be improved if variables other than dietary intake that influence the values of measurements can be identified and controlled. For example, the lipid-soluble vitamin E is carried by plasma lipoproteins, and its level in serum or plasma is influenced by the concentration of cholesterol in the blood. Adjusting for cholesterol concentration can improve the ability of the vitamin E concentration to reflect vitamin E intake and uptake.

As to sensitivity, many physiological variables can be measured and may be of interest *per se*, but they may not be sensitive to the uptake of dietary components. For instance, experiments in metabolic wards demonstrate that dietary intake of cholesterol affects plasma cholesterol concentration. However, large changes in cholesterol intake produce small changes in its plasma concentration, so that in any cross-sectional study, given the presence of other factors affecting cholesterol concentration, the correlation between intake and blood concentration is bound to be weak (Willett 1987). Similarly, the plasma concentration of retinol reflects vitamin A intake poorly, except in severe nutritional deficiency, being controlled mostly by strict homeostatic mechanisms (Peto 1983).

It is plausible that the cumulative effect of diet over some prolonged period of time (months or years) is more relevant to the aetiology of diet-related disease than diet over shorter spells. Thus good measurements of diet ought preferably to reflect the integrated uptake over prolonged timespans.

While the range of feasible biological measurements bearing some kind of relationship to diet is broad, good measurements of dietary uptake are still very few. For example, there are as yet no satisfactory measurements for key macronutrients such as total fat, fibre, and sucrose. Protein, on the other hand, offers an example of the advantages and limitations of a reasonably good measurement, urinary nitrogen. After allowing for extra-urinary losses, 24-hour urinary nitrogen excretion correlates well with intake of protein during the preceding 24 hours. Repeated measurements are necessary, however, to accurately assess *usual* protein intake which varies from day to day. Results of some long-term studies indicate that measurements of urinary nitrogen on 6–8 days allow a valid estimate of the usual protein intake of an individual.

A further problem that the measurement of urinary nitrogen shares with others is the need for a complete 24-hour collection of urine. Prolonged collection of urine is always difficult, and may be a source of major errors when attempted on a large population rather than in the more tightly controlled conditions possible in a small-scale study. Measurement of urinary creatinine with expression of the results of other measurements as units of the substance excreted per unit of creatinine excreted has been the tool usually employed to take into account possible losses in the collection of urine. This adjustment may not work well, however, due to intra-individual variation in creatinine excretion. A method of evaluating the completeness of collection of urine, based on the administration of 250 mg of para-aminobenzoic acid, has been proposed (Bingham and Cummings 1983). Para-aminobenzoic acid is completely recoverable in the urine over the 24 hours following administration and thus appears to be a good check for the completeness of collection.

A summary of the measurements of dietary uptake available today for use in epidemiological studies is presented in Table 9.1. This table was prepared bearing particularly in mind studies of the aetiology of cancer, and this orientation has been particularly reflected in the assessment of acceptability to the subjects; for example, it is not usually feasible to approach cancer patients repeatedly to assess their past diet. The paper from which this table is taken (Riboli *et al.* 1987) presents a detailed discussion of biochemical markers of nutritional intake. A similar discussion with a description of the essentials of assay procedures can be found in Hunter (1990).

QUALITY CONTROL IN BIOLOGICAL MEASUREMENTS

'Quality control . . . begins before the sample is collected . . .' (Pickard 1989) and extends from a systematic scrutiny, in consultation with specialists in laboratory methods, of the materials and procedures for specimen collection, storage, and analysis, through their implementation to the review of results before they are accepted and incorporated into a study database.

Collection of specimens

Epidemiological studies make use of biological specimens specially collected for the purpose of the study or make secondary use of materials, or portions of materials, collected for other reasons, usually for diagnostic or therapeutic purposes. Clinical activities may be an easy source of biological materials but the specimens may be inadequate for an epidemiological investigation, particularly if collected by a number of different persons only remotely connected with the study. For example:

- 'leftovers' of blood and tissues may be insufficient in volume or quality (e.g. fragments of normal tissues mixed with adjacent pathological tissue, when only the former was required for the study)
- specimens may have remained too long in less than optimal conditions of preservation
- contamination with extraneous materials may also have occurred.

If, for ethical or practical reasons, certain specimens can be obtained only as by-products of clinical procedures (typically surgical or diagnostic specimens) it is advisable that a person belonging to the epidemiological study team and thoroughly familiar with the collection protocol be present in the biopsy room or operating theatre. This was done, for example, in a study of carcinogen activation that made use of lung tissue specimens from lung cancer cases and controls (Petruzzelli *et al*. 1988).

Members of the epidemiological study team should also be directly responsible for the collection, initial processing, and storage of the specimens collected expressly for an epidemiological study. At these stages, a number of variables should be controlled by way of standard procedures and any departure from these procedures immediately recorded in a log-book indicating the specimens affected. These records will permit departures from accepted collection procedures to be addressed during analysis of the data.

To illustrate the matters that should be addressed in developing the measurement procedures, the following are variables that should be controlled during the collection of blood (Young and Bermes 1986; Pickard 1989).

Contamination of collection tubes

A large variety of collection and storage tubes are now commercially available. Especially for measurement of substances that are at low concentration in blood and common in the environment, such as trace metals, it is necessary to ensure that all materials (needles, tubes, pipettes, stoppers, additives if any, etc.) do not release the substance and that manipulations are conducted in a way that no contamination from the ambient environment occurs.

Table 9.1 Summary of biological measurements of dietary uptake available for use in epidemiological studies (adapted and updated from Riboli et al. 1987)

Measurement	Value as an indicator of dietary intake	Useful for Short or long-term diet[a]	Useful for Prospective or retrospective studies	Number of measurements required	Acceptability To researcher[b]	Acceptability To subject
Protein						
24 h urinary nitrogen	Very high	Short	Prospective	2 +	Medium	Low
24 h urinary 3-methylhistidine	Very high	Short	Prospective	2 +	Medium	Low
Fat						
Fatty acids in adipose tissue	Very high	Long	Both	1	High	Medium
Fatty acids in red cell membranes	High	Long	Both	1	Very high	Very high
Fatty acids in other cell membranes	High	Long	Both	1	Low	Very high
Fatty acids in plasma lipids	Very high	Short	Prospective	2 +	Very high	Very high
Vitamins						
Vitamin A in plasma	Low	Uncertain	Uncertain	Uncertain	High	Very high
Carotenoids in plasma	High	Both	Both	1	High	Very high

Ascorbic acid in:						
Plasma	Medium	Short	Prospective	2 +	Very high	Very high
Leucocytes	Medium	Both	Both	1	High	Very high
Lingual ascorbic acid test	Low	Uncertain	Uncertain	Uncertain	High	Very high
Saliva	Low	Uncertain	Uncertain	Uncertain	High	Very high
α-tocopherol in plasma	Medium	Both	Prospective	1	High	Very high
Trace Minerals						
Selenium in:						
Plasma	Low (?)	Short (?)	Prospective	2 + (?)	High	Very high
Red cells or whole blood	High (?)	Both	Both	1	High	Very high
Nails or hair	High (?)	Long	Both	1	High	Very high
24 h urine	Medium (?)	Short (?)	Uncertain	2 +	Medium	Low
Glutathione peroxidase activity	Medium (?)	Long	Uncertain	1	Low	Very high
Zinc in:						
Plasma	Low	Uncertain	Prospective	Uncertain	High (?)	Very high
Saliva	Low	Uncertain	Prospective	Uncertain	High (?)	Very high
24 h urine	Medium (?)	Short	Uncertain	2 +	Medium	Low
Hair	High	Long	Both	1	High	Very high
Tolerance test	Low	Uncertain	Uncertain	Uncertain	Medium	Low

[a] Short = days; long = weeks to months or more.
[b] Acceptability taking into account complexity and cost of the analysis.

Type of additives

Serum, requiring no additive, and plasma, collected with added heparin, are the most commonly used 'all-purpose' materials. Other additives may be needed depending on the desired analytical determinations; for example, citrate or EDTA for coagulation and fibrinolysis measurements. In the choice and control of additives, the comments made above clearly apply.

Order of collection tubes

When several tubes are filled, one should first proceed with those with no additive, then with those with additives (say, heparin) leaving to the last the ones with the chelating agent, EDTA. This procedure is designed to avoid carry-over of additives from tubes with additives to others without.

Time of venepuncture

The importance of the timing of blood collection, with reference to the time of the external exposure and the time of day, has been discussed above. Time factors that may affect the value of exposure measurements (e.g. time since exposure to a xenobiotic agent, time within the mestrual cycle, time since the last meal) should, preferably, be controlled by the protocol, and/or be recorded and accounted for in the analysis of the data.

Subject posture

Posture has been shown to influence the plasma concentrations of several physiological compounds (e.g. total protein, iron, total cholesterol and its fractions) which can be increased by as much as 5–15 per cent in the standing position in comparison with the supine position due to orthostatic reduction in plasma volume.

Use of tourniquet

Tourniquets should be applied only very briefly, as a stasis of more than a couple of minutes may alter the concentration of many blood components, particularly proteins and protein-bound compounds.

Haemolysis

Smooth, gentle manipulations are required to avoid visible or occult, and therefore uncontrollable, haemolysis which alters the concentrations of many compounds. Haemolysis may also occur during transport of tubes if they are incompletely filled.

Transport and storage conditions

The optimal transport and storage conditions vary according to the substances to be measured. The prevention of oxidation caused by contact with air or the action of light is a prime requirement. Under normal circumstances, cells should be separated from serum or plasma within 2 hours after venepuncture. During this period, the specimens can be left at room temperature, but preferably held at 4°C. Immediate treatment with an appropriate additive, centrifugation, and deep freezing are necessary for some substances such as, for example, vitamin C (Galan *et al.* 1988).

Similar guiding principles apply to the collection, initial processing, and storage of specimens other than blood. Particular care is necessary in instructing study subjects, and in checking that instructions have been followed, when specimen collection depends on them (e.g. urine collection).

Laboratory quality control

Laboratory quality control (Westgard and Klee 1986; Copeland 1989) is the responsibility of the laboratory staff and is substantially beyond the scope of this book. An epidemiologist depending on laboratory-based measurements of exposure, however, should be familiar with laboratory control procedures and be assured that they are being applied in the laboratory being used.

For the purpose of an epidemiological study the following are essential.

(a) If any specimen is rejected by the laboratory as 'unacceptable' for analysis, the reasons should be stated, as they may point to faults in collection, initial processing, storage, or transport which may be amenable to correction.

(b) Time from collection of the specimen to analysis should be known and, as a rule, controlled, either at the stage of allocating specimens to days of analysis or during statistical analysis of the study. As specimens generally accrue over long periods of time and a laboratory can only process a limited number of specimens each day, it is neither correct nor feasible to have all specimens analysed on a single occasion. The interval between collection and analysis should be kept to a minimum, unless a long-term storage approach, with its additional requirements (see below), is adopted.

(c) The imprecision and bias of the measurements of interest due to variations in the laboratory procedure should be known and monitored at regular intervals (as a rule, daily) and maintained within the laboratory's acceptable limits. These limits can be quite narrow for the best methods of analysis. For example, measurements of electrolytes (sodium, potassium, and calcium) may have day-to-day coefficients of variation (see page 110) of less than 2 per cent (Copeland 1989). For plasma total cholesterol concentration, most current assays have a day-to-day coefficient of variation of 3–6 per cent (Naito 1989). Even higher values, 5–10 per cent or more, may apply to other measurements, for example, of oestriol (Kaplan 1989) or of other hormones in serum. Imprecision leads to random misclassification of subjects, and variable accuracy over time has the same effect. Moreover, bias, if unknown, prevents comparison of absolute values of biological measurements made in different places or at different times.

Imprecision is monitored through control measurements on replicate samples from a standard specimen or reference material made without the analyst being aware of their identity as replicates. Bias can also be assessed if the reference material contains a known concentration of the substance of interest. For example, frozen aliquots from a pool of sera can be used for reference. The reference concentration is determined under optimal conditions by use of the best available reference method, and the sera can be stored and used for up to about a year. If a reference material is not available, accuracy (inter-method reliability) can be monitored by double assaying some specimens with the current method and with a reference method. It may also be possible to carry some specimens over for some them and assay time repeatedly. A sufficient number of control measurements should be taken to provide sufficient statistical power to promptly detect increasing imprecision or trends in bias over time (Saracci 1974).

It is the epidemiologist's responsibility to ensure that statistical quality control procedures are being applied by the responsible laboratory scientists to biological measurements of exposure. Usually there will be no difficulties with well-established methods of measurement, for which good laboratories routinely apply intra-laboratory quality control, often supplemented by inter-laboratory controls. Problems may arise, however, for methods still in development, as are many of those used for measuring exposure, because requirements for a regular quality control may be difficult to meet: the assay may be time-consuming and cumbersome, an accepted reference method may not exist, reference materials may not be available, etc. Compromise approaches may then be necessary varying from mere 'spot checking' for inaccuracy and imprecision to a systematic quality control programme. As a rule, however, no large series of biological measurements should be started until regular quality control procedures are applicable.

A final requirement, more in a nature of the safety precaution than a quality control procedure, is to ensure that study staff and subjects are protected against the risk of infection from microbiological contamination of specimens, notably with HIV and hepatitis viruses. The 'universal precautions' recommended by the US Centers for Disease Control are relevant to all persons dealing with human biological specimens (US DHHS 1987).

BANKS OF BIOLOGICAL SPECIMENS

Epidemiological investigations of exposure–disease relationships can make use of banks of biological specimens collected from large groups of easily identifiable subjects. For example, the relationship between breast cancer and selenium intake could be studied by comparing subjects with breast cancer and control subjects from a population from which blood, hair, or toenail specimens had been collected in the past. Obviously, the investigation would be much more informative and its results more clearly interpretable if, in addition to the collection of biological specimens, other information had been gathered, such as food habits, reproductive history, etc.

The banking approach has three main advantages.

(a) It avoids having to perform the biological measurements of exposure after a disease has been diagnosed. Measurement after onset of disease may be useless if the aetiologically relevant period of exposure goes back decades and the exposure level has changed with time. In addition, it may result in a misleading measurement of exposure if the presence of the disease has altered the metabolism of the substance to be measured or has made the subjects change their exposure (e.g. their food habits).

(b) By restricting the number of biological determinations to, say, a few hundred cases and controls rather than to the tens of thousands of subjects in the source population it can make an investigation feasible that would be impracticable otherwise.

(c) As new analytical techniques are developed they may be applied to specimens in existing banks and thus greatly shorten the time needed to obtain results relating outcome to newly measurable exposures.

Against these advantages must be weighed the disadvantage of the cost of establishing and maintaining a large bank of specimens and the potential problems arising from the fact that the analytical procedures have to be applied to stored rather than fresh materials.

Long-term preservation of biological specimens is made possible by freezing or freeze-drying, the former being the method more generally applicable to samples of blood, serum, plasma, urine, cells, and tissues. For long-term preservation, temperatures of at least $-70°C$ to $-80°C$ (in an electrically operated deep freezer) or $-130°C$ to $-196°C$ (nitrogen vapours and liquid nitrogen) are currently used. The results, in terms of maintaining all the properties of the fresh sample qualitatively and quantitatively, usually vary inversely with the biological complexity of the stored material. For example, urine is an easier material to preserve than tissue.

While $-70°C$ may be adequate for many purposes, several biological degradation processes still go on at that temperature and, indeed, some enzymatic activity is even present at $-196°C$. Degradation is also influenced by the frequency with which a specimen has been left to withstand temperatures above the nominal storage temperature (say, $-70°C$), whether this is through a failure of the freezing system or because the specimen was thawed and refrozen when part of it was used in the past. In fact, some of the changes resulting from storage at low temperatures only come about during thawing. If thawing is not rapid (as it would be by transferring the specimen directly from the freezer to a 37°C bath), micronuclei of ice formed within cells during freezing act as starting points for crystal growth capable of seriously damaging biological structures.

These general considerations point to four requirements.

(a) Any freezing system must incorporate back-up facilities, adequate in size and performance, to overcome the effects of failure of the main system. In this respect liquid nitrogen, which does not depend on an electrical power supply, has a definite advantage.

(b) Specimens should be stored in aliquots so that sub-specimens can be easily and correctly identified and retrieved with minimal change in the temperature of the other specimens and without the need for thawing and refreezing of the whole material from the subjects to be studied.

(c) A 'history' or chart of the storage conditions should be kept for all specimens. This chart should include, in particular, the speed of freezing, the speed of thawing, and the temperature of storage, which may vary in different positions within a freezer.

(d) Several specimens containing different concentrations of a number of substances of interest should each be stored in multiple small aliquots and then analysed at regular intervals (say every 3 months initially and then every year) to monitor time-related changes in concentrations.

Actual experience in dealing with the technical and logistic problems of large biological specimens banks set up specifically for epidemiological purposes is very limited (Fondation Marcel Mérieux 1987), and published descriptions giving details (Jellum *et al.* 1987) are rare. Several bank projects are, however, currently being developed, especially for the purpose of long-term prospective studies on diet and cancer (Riboli and Saracci 1988). When developing a bank project, direct contact and consultation is advisable not only with laboratory specialists, but also with professionals in charge of banks maintained for medical care purposes (blood, bone marrow, organs, semen, etc.).

Biological specimen banks can be used for measuring exposure at both the individual level and at the group level. At the group level, it has been proposed that specimens from various subjects be mixed together and the measurements made on the pool of blood instead of on each specimen individually, particularly when a large number of different measurements (say of a variety of vitamins in blood) are to be made (Peto 1983). The groups for which the pooling is done could be defined by sex or age, or geographically, or might be the cases and controls in a case-control study. The former would be a special case of the 'ecological' approach to the investigation of exposure–disease relationships, which has both advantages and disadvantages. In a case-control study the pooling approach might be used to screen a large number of variables for differences between cases and controls, with advantages both in terms of cost and amount of blood used. It would then be necessary to proceed to measurements in individuals for the variables found to differ between cases and controls so that a full statistical analysis of the study, including consideration of confounding variables, could be undertaken.

At the individual level, biological measurements are increasinly being made in case-control studies nested within cohort studies. This is an efficient way of processing specimens and analysing data from large cohorts of subjects followed up prospectively (Breslow and Day 1987). Samples are formed consisting of the cases of the disease under study and random samples of controls from each 'risk set' of subjects under observation at the same age and calendar period in which a case occurs. Biological measurements are then made on specimens from the cases and the selected controls. A loss of statistical power is unavoidable in comparison with the results that would have been obtained if the measurements and statistical analysis had been carried out on the whole cohort rather than on the cases and selected controls. To make this loss negligible, particularly for categories of exposures within which few cases are observed (e.g. those with extreme exposure levels) as many as 20 controls per case may have to be selected. This approach still usually produces a large saving in cost and other resources in comparison with making measurements on specimens from every individual in the cohort.

SUMMARY

Measurements made directly in the human body or on its products represent, in principle, the ideal approach to measuring exposure. They can be:

- objective, that is, independent of the observed persons' perceptions and of the observer, if instrumental or laboratory methods are used
- individualized, that is, exactly targeted on each subject at times relevant to causation of the disease under study
- quantitatively specific and sensitive to the exposure of interest.

In practice, these valuable chracteristics are realized to a variable extent depending on the exposure to be measured and the methods employed.

It is essential to sample the correct site within the body (or the correct body product) at the appropriate time, lest an exposure go undetected which could have been correctly identified by a cruder measurement in the environment or even by a simple answer to a questionnaire. Sampling which varies from subject to subject with respect to the choice of site and time of sampling may introduce a large amount of error.

For xenobiotic compounds, correct sampling implies a knowledge of the kinetics of absorption, distribution, transformation, and elimination (or storage) of the compound of interest. For endobiotic substances, like hormones, the distribution in tissues and in time is substantially influenced by homeostatic mechanisms as well as important day-to-day variations reflecting changes in diet. This within-person variation, which is often of the same size or larger than the between-person variation, causes substantial misclassification of subjects with respect to the exposure when only a single measurement of exposure is made. Multiple measurements can reduce this sources of variation.

The materials used for sampling, the sampling procedures, and the storage and analysis of biological specimens, require systematic quality control. Even though many methods for measuring exposure in the human body or its products are today still in a developmental stage, no large series of biological measurements should be embarked upon until a regular quality control programme can be set up.

The expectation that in the near future it will be possible to expand the range of exposures accessible to measurement in biological materials is one of the reasons behind the establishment of banks of biological specimens from large groups of subjects from whom other information has also been gathered (on personal characteristics, habits, etc.). Typically, the stored specimens can be analysed for selected exposures when new cases of a disease of interest occur and compared with similar measurements on a sample of the specimens from the whole population.

The development of methods of measurement of exposures in biological materials is a rapidly advancing front. The epidemiologist can contribute, in collaboration with laboratory scientists, to ensure that these methods acquire properties of objectivity, individualization, specificity, sensitivity, and technical and economic practicability to a sufficient degree to make them usable and to have an advantage over other methods in epidemiological studies.

REFERENCES

Bartsch, H., Hemminki, K., and O'Neill, I.K. (1988). *DNA damaging agents in humans: applications in cancer epidemiology and prevention.* IARC Scientific Publications No. 89. International Agency for Research on Cancer, Lyon.

Berlin, A., Wolff, A.H., and Hasegawa, Y. (1979). *The use of biological specimens for the assessment of human exposure to environmental pollutants.* M. Nijhoff, The Hague.

Berlin, A., Draper, M., Hemminki, K., and Vainio, H. (1984). *Monitoring human exposure to carcinogenic and mutagenic agents.* IARC Scientific Publications, No. 59. International Agency for Research on Cancer, Lyon.

Bingham, S. and Cummings, J.H. (1983). The use of 4-aminobenzoic acid as a marker to validate the completeness of 24h urine collections in man. *Clinical Science*, **64**, 629–35.

Bloom, A.D. (1981). *Guidelines for studies of human populations exposed to mutagenic and reproductive hazards.* March of Dimes Birth Defects Foundation, White Plains, New York.

Breslow, N.E. and Day, N.E. (1987). *Statistical methods in cancer research, Vol. 2. The design and analysis of cohort studies.* IARC Scientific Publications No. 82. International Agency for Research on Cancer, Lyon.

Copeland, B. (1989). Quality control. In *Clinical chemistry: theory, analysis and correlation*, (2nd ed), (ed. L. A. Kaplan and A. J. Pesce), pp. 270–89. C. V. Mosby, St Louis, Missouri.

Droz, P. O., Berode, M., and Wu, M. M. (1991). Evaluation of concomitant biological and air monitoring. *Applied Occupational and Environmental Hygiene*, **6**, 465–74.

Galan, P., Hercberg, S., Keller, H. E., Bellio, J. P., Bourgeois, C. F. and Fourlon, C. H. (1988). Plasma ascorbic acid determination: is it necessary to centrifuge and to stabilize the blood sample immediately in the field? *International Journal of Vitaminology and Nutritional Research*, **58**, 473–4.

Haugen, A., Becher, G., Benestad, C., Vahakangas, K., Trivers, G. E., Newman, M. J. *et al.* (1986). Determination of polycyclic aromatic hydrocarbons in the urine, benzo(*a*)pyrene diolepoxide-DNA adducts in sera from coke oven workers exposed to measured amounts of polycyclic aromatic hydrocarbons in the work atmosphere. *Cancer Research*, **46**, 4178–83.

Holman, C. D. J. and Armstrong, B. K. (1984). Cutaneous malignant melanoma and indicators of total accumulated exposure to the sun: an analysis separating histogenetic types. *Journal of the National Cancer Institute*, **73**, 75–82.

Hulka, B. S., Wilcosky, T. C., and Griffith, J. D. (1990). *Biological markers in epidemiology*. Oxford University Press, New York.

Hunter, D. (1990). Biochemical indicators of dietary intake. In *Nutritional epidemiology*, (ed. W. Willett), pp. 143–216. Oxford University Press, Oxford.

IARC (International Agency for Research on Cancer) (1990). *Chromium, nickel and welding*. Monographs on the Evaluation of Carcinogenic Risks to Humans, Vol. 49. International Agency for Research on Cancer, Lyon.

Jellum, E., Andersen, A., Orjasaeter, H., Foss, O. P., Theodorsen, L., and Lund-Larsen, P. (1987). The JANUS serum bank and early detection of cancer. *Biochimica Clinica*, **11**, 191–5.

Kaplan, L. A. (1989). Estriol. In *Clinical chemistry: theory, analysis and correlation*, (2nd edn), (ed. L. A. Kaplan and A. J. Pesce), pp. 944–50. C. V. Mosby, St Louis, Missouri.

Klaassen, C. D. (1980). Absorption, distribution, and excretion of toxicants. In *Casarett and Doull's toxicology*, (2nd edn), (ed. J. Doull, C. D. Klaassen, and M. O. Amdur), pp. 28–55. MacMillan, New York.

Lauwerys, R. (1984). Basic concepts of monitoring human exposure. In *Monitoring human exposure to carcinogenic and mutagenic agents*, (ed. A. Berlin, M. Draper, K. Hemminki, and H. Vainio), pp. 31–6. IARC Scientific Publications, No. 59. International Agency for Research on Cancer, Lyon.

Liu, K., Cooper, R., McKeever, J., McKeever, P., Byington, R., Soltero, I. *et al.* (1979). Assessment of the association between habitual salt intake and high blood pressure: methodological problems. *American Journal of Epidemiology*, **110**, 219–26.

Lucier, G. W. and Thompson, C. L. (1987). Issues in biochemical applications to risk assessment: when can lymphocytes be used as surrogate markers? *Environmental Health Perspectives*, **76**, 187–91.

Naito, H. K. (1989). Cholesterol. In *Clinical chemistry: theory, analysis and correlation*, (2nd edn), (ed. L. A. Kaplan and A. J. Pesce), pp. 974–83. C. V. Mosby, St Louis, Missouri.

Peto, R. (1983). The marked differences between carotenoids and retinoids: methodological implications for biochemical epidemiology. *Cancer Surveys*, 2, 327–40.

Petruzzelli, S., Camus, A.M., Carrozzi, L., Ghelarducci, L., Rindi, M., Menconi, G., Angeletti, C.A., Ahotupa, M., Hietanen, E., Aitio, A., Saracci, R., Bartsch, H., and Giuntini, C. (1988). Long-lasting effects of tobacco smoking on pulmonary drug-metabolizing enzymes: A case-control study on lung cancer patients. *Cancer Research*, 48, 4695–700.

Pickard, N.A. (1989). Collection and handling of patients specimens. In *Clinical chemistry: theory, analysis and correlation*, (2nd edn), (ed. L.A. Kaplan and A.J. Pesce), pp. 40–8. C.V. Mosby, St Louis, Missouri.

Randerath, K., Reddy, M.J., and Gupta, R.C. (1981). ^{32}P-labelling test for DNA damage. *Proceedings of the National Academy of Science USA*, 78, 6126–9.

Randerath, K., Miller, R.H., Mittal, D., and Randerath, E. (1988). Monitoring human exposure to carcinogens by ultrasensitive post-labelling assays: application to unidentified genotoxicants. In *DNA damaging agents in humans: applications in cancer epidemiology and prevention*, (ed. H. Bartsch, K. Hemminki, and I.K. O'Neill), pp. 361–7. IARC Scientific Publications, No. 89. International Agency for Research on Cancer, Lyon.

Riboli, E. and Saracci, R. (1988). *Diet, hormones and cancer: methodological issues for prospective studies*. IARC Technical Report No. 4. International Agency for Research on Cancer, Lyon.

Riboli, E., Rönnholm, H., and Saracci, R. (1987). Biological markers of diet. *Cancer Surveys*, 6, 685–718.

Rowland, M. and Tozer, T.N. (1980). *Clinical pharmacokinetics*. Lea and Fibiger, Philadelphia.

Saracci, R. (1974). The power (sensitivity) of quality control plans in clinical chemistry. *American Journal of Clinical Pathology*, 62, 398–406.

Saracci, R. (1984). Assessing exposure of individuals in the identification of disease determinants. In *Monitoring human exposure to carcinogenic and mutagenic agents*, (ed. A. Berlin, M. Draper, K. Hemminki, and H. Vainio), pp. 135–42. IARC Scientific Publications No. 59. International Agency for Research on Cancer, Lyon.

Sébastien, P., Bégin, R., Case, B.W., and McDonald, J.C. (1986). Inhalation of chrysotile dust. In *The biological effects of chrysotile. Accomplishments in oncology*, Vol. 1, No. 2, (ed. J.C. Wagner), pp. 19–29. J.B. Lippincott, Philadelphia.

Fondation Marcel Mérieux (1987). *Sérothéque Rhône-Alpes*, 9ème Séminaire Y. Biraud. Fondation Marcel Mérieux, Lyon.

Shekelle, R.B., Shryock, A.M., Paul, O., Lepper, M., Stamler, J., Liu, S. *et al.* (1981). Diet, serum cholesterol and death from coronary heart disease. *New England Journal Medicine*, 304, 65–70.

Tangney, C.C., Shekelle, R.B., Raynor, W., Gale, M., and Betz, E.P. (1987). Intra- and inter-individual variation in measurements of β-carotene, retinol and tocopherols in diet and plasma. *American Journal of Clinical Nutrition*, 45, 764–9.

Teeuwen, H.W.A. (1988). Clinical pharmacokinetics of nicotine, caffeine, and quinine. Thesis. University of Nijmegen. CiP-DATA. Koninklijke Bibliotheek, Den Haag.

US DHHS (US Department of Health and Human Services) (1987). Recommendations for prevention of HIV transmission in health care settings. *Morbidity and Mortality Weekly Report*, **36**, (2S), 1S–18S.

Van Vunakis, H., Gjika, H.B., and Langone, J.J. (1987). Radioimmunoassay for nicotine and cotinine. In *Environmental carcinogens: Methods of analysis and exposure measurement*, *Vol. 9, Passive Smoking*, (ed. I.K. O'Neill, K.D. Brunnemann, B. Dodet, and D. Hoffmann), pp. 317–330. IARC Scientific Publications, No. 81. International Agency for Research on Cancer, Lyon.

Vine, M.F. (1990). Micronuclei. In *Biological markers in epidemiology*, (ed. B.S. Hulka, T.C. Wilcosky, and J.D. Griffith), pp. 125–46. Oxford University Press, New York.

Westgard, J.O. and Klee, G.G. (1986). Quality assurance. In *Textbook of clinical chemistry*, (ed. N.W. Tietz), pp. 424–58. W.B. Saunders, Philadelphia.

Willett, W. (1987). Nutritional epidemiology: issues and challenges. *International Journal of Epidemiology*, **16**, 312–7.

Willett, W. (1990). *Nutritional epidemiology*. Oxford University Press, New York.

Young, D.S. and Bermes, E.W. (1986). Specimen collection and processing; sources of biological variation. In *Textbook of clinical chemistry*, (ed. N.W. Tietz), pp. 478–518. W.B. Saunders, Philadelphia.

Zielhuis, R.L. (1985). Biological monitoring studies in occupational and environmental health. In *Epidemiology and quantitation of environmental risk in humans from radiation and other agents*, (ed. A. Castellani), pp. 291–306. Plenum Press, New York.

10

Measurements in the environment

In the last decade, recognition of the complexity of the determinants of individual exposure to air pollutants and the impact of misclassification has led to the need for a new conceptual framework for exposure assessment. (National Research Council 1985)

INTRODUCTION

Environmental agents include physical, chemical, and biological components or contaminants of the general environment (soil, air, water), the local environment (home, workplace, recreational sites), or the personal environment (food, drinks, cosmetics, drugs). Frequently, exposure to these agents is unknown or unsensed by the exposed individual. Under these circumstances, the exposure as such cannot be recalled or recorded by the study subject, so it can only be documented through measurements in the environment. In other circumstances measurements in the environment represent an alternative or a complementary approach to questioning the subject.

Methods of making measurements in the environment vary in sophistication from rating by skilled observers (e.g. of the dustiness of air in the workplace) through measurements made in the field by simple or complex instruments (e.g. concentration of dust in the atmosphere measured by nephelometry) to measurements in the laboratory of the concentration of substances in samples taken from the environment (e.g. the counting of specific mineral fibres in air samples by electron microscopy). The choice of a method depends on the environment to be sampled, the agent to be measured, the availability of the appropriate technology, and its cost.

This choice, together with the development and application of the relevant technical methods, belongs mainly to the disciplines of industrial and environmental hygiene rather than to epidemiology. For this reason, the emphasis of this chapter, like that of the last, is on those aspects of these methods of measurement that most demand the epidemiologist's attention and action.

In this chapter, we outline the characteristics, value, and limitations of measurements in the environment, and address issues of measuring both present and past exposure by way of examples taken mainly from the occupational environment. For present exposure, the selection of exposures to be measured and places and substances to be sampled, the extent of sampling, and some analytical aspects are discussed. Reconstruction of measurements of past exposure are considered in circumstances in which complete, incomplete, or no actual measurements of the relevant past environment are available. The use of conversion tables with data derived from questionnaires, as a substitute for direct measurements in the environment, is also considered.

THE VALUE AND LIMITATIONS OF ENVIRONMENTAL MEASUREMENTS

Measuring an exposure in the external environment by instrumental and laboratory methods may render exposure assessment objective, individualized, and quantitatively specific and sensitive. Because of these desirable characteristics, the use of these methods for measuring environmental exposures in epidemiological studies is becoming more common. In addition, there is an increasingly popular belief that they are methods of choice for exposure measurements, intrinsically superior to questionnaires and related subjective approaches on every occasion that they can be applied. While this may be attractive in theory, it has no general validity in practice. The extent to which the potential superiority of instrumental and laboratory methods can be achieved depends on circumstances particular to each epidemiological study. Also particular to the design and conduct of each study are the consequences of deficiencies in objectivity, individualization, sensitivity, and specificity of environmental measurements. Two such consequences occur most commonly:

- non-differential misclassification of subjects with respect to exposure (see Chapter 3)
- systematically incorrect estimation of exposure levels.

The latter error has recently been found for the earlier estimates of radiation exposure following atomic bombing in Hiroshima and Nagasaki (Preston and Pierce 1987). This kind of error may lead to overestimation or under-estimation of the risk per unit of exposure, a major problem in public health terms, especially when control limits for exposure to an environmental agent must be established.

The *objectivity* of a measurement in the environment depends on two steps: first, the sampling of the environment and, second, the measurement procedure proper. Both steps can be highly objective as, for example, when a personal sampler is used to take a sample of air during a working shift for subsequent automated measurement of the concentration of a gaseous pollutant. Often, however, only the second step can be objective, while identification and selection of the sample involves substantial subjectivity. Typically, reliance must be placed on information provided by the study subject to identify environmental materials to be sampled. For example, the subject must identify recently consumed food and drinks to be tested in the laboratory for chemical and microbiological contaminants when investigating an outbreak of diarrhoea. Similarly, when studying lung cancer in relation to inhaled carcinogens (other than those from active tobacco smoking) the work and residentials histories gathered from the subjects, sometimes corroborated by pre-existing records, identify the part of the environment to be searched for records of past measurements of airborne contaminants. Subjectivity also enters into the second step, the analytical procedure, to the extent that it is not totally automated, but demands the intervention of human operators in the form of manipulation of samples, taking readings, and recognition of objects to be measured or counted (e.g. asbestos fibres in a microscopic field).

Individualized measurement can be achieved fully only when personal sampling is practicable over repeated and extended periods of time. In many circumstances it can only be approximated by average measurements over time or groups of persons (or personal space), as when an area sample of air is taken with a static sampler in the workplace. The approximation is even more distant when only a few haphazardly collected spot samples of the environment are available. Measurements on such samples, however accurate analytically, may be only rough guides to the amount of exposure and cannot be regarded as unbiased estimates of either individual or average values. Error in obtaining the original specimens from the environment and in sub-sampling for laboratory analysis may be the main source of loss of individualization and, therefore, error in environmental measurements. For example, in control of food contamination, random samples of kernels are drawn from commercial lots of shelled peanuts and comminuted in a mill to produce sub-samples. These sub-samples are then tested for aflatoxin, a highly hepatotoxic and carcinogenic mycotoxin. In one investigation it was found that, at a concentration of 20 parts per billion of aflatoxin, 66 per cent of the random measurement error could be attributed to the initial sampling of kernels, 21 per cent to sub-sampling, and only 13 per cent to the analytical method (Whitaker and Dickens 1974). This example emphasizes the importance of an adequate sampling strategy when aiming at accurate measurements of individual exposures, especially when the concentration of the agent of interest varies widely. This is the case for aflatoxin in batches of peanuts, where a few peanuts account for most of the contamination.

Specificity and *sensitivity*, which jointly describe the accuracy of a method, also deserve careful consideration before choosing instrumental or laboratory-based measurements of the environment in preference to some alternative method of exposure measurement. If the exposure relevant to the epidemiological study is a mixture of chemicals (e.g. air pollutants), measurements specific for a single chemical may be inappropriate if that chemical is not the one, or is not on its own, responsible for the biological effect under study and its concentration is not highly correlated with that of the active agent(s) or with the total activity in the mixture. For example, in attempting to evaluate the possible carcinogenicity of chlorination of by-products in water, a number of epidemiological studies have used measurements of concentrations of particular trihalomethanes (e.g. chloroform) to indicate the exposure. The chemical or chemicals measured may not, however, be the only potentially carcinogenic by-products of chlorination of water. High sensitivity is never a disadvantage, but there is little point, at least for epidemiological purposes, in pursuing it to concentrations of the agent much below those likely to produce epidemiologically detectable effects.

Whether or not measurements in the environment will be useful in practice also depends on their cost and the feasibility of their use on a large scale, as is usually required in epidemiology. Neither cost nor logistic feasibility will usually present insurmountable difficulties if the number of measurements can be restricted to the range of hundreds rather than thousands or tens of thousands. This restriction may be achieved by limitation of the collection and analysis of environmental specimens to a sample of all subjects in the study for the purpose, for example, of validating some less expensive measure of exposure. Alternatively, if the cost of obtaining and storing the samples compares favourably with the cost of the analysis, one or more environmental specimens may be collected and preserved for each study subject while only a proportion is later analysed; or specimens from subgroups of subjects may be pooled so that the exposure of the subgroup can be characterized by measurements in the 'pool'. The application of these 'banking' and 'pooling' approaches has been discussed in Chapter 9.

Whatever the part of the environment to be studied, the exposure to be assessed, and the properties (chemical, physical, or biological) by which it is measured, several issues require detailed consideration. They include sampling of and measurements in present and past environments, and the use of records or questionnaires in place of actual measurements to estimate environmental exposures. These issues are considered below, mainly focusing, by way of example, on measurement of exposure to an airborne agent in the working environment. The principles outlined are general, however. They can be applied, with modification, to measurements of different kinds of agents in a variety of general, local, or personal environments. Several issues of quality control of measurements have been considered already, particularly in Chapters 5 and 9. Their specific application to measurements in the environment should be developed in collaboration with environmental hygienists, and will not be dealt with here.

SAMPLING AND MEASURING PRESENT EXPOSURES

In epidemiology, measurements of present environmental exposures are made for two main purposes:

(a) To be used as such in prospective cohort studies aimed at relating present exposure to future disease occurrence.

(b) To be entered as one element in the process of estimating past exposure within cross-sectional, retrospective cohort, or case-control studies.

In principle, use can be made in epidemiology of measurements of present exposure gathered for other purposes, such as measurements of workplace contaminants carried out for checking compliance with regulatory standards or monitoring process leakages, the effect of process changes, or the success of technical control measures. Such measurements, however, usually cannot be used to define the exposure of individual subjects. An *ad hoc* environmental survey is desirable, especially in a prospective cohort study. Even such a survey cannot possibly characterize *all* the environmental exposures of every member of a population, and it is necessary to determine how the scope of an environmental survey can be focused and restricted with respect to both the number of agents to be measured and the number of measurements to be made of each agent.

Selecting the exposures to be measured

Taking airborne agents in the workplace as an example, the first step is to make an inventory of all airborne agents present in the workplace. It is not uncommon, in moderate-sized production plants (500 workers or so), for the total inventory to include 500–1000 chemicals (Corn 1981). A full inventory requires first the listing of all incoming materials, which is best undertaken by systematic review of the purchase records for the last 1–2 years. Sole reliance on data provided informally by key informants (managers, engineers, other staff) is best avoided, because important items may be missed. If records are not available then, at the very least, data from key informants should be elicited by means of a standard questionnaire. Next, a department-by-department review of the plant is made to list all the products, both intermediate and final, derived from the incoming materials. The exposure variables to be measured are then selected from the lists of incoming materials and their transformation products. In a less structured situation, for example when the environment to be measured is a water supply rather than workplace air and a complete inventory of chemical or biological inputs and transformation products cannot be prepared, a complete list of likely constituents and contaminants should still be prepared with reference to relevant empirical data and theory.

Which variables are selected for measurement depends critically on the objectives of the study being undertaken. For example, in a cohort study of lung cancer in relation to exposure to ceramic fibres, a decision would have to be made whether to limit the measurements to ceramic fibres, or to include established and suspected carcinogens for the human lung which may also be present as potential confounders, and biologically plausible effect modifiers, should any be present. The selection of the agents to be measured may need to be more extensive if several endpoints are to be investigated, such as cancer at several sites, as each may call for measurement of some additional confounding variables.

Methods of environmental sampling

As the purpose of sampling is to measure the exposure of individuals, a sampling strategy, centred on individuals rather than on broad sections of, for example, a plant, should be adopted. There are two broad approaches to sampling the environment.

(a) Measurement at fixed points (static sampling) within the environment and inferring individual exposure from the concentrations of contaminants measured in the parts of the environment covered by each sampler.

(b) Measurement of the immediate and continually changing environment of individual subjects by some form of personal sampling.

The latter is the preferred approach because it takes into account the subject's position in the environment, the concentrations of the environmental agent there, and behaviours that may modify exposure in particular circumstances (e.g. avoidance of sudden increases in emissions at particular points, use of protective devices, etc.).

In the case of sampling for airborne contaminants in the workplace, a personal sampler is worn by each worker whose environment is to be sampled. The sampler consists of a power source and a pump connected to an aspirating head containing, for example, a filter membrane on to which the substance to be tested is deposited. The aspirating head is placed anywhere within the breathing zone, a zone of air extending to 30 cm from the head of the sample individual. Unless the pump is of a self-correcting type, the flow of air is checked regularly, during sampling periods extending over several hours, lest the quantity of air captured and filtered should vary and cause error in measurement of the concentration of the substance under study. Wearing a pump and a battery for hours may be considered a nuisance, and a high participation rate in measuring sessions may be difficult to maintain. 'Passive' samplers (Thain 1980) based on the diffusion or permeation of gases and vapours into some chemical trap have been developed in recent years. These minimize the weight and eliminate the noise of the sampler, but they do not yet seem to be capable of matching the accuracy of aspiration samplers.

The measurement of dietary intake of nutrients and other components of food by sampling and analysis of the diet provides a very different example of personal sampling. Three techniques may be used.

(a) In the *duplicate portion technique*, portions of all foods and beverages (except for water) identical to those consumed by the individuals are collected and analysed chemically.

(b) In the *aliquot sampling technique*, all foods and beverages (except for water) consumed by an individual during the survey period are weighed and aliquot samples, for example one-tenth of all foods and beverages consumed, are collected daily for chemical analysis.

(c) In the *equivalent composition technique*, the weights of all foods and beverages (except for water) consumed by an individual are recorded during the whole survey period. Afterwards, a sample of raw foods equivalent to the foods eaten by the individual during the survey period is analysed chemically.

The highly intrusive nature of these methods may discourage participation and is likely to alter the normal eating patterns. These problems, together with the cost of direct chemical analyses, limit the use of these methods to small-scale studies.

Selecting subjects for environmental sampling

At one extreme, measurement of the environment could entail continuous sampling of the environment of each subject throughout all periods of exposure relevant to the study. While in some circumstances this is comparatively simple (e.g. film-badge monitoring of exposure to ionizing radiation), in most cases it is neither practicable nor necessary. To make the measurements logistically and economically feasible, and to ensure that quality is not sacrificed to quantity, sampling both of subjects and of exposure time is usually undertaken.

Two main approaches have been used for the sampling of subjects in the workplace.

(a) Random selection of subjects and then grouping those appearing to share common levels of exposure to the environmental agent (Woitowitz *et al.* 1970).

(b) More efficiently, pre-definition of strata presumptively homogeneous with respect to the exposure and sampling randomly within the strata.

Measurements of environmental exposures in these samples are then used to estimate the exposure of all subjects in the classes into which the sampled subjects were grouped or from which they were taken. The former approach requires definitions of statistical criteria to separate groups of measurements into classes, the latter stands on the assumption that relatively homogenous strata can be identified *a priori*. These strata have been defined as 'exposure zones' (Corn and Esmen 1979; Corn 1981; Corn 1985) and their definition is a valuable approach to the sampling of subjects for environmental measurements.

In the occupational environment, an exposure zone is defined with reference to knowledge of the production or other process, work tasks, sources of contaminants, and devices used for their removal. The procedure for selecting zones involves an examination of all processes, job classifications, material inventories, and ventilation and exhaust facilities in the plant. The definition of exposure zones should rely purely on these *a priori* criteria. Any measurements that may be available should not be used for definition of the zones because they will rarely, if ever, have been derived from a previous random sampling survey. For example, knowledge of high concentrations of a contaminant found at some of the few sites in a plant checked during a compliance control survey may lead to their grouping together to form a zone, removing them from the zones to which they would have been assigned on the basis of the *a priori* criteria used to classify all other sites. A zone can be, but is not necessarily, a definable area or volume of the physical plant space that might be suitable for static sampling. Indeed, it is commonly found that a proportion of the workers in a given plant area belong to a zone they share with a proportion of the workers in another area; for example, workers undertaking the same tasks but on another production line, differently located. Conversely, some workers sharing physical space may not belong to the same zone because of different tasks, and different positions with respect to sources of pollutants, and exhaust and ventilation devices.

Each zone should meet four basic criteria (Corn 1981, 1985).

(a) *Work similarity*. Employees in the zone must perform similar tasks, so that similar mechanisms generating environmental contaminants exist.

(b) *Similarity with respect to hazardous agents*. Zone members must use the same agents (chemicals, heat, electricity), and the potential for exposure to the agents under investigation must be similar. Where multiple agents are present the potential for exposure to all of them must be similar for all persons included in the zone.

(c) *Environmental similarity*. Process equipment and ventilation must be similar for all zone members.

(d) *Identifiability*. The same employee must not be classifiable to more than one zone. This requirement is important for the subsequent random selection of workers from a zone. Employees classified to a zone must be identifiable in company records as belonging to that zone by, for example, job title and plant department. It is not uncommon to see that in some departments there is no distinct job classification and all workers may be involved in the different phases of the operation on a non-specific schedule; that is, while tasks can be distinguished, workers cannot be readily identified with them. In this situation, the number of different zones will be small, the heterogeneity of exposure within them potentially great, and error in individual measurement more likely.

Once employees have been preliminarily assigned to zones they are observed individually to see whether changes in zone assignments are needed.

The zoning process characterizes the work with respect to exposure in such a way that any person with any job title identified as belonging to a given zone can be expected to experience the exposure value representative of that zone. This marks the limit of the degree of individualization possible in the zoning approach. Such a limit reflects the trade-off between direct measurement of the environment of every exposed person and feasibility, cost, and the assurance of quality.

The definition of zones requires close cooperation between the industrial hygienist primarily responsible for making the measurements on workers, plant engineers, and other staff. It is also highly desirable that the epidemiologist who is going to use the exposure measurements in the analysis of health effects be present at some time during the assessment of exposure in zones, to become familiar with the source of the exposure data and the errors that may affect it, such as biased selection of subjects, poor response rate among those selected, failure to follow instructions, etc.

The concepts of exposure zones and personal sampling, intuitively straightforward and developed for sampling the occupational environment, can be extended and adapted to sampling current exposure to a variety of agents in other parts of the environment. The essential elements for defining zones, prior to any measurements, are similarity of the subjects' activities, the hazards present and the environmental conditions, and unique identifiability, that is assignment of each subject to one zone only. These criteria can be readily applied when sampling indoor environments as well as some features of the general environment. For example, a proportional sampler can be used to sample tap water in the home (5 per cent of water flowing through the tap) so that measurements of the constituents of water can be made and related to individuals or, at least, household consumption of water for different purposes. The households to be sampled would be selected according to 'zoning criteria'.

It may not be possible to employ the exposure zone approach when sampling the general environment over a relatively large area because only scanty information may be available to characterize a large non-captive population according to the zoning criteria. In these circumstances, a topographical approach to sampling may be used (Gilbert 1987). In the case of general air pollution, for example, a grid would be superimposed on the area to be studied and cells of the grid selected by simple random, multistage random, or stratified random sampling. It may be desirable, for example, to stratify by topographical orientation, dominant wind direction, and proximity to a particular point source of pollution. Systematic sampling may also be considered, as it is usually easier to implement under field conditions, although it may lead to substantial bias to the extent that the surveyed population is not randomly distributed in space. Within each cell selected for the sample, measurements would be carried out by choosing, at random, a number of subjects to wear personal samplers, or by use of fixed area samplers, or both. Other approaches may be used to define zones in the general environment. For example, with respect to contamination of water, zones may be defined by characteristics such as town area, socioeconomic status, features of housing, water supply and plumbing, and family size, which may be readily ascertainable through a simple questionnaire.

Special sampling schemes have been suggested for the case in which, prior to any consideration of zones in the general environment, a pollution source or 'hot spot' must be located; for example, buried waste or a point source contaminating a water distribution network (Gilbert 1987).

Extent of sampling

The extent of sampling within each exposure zone is defined in terms of the number of measurements to be made, the duration of collection (or size) of each sample, the period during which the measurements are taken, and the distribution of the measurements over this survey period.

The number of measurements made usually corresponds to the number of subjects whose environment is to be sampled. Subjects are chosen at random from all members of each exposure zone. The number to be chosen is decided, in principle, on the basis of the desired degree of reliability obtainable through repeated measurements in time, along the lines of the example on page 214 in which the number of days a subject needs to keep an exposure diary is discussed. This approach has not yet been applied to zone measurements, however. These measurements are affected not only by intra-subject variation in exposure over time but also by between-subject variation within a zone, and few data are available that would allow simultaneous assessment of these two sources of variability (Rappaport 1991). At present the number of subjects is chosen either arbitrarily or, preferably, through specification of the precision with which the average concentration of the environmental agent is to be measured.

As the survey will extend over several days or weeks, the selection of zones for measurement, and of subjects within zones, should be random with respect to time. In the case of airborne contaminants, a reasonable assumption is that the measurements will be log-normally distributed and, if no preliminary measurements are available, a geometric standard deviation of between 2 and 3 can be assumed (Corn 1985). Table 10.1, which has been derived by standard methods of sample size calculation (Mace 1964; Hale 1972), shows the number of measurements required to estimate their median value or geometric mean (assuming a log normal distribution) with

Table 10.1 Approximate number of measurements required to estimate the median with given precision

90% confidence interval	Number of measurements	
(in % of median)	GSD^a = 2	GSD = 3
10	145	360
20	40	100
30	20	50
40	15	30
50	10	20
60	8	15

^{a} GSD is the geometric standard deviation of individual determinations

a given precision: for example, with an approximate 90 per cent confidence interval of given width. Thus, for example, with 10–20 measurements in each zone, the true median will be included in an interval equal to 50 per cent of the observed median in 90 per cent of the zones. A similar precision will be achieved for the estimate of the arithmetic mean. Taking 10–20 measurements will also give 90 per cent confidence that the sample range covers 75–80 per cent of the possible values of individual measurements in a zone.

The duration of sampling is first determined by the need to obtain enough material for accurate analysis; this entails consideration of the likely concentration of the contaminant, the efficiency of its collection, and the sensitivity of the analytical method. Second, the nature of the biological effect expected and its relationship to onset of exposure and the amount of the agent absorbed and retained in the body must be considered. The latter depends, in turn, on the airborne concentration of the substance, the time a given concentration is maintained, and the biological half-life of the agent. For irritants, asphyxiants, sensitizers, and allergenic agents, that is, agents which produce rapid biological responses, short-term sampling of, say, 15 minutes or less may be used. In general the sampling time should be in proportion to the biological half-life of the substance. It has been proposed (Roach 1966) that an optimum duration is about one-tenth of the half-life. This turns out to be neither so short as to miss fluctuations in airborne concentration capable of being reflected in important variations in body burden, nor so long as to dampen and mask such variations. When the objective is to study late effects of exposures, like pneumoconiosis or cancer, sampling over a full working shift (8 hours) is usually adopted, as variations in exposure which may occur within this interval are regarded as being of negligible relevance.

The choice of the period of the year in which to perform the measurements must take into account the fact that concentrations of environmental agents may vary not only within a day (e.g. between shifts) but also from season to season. While the variability from hour to hour and between shifts can be accommodated in a single survey lasting from several days to a few weeks, documentation of seasonal or yearly variation may necessitate repetition of the survey. If resources are limited it is better to target the survey on periods when the highest concentrations can be found (e.g. winter, when there is less ventilation of the workplace in the case of an airborne contaminant). Repetition might then be limited to sub-samples, to ascertain the stability or variability of the concentration established in the survey.

The exact programme of sampling adopted depends on the objectives and type of the epidemiological study proposed. For any kind of study of a disease or other biological effect with a short induction period (i.e. a short period from commencement of exposure to onset of the effect) it is desirable to sample close in time to the period during which occurrence of the effect is being determined. In the case of a prospective cohort study, or a case-control study within a cohort study, repetition of sampling at intervals within the period over which cases are determined is desirable. The frequency of repetition should be determined by the length of the induction period and the day-to-day, week-to-week, or month-to-month variability of the exposure. At one extreme, if the induction period is very short (e.g. of the order of a few hours), variability is high, and there is little discrimination between exposure zones, useful measurements may be obtained only be very frequent sampling. At the other extreme, if the exposure varies little with time or there are substantial and stable differences in level of exposure between zones, a single survey of exposure may suffice even where the induction period is very short.

For cohort studies of an effect with a long induction period, a survey extending, preferably, over a period of about a year will be necessary, with at least partial repetition periodically over the period of follow-up.

Analytical aspects

Repetition of a survey means that the collection of specimens and the analytical procedures are carried out at intervals of months or years. To ensure uniformity of the whole measurement process, strict attention to quality control is essential. At the very least, this requires that all procedures are carried out according to a written protocol and that reference samples are included in all batches of analyses. When measurements are done at different laboratories, there is a need for inter-laboratory, as well as intra-laboratory, comparisons to monitor and maintain accuracy and precision within fixed limits.

Some methods of measurement involve substantial subjectivity and analyst fatigue (e.g. counting fibres by optical microscopy, for which the advice is that no operator should do more than six counts a day). These methods may have coefficients of variation (see page 110) for repeated measurements of the same sample of 20 per cent or more (Rajhans and Sullivan 1981). For chemical methods, substantially lower coefficients, below 10 per cent and down to 2–3 per cent or lower, may be found (Horwitz 1977). However, beside the analytical errors, a variability between parallel replicates of some 5 per cent for example, in obtaining an air sample by pump and filter, has to be taken into account. This brings the total error (coefficient of variation) for repeated measurements of the same part of the environment to near 10 per cent. Further non-negligible variability is introduced if several different laboratories are used.

Whereas the size of the total error and its components are of direct interest to the epidemiologist who is going to use the environmental measurements, technical aspects relevant to its minimization are the province of the environmental hygienist and the analyst. These aspects include choice of equipment and procedures for collecting, handling, and storing specimens (by definition, if an agent is present in the environment it has the potential for contaminating containers, equipment, hands, and clothes), analytical methods and quality control procedures.

A point worth noting is that, depending on the concentration of the agent to be measured and the concurrent presence of other agents, different methods of measurement may need to be used, even for the same medium (e.g. air or water). For example, the number of fibres $>5 \mu m$ in length counted on membrane filters by phase contrast microscopy is today used as a measure of exposure to asbestos in the occupational environment (Rajhans and Sullivan 1981), although these fibres form only a small proportion of the total number of fibres present, and the method is not specific for asbestos fibres. This lack of sensitivity and specificity is not a problem at the level of contamination which is the subject of control in the occupational environment, and where asbestos is the predominant fibre present. Measurements in the general environment, however, are complicated by the low concentration of asbestos and by the predominance of other mineral particulates. Under these circumstances it has proved necessary to resort to examination of the sampled material by electron microscopy, which permits both sensitive and specific identification of asbestos fibres at the levels found in urban air, although it produces measurements that are not directly comparable with those derived by optical microscopy from the higher concentrations present in the occupational environment (Dupré *et al.* 1984; Nicholson 1989).

Sampling strategies and analytical methods for different agents are dealt with in reference books such as *Patty's Industrial Hygiene and Toxicology* (Clayton and Clayton, 1978, 1979, 1981). The series of volumes *'Environmental Carcinogens: Methods of Analysis and Exposure Measurement'*, published by the International Agency for Research on Cancer (IARC

1978–88), gives a detailed account of the measurement of carcinogens in the environment.

SAMPLING AND MEASURING PAST EXPOSURES

Measurements of present exposure to agents in the environment are applicable to cross-sectional, case-control, and retrospective cohort studies only when it can be reasonably assumed that measurements of concentrations of agents in the present environment are highly correlated with the concentrations present at aetiologically relevant periods in the recent or remote past. As an alternative to making this often unrealistic assumption, records of measurements of relevant exposures may be sought. These can be used, alone or in combination with results from surveys of present exposures, to infer 'best estimates' of past exposure for each subject in an epidemiological study. While usually useful to some degree, the records and the measurements they document are frequently far less than ideal for epidemiological purposes. Their use therefore requires the utmost care.

The reconstruction of measurements of past exposure in the environment can be conveniently divided according to whether past records are complete, incomplete, or unavailable. The epidemiologist is confronted today, and will continue to be confronted in the future, with all three situations, as it is practically impossible to adequately monitor *all* agents present in the environment, including those which may one day turn out to be worthy of epidemiological investigation.

Complete past measurements

When a complete set of measurements in exposure zones or similar strata are available, carried out in the past for epidemiological purposes by methods still judged as acceptable, they are as good as measurements obtained in contemporary surveys. The position is different, however, when the measurements were collected for purposes other than an epidemiological investigation. Commonly, the measurements available were collected to check compliance with regulatory standards. Care is required in the use of such data. It is important to ascertain the purpose of the measurements and the frame within which they were collected, as these two factors determine the way in which the samples were selected and the way they reflect the pattern of exposure of the study subjects. For example, compliance may have been monitored by measurement of some readily measurable substance, which may have represented only a fraction (e.g. the water-soluble part) of the mixture of interest. Compliance control may also have concentrated on measurements in 'maximum risk employees', that is, the employees judged to have had the highest potential for exposure at a given time. Attributing their levels of exposure to everyone would be likely to introduce substantial errors.

Incomplete past measurements

Past measurements may be incomplete because they were made only in selected exposure zones, they were made by methods that are sub-optimal according to present-day knowledge, or they were only of some correlate of the exposure of interest (e.g. total dust concentration when only the concentration of mineral fibres is of interest).

In principle, incomplete past measurements may be used in the same way as complete past measurements or present measurements to reconstruct past exposure to environmental agents. Detailed estimates are made of the exposure levels in each exposure zone, or like stratum, at a single point or at different points in time in the past. Individual subjects are then assigned to zones in the usual way, that is, in the case of an occupational exposure, by matching job histories (by job titles and plant department) to jobs and areas included in a zone.

This approach was adopted by Stewart *et al.* (1986) to estimate past exposure to formaldehyde in a retrospective cohort study of the mortality of some 30 000 workers employed by 10 companies. The procedure consisted of estimating the concentration of formaldehyde in inhaled air in each exposure zone as belonging to one of six 8-hour, time-weighted average levels:

- *trace* (it was assumed that regardless of where a person worked in a formaldehyde plant their exposure would be greater than that of a person not working in such a plant);
- < 0.1 *p.p.m.* (for example, an employee who occasionally went into the production area);
- 0.1–0.5 *p.p.m.* (odour noticeable occasionally in each eight-hour day);
- 0.5–2.0 *p.p.m.* (odour consistently present throughout the eight-hour day)
- > 2.0 *p.p.m.* (eye irritation or lacrimation and odour occuring throughout the 8-hour day)
- *unknown*.

These categories were developed before the estimation process was carried out.

The estimation process involved several steps. First, personnel records were abstracted to list, standardize, and aggregate the job titles held by cohort members and the areas in which they worked (the components of allocation to exposure zones). Next, other plants were walked through to gather historical and current production, control, and air-monitoring data. From these data a matrix of exposures by job and time was then developed, which took detailed account of the tasks performed within each job at each time and the effects of engineering controls and production or process changes. Exposure estimates made by industrial hygienists belonging to the plant were then reviewed and the present-day operation monitored to a total of about 2000 measurements of formaldehyde concentrations in air. In addition to supplementing historical monitoring data, these measurements allowed standardization of measurements across the different plants. Finally, the information from these sources was integrated to produce the estimates of historical exposure levels by job and area used for the study. These estimates fully characterized past exposures at particular points in time, and were matched to the workers' job history files to provide individual estimates of exposure.

A more general approach to the estimation of past exposure was proposed by Esmen (1979). In essence he broke down each job or occupational title into component, elementary tasks called 'uniform tasks' which, unlike job titles, applied to the whole of an industry in a relatively uniform way, independently of plant. A set of uniform task units, adaptable to several kinds of production industries, is shown in Table 10.2. The major objective of this breakdown was the reduction of variability in exposure within these units.

Estimates of exposure levels were then made for each uniform task category at appropriate times in the past. If only current measurements were available, possibly supplemented by a few measurements in the past, they were extrapolated back correcting for four factors:

- changes in the process
- changes in the physical characteristics of the agent
- periodic use of personal protective devices
- rate of output of the product.

If, instead, there were only current measurements for the agent of primary interest, but current and past data existed for some other agent, the two sets of current measurements were correlated, always within uniform task units, to permit estimation of past exposure to the agent of primary interest. Once estimates of exposure had been made for the uniform tasks, exposures for each job in each plant were estimated as weighted averages of exposure levels in uniform tasks, with the time each task contributed to a job used as its weight.

The work of both Stewart *et al.* (1986) and Esmen (1979) indicates that estimation of levels of exposure, whether in exposure zones or similar strata, is a painstaking endeavour, requiring a combination of search of documents, interviews with key informants, inspection of plants, and current measurements. The person-time required to make the exposure estimates for the study of Stewart *et al.* (1986) is summarized in Table 10.3 and gives an idea of the amount of work involved. It is a safe general rule that a feasibility

Table 10.2   Uniform task categories in which separate estimates of exposure can be made (Esmen 1979)

Making A
  Tasks which involve direct contact with the agent or precursors of the agent in operations that 'make' or 'get' the product, i.e. direct mining, mixing ingredients, loading raw material to processor.

Making B
  Tasks which involve indirect contact with the agent or precursors of the agent in operations that 'make' or 'get' the product, e.g. indirect mining, joy loader operating, controlling mixers, kettles, or process ovens.

Production A
  Tasks which involve direct contact with the agent as the material is produced to be formed by a manufacturing process or formed to be shipped as is, e.g. moulding operations, process helping, mill operations, and process machine operations.

Production B
  Tasks which involve direct or indirect contact with the agent through the manufacture of a finished product from the material containing the agent by the use of cutting or abrasive tools, e.g. trimming, sawing, weaving, and sending operations.

Production C
  Tasks which involve direct or indirect contact with the agent through the manufacture of a finished product from the material containing the agent using heated tools, e.g. welding, hot joining, soldering, heat treating, and drying operations.

Production D
  Tasks which involve general manufacturing operations where exposure to the agent is less likely than in tasks A, B or C, e.g. painting finished product, handling packaged material, packaging finished product (foremen and floor supervisors).

Clean up A
  Tasks which involve general cleaning of non-production areas.

Clean up B
  Tasks which involve cleaning production machinery and production areas, e.g. sweeping floor in production areas, cleaning particulate control devices.

Maintenance
  Tasks which involve the repair and upkeep of production machinery.

Quality control
  Tasks which involve sampling the product and performing tests to ascertain product quality.

Table 10.2 *cont.*

Shipping
Tasks which involve transportation of packaged material, forklift, truck operations, and shipping yard operations

Isolated tasks
Tasks which are isolated from production areas and do not involve contact with the agent except for general plant exposure, e.g. boiler operations, tool crib, and shipping yard supervision.

Table 10.3 Time taken to estimate exposure to formaldehyde from an incomplete set of past exposure measurements in a cohort of some 30 000 workers employed by 10 companies (Stewart *et al.* 1986)

Activity	Participants	Time (person-months)
Abstracting 30 000 personnel records	Abstracting team	45
Development of protocol and form	Industrial hygienists	5
Standardization of job titles	Industrial hygienists	9
Walk-throughs	Industrial hygienists	3
Estimation of exposures	Industrial hygienists	15
Monitoring	Industrial hygienists	9
Review of jobs	Company personnel	7
Integration to make final estimates	Industrial hygienists	2

investigation should be carried out as the first step to find out what type of information can be obtained at what cost, and what this may yield in terms of validity and precision of risk estimates.

Estimation of past exposures is apparently simpler when a set of measurements is available which is incomplete only in that it was obtained by methods different from those now regarded as acceptable or optimum. In principle, the establishment of some form of equivalence between measurements taken with the different methods is all that is required. However, that objective may prove to be difficult to achieve.

Measurement of exposure to asbestos (Doll and Peto 1985) illustrates the difficulty of establishing equivalence of measurement methods. Table 10.4 shows the main changes that took place in the methods of measuring asbestos dust in one British asbestos textile factory over a 30-year period. They reflect the evolution of measurement technology over that period.

Table 10.4 Methods used to measure asbestos dust concentrations in a British asbestos textile factory in different time periods (Doll and Peto 1985)

Period	Instrument	Method of evaluation	Object measured	Unit[a]
1951–60	Casella thermal precipitator (CTP)	Incinerated, × 1000 dark field	Particles (including fibres)	p ml^{-1}
1961–64	Ottway long running thermal precipitator (LRTP)	Not incinerated, × 500 light field	Fibres >5 μm long, length diameter ratio >3:1	f ml^{-1}
1965–74	Membrane filter sampler	× 500 Phase contrast, full field	Fibres >5 μm long, length diameter ratio >3:1	f ml^{-1}
	or			
	Royco automatic particle counter (RPC)	Automatic	Fibres >5 μm long, length diameter ratio >3:1	f ml^{-1}
1975 to date	Membrane filter sampler	× 600 Phase contrast, graticule grid count	Fibres >5 μm long, length diameter ratio >3:1	f ml^{-1}

[a] Particles counted down to a diameter of 0.5 μm; 35 particles per ml are equivalent to one million particles per cubic foot (mppcf); f ml^{-1} = fibres (as defined by regulations) per ml.

There were several changes in the approach to measurement, instrumentation, and sensor devices; and in different periods different components of the dust were measured. In addition, personal sampling gradually replaced area sampling after 1975, thus introducing a further difference. That the measurements obtained with different techniques are not directly comparable is obvious, but is it possible to find valid factors for conversion from one method to the other? The key conversion is from measurements in the form of particles per unit volume made by the older particle counting methods (midget impinger, used in North America, and thermal precipitator used, for example, in Britain) to measurements in terms of 'regulated' fibres (i.e. particles longer than $5\,\mu m$ and with a length diameter ratio of at least 3) counted by optical microscopy. Unfortunately, no simple conversion is possible. Fibre counts ranging from 3 per cent to more than 50 per cent of the particle counts have been obtained in different processes (mining and milling and manufacture of textiles, friction materials, and asbestos cement) and a similar range of variation has been found among areas within a single plant. No comparable measurements of particles and fibres are available at all for exposure during the use of asbestos insulation. Moreover, when measurements have been made simultaneously by different methods in the same environment, the correlations obtained have invariably been weak (correlation coefficients of 0.3–0.6) and the relationship between particles and regulated fibres has not always been linear on an arithmetic scale.

The difficulty in finding a valid conversion factor is clearly shown by data from the Quebec mines and mills, where a large series of parallel measurements was available of particles counted by the midget impinger and fibres collected on membrane filters and counted by use of an optical microscope. A logarithmic transformation of both sets of measurements was chosen and a linear relationship sought between them. Estimates of the arithmetic conversion factor were derived from the regression line. Three selected values corresponding to typical counts (0.1, 1 and 10 millions of particles per cubic foot) are shown in Table 10.5.

Table 10.5 Values of the multiplying factor to convert measurements of asbestos particle concentrations into asbestos fibre concentrations $(f\,ml^{-1})$ (Dagbert 1976)

Particle concentration (mppcf)[a]	Multiplying factor to convert to $f\,ml^{-1}$	95% confidence interval about factor
0.1	23	1.2–116
1.0	11	0.6– 58
10.0	5	0.3– 27

[a] mppcf = millions of particles per cubic foot

As expected from a linear relationship, on a log-log scale the arithmetic conversion factor systematically decreases with the increasing values of the particle concentrations. Also, the arithmetic 95 per cent confidence intervals about the conversion factors were very wide due to the large scatter of the points from which the regression line was calculated.

The regression line summarized in Table 10.5 can be regarded as correctly predicting the fibre concentrations from the particle concentrations under the conditions in which this limited series of parallel measurements was obtained. However, the very reason for deriving a conversion factor is to use it outside these strict circumstances, and this requires estimating a regression line corrected for the biasing effect of the measurement error in the 'independent' variable (particle concentration). This error has the effect of flattening the slope and increasing the intercept, with the consequence that at low concentrations the fibre concentrations would be overestimated from the particle concentrations, while at high concentrations they would be underestimated. One possible way of correcting for this bias is to force the regression line through the origin. If, in addition, a logarithmic model is not assumed and, instead, the assumption is made that the variance of the estimated fibre counts increases in proportion to the values of the particle counts on an arithmetic scale, the estimator of the regression coefficient reduces to the simple ratio of the two mean values (Snedecor and Cochran 1980). This estimator, which is relatively insensitive to large random errors and to outliers, has been used (Doll and Peto 1985) to derive a single conversion factor from a series of British measurements made with the Casella thermal precipitator (particles) and a membrane filter and optical microscopy (fibres). The value of the factor turned out to be 35.

Equivalence approaches, which use single conversion factors or regression equations, are virtually unavoidable if maximum use of available exposure measurements, obtained with different methods and under different conditions, is to be made for quantitative risk assessment. It is clear, however, that they are subject to substantial error. Similar approaches are used when one agent is measured as a surrogate for another or for a mixture.

No past measurements

When no past measurements of the environment are available, any characterization of subjects according to their likely past exposure to environmental contaminants will of necessity be crude and at the level of broad groups of subjects rather than individuals. A simple solution, often adopted in retrospective cohort studies of occupational exposures, is to group subjects according to their dates of first employment or, better, first exposure after employment (the two do not necessarily coincide). This calendar classification should reflect trends in exposure levels: decreasing because of improved hygiene and environmental control or, perhaps, increasing because of new exposures being added to the environment, or more activity being carried out within the same factory area. The dates defining different levels of exposure can be selected according to whatever knowledge is available on secular trends affecting the exposure of interest. The more extensive and specific this information, the more detailed will be the chronological criterion.

This approach can be illustrated from a retrospective cohort study of workers in the synthetic mineral fibre industry in 13 production plants located in seven European countries (Saracci *et al.* 1984). Once it became clear that the data obtained in an *ad hoc* survey of present concentrations of airborne fibres (Cherrie *et al.* 1986) were not representative of past conditions, a reconstruction of past exposure was attempted (Dodgson *et al.* 1987). No past measurements being available, information about the technical history of each factory was obtained by means of a self-administered questionnaire first introduced in a meeting with staff of the plant, completed by the staff, and then discussed at an interview with the research team. Great care was taken in the design of the questionnaire so that experienced plant managers could provide the best possible information on factors likely to affect exposure to fibres or other potential risk factors. Table 10.6 lists the major factors relevant to changes in fibre concentrations in the air.

Table 10.6 Factors considered to influence airborne fibre concentrations when estimating airborne fibre concentration of synthetic mineral fibres in 13 plants in Europe for which no past measurements were available (Dodgson *et al.* 1987)

- Fibre size in the bulk product
- Binder and oil content
- Type of process
- Size of building
- Production rate
- Ventilation
- Use of respirators
- Cleaning of workplace
- Secondary production processes

Reduction in nominal fibre size (i.e. length-weighted average fibre diameter in the bulk product) could produce an increase in emission of respirable fibres by up to 10 times. Addition of oil to the fibrous material would, on the other hand, reduce the concentration of airborne fibres by a factor of about 10, by causing them to form larger conglomerates which are non-respirable and settle rapidly. Change from a discontinuous, manually intensive process to a continuous one was also judged to reduce dust levels, by a factor of somewhat less than 10. Each of the other listed factors, some of which are interrelated (size of factory building, production rate, and ventilation) were judged not to contribute more than twofold variation to concentrations.

By use of this information on the presence and likely size of the effects of the main factors affecting fibre concentrations, it was possible to subdivide the production history of *each* plant into three technological phases:

(a) *early phase*, when a discontinuous production system was in use and/or no oil was added to the fibres during production.

(b) *late phase* when continuous modern techniques were used to manu-facture the fibres and oil was added.

(c) *intermediate phase* in which a mixture of these techniques operated.

Critical dates were established separately for each of the 13 plants so that workers could be classified according to the phases in which they had worked and, in particular, to the phase in which they were first employed. Although seemingly crude, this classification was employed to relate exposure to health outcomes (Simonato *et al.* 1987), and was regarded as being able to rank workers according to their exposure to fibres more accurately than the much more refined, but much less relevant, measurements of airborne fibres under present-day conditions. A small-scale simulation experiment of an early production process was also performed to gauge the airborne fibre concentrations more directly (Cherrie *et al.* 1987). This experiment provided data broadly supportive of the ranking classification.

Use of conversion tables with data derived from questionnaires

In the absence of actual measurement of the concentration of agents in the present or past environments, an attempt may be made to quantitate expo-sure by the use of conversion tables constructed from data external to the population under study and linked to data derived from records or questionnaires.

Some points on the use of conversion tables can be illustrated with reference to 'job-exposure' matrices used in studies of occupational epidemiology, and food tables used in studies of nutritional epidemiology.

The term *job-exposure matrix* has been loosely used to cover any method for converting job titles into exposures. An *a priori* job-exposure matrix is an instrument prepared prior to or separately from any data collection for the study in which it is used, and consisting of a typical two-entry conversion table with job classification along one axis, a list of potential exposures along the other axis, and an indication in the cells of the matrix of whether the par-ticular exposure occurs or occurred in the particular job. Thus, knowledge of the occupations of subjects allows an automatic coding of their possi-ble exposures. The exposure classifications for each job all build on what is generally known about exposures associated with particular tasks in par-ticular industries. This approach is necessarily limited by the fact that, even within narrowly defined occupational groups, exposure may vary from worker to worker according to their specific tasks, from country to country, from plant to plant, and from period to period.

The main features of this approach are that exposures are assigned at the group level, that is, at the level of occupation, industry, or a combination of the two, without reference to the particular exposure circumstances of individual workers. Exposure may be assigned by a subject-by-subject approach (sometimes, and confusingly, called the *a posteriori* matrix approach) involving the examination of each subject's work history by a team of trained experts who use their expertise and other sources of information to infer the exposures for each subject (Gérin *et al*. 1985). This approach is similar to what we have described above for reconstruction of exposures in workplaces when past measurements are incomplete or absent. However, here it is applied to individual workers in different industries rather than groups of workers in one industry. Both the *a priori* matrix and the subject-by-subject method have been developed mainly for reconstructing past exposures in case-control studies. The *a priori* job-exposure matrix is particularly useful when only minimal information on occupation is available to the epidemiologist, although its use in these circumstances makes it correspondingly prone to error.

Tables of composition of food have been in use for many decades. In essence, they are two-entry conversion tables with food items on one axis, nutrients on the other axis, and the amounts of given nutrients per unit weight of each food item in the cells of the table. The tables are used to convert estimates of amounts of food items eaten by a subject during a specified time into estimates of intake of water, nutrients, and nutrient-derived energy. They are based on analyses of samples of foods obtained in particular countries at particular times, but are commonly applied to the equivalent foods eaten in other countries and at other times.

There are a number of problems in the use of food tables. First, they rarely cover exactly the same list of food items as the dietary questionnaire, so some pooling and averaging of the values from different foods may be needed. This process increases the measurement error for the subjects under study (i.e. reduces the degree of individualization of the measurements of nutrients) and reduces the power of the study to detect diffferences between groups.

A second important approximation in the use of food tables derives from the way the nutrient concentrations are estimated. The concentrations are derived either from review of the literature on composition of foods or from *ad hoc* analyses. The tables available today are compiled from a mixture of these two sources. Unfortunately, one food item may vary substantially in its chemical composition. For example, composition may depend on the geographical origin (soil conditions, climate, fertilizer, method of husbandry and slaughter, etc.), the sampling procedure (time of collection, whether sample taken fresh, frozen, raw, etc.), and the treatment of samples before analysis (Paul and Southgate 1988). Composition may also change over time, making periodical revision necessary. The variability in nutrient composition of one food item is inadequately captured by the fixed conversion values of the table.

A third problem with food tables is lack of standardization of their methods of analysis and expression of concentrations of nutrients. For example, concentrations of nutrients may be expressed per unit of 'food as purchased', 'edible matter', or 'dry matter'. This lack of standardization can lead both to incorrect application of the tables (e.g. estimation of intake based on 'edible' quantities of food when the table refers to food 'as purchased') and to artefactual differences in the results of studies based on different food tables. A further source of variability between food tables results from the factors used to convert nitrogen into protein, when nitrogen content of an item has been determined to estimate protein content, and to convert carbohydrate, fats, and proteins into energy values.

Affected, as they are, by a number of limitations ('Anyone who uses a table of food composition as an oracle is misleading himself.' Paul and Southgate 1978), food tables are employed as an almost universal tool in studies of nutritional epidemiology. The tables to be used should be examined with the same detailed and critical attention as would be given to methods of direct chemical determination for which they are substitutes. In addition, Kaldor (1991) noted that whereas the exposure variables measured directly in a study may be crude, they have the advantage that they can be interpreted unambiguously. They are independent of the conversion table, and do not contain the additional error arising from use of the tables which, in some cases, could overwhelm the reduction in error obtainable through more specific identification of the exposure of interest. Thus, analyses based on derived variables (e.g. nutrients) should not be carried out to the exclusion of analyses based on the measured variables (e.g. foods or food groups). This may be of particular importance in exploratory studies aimed at finding aetiological clues.

SUMMARY

Components of the external environment which may be measured include physical, chemical and biological constituents or contaminants of soil, air, water, food, drinks, cosmetics, and drugs occurring specifically in homes, workplaces, or recreational sites, or in the general environment. The exposed individual may not sense these exposures, or even be aware of their existence, and in these circumstances the exposures can only be documented by measurements in the environment.

Objectivity and individualization of measurements in the environment are best achieved by personal sampling over extended periods of time, using fully automated sampling and measuring devices. Most often, however, reliance must be placed on samples collected over relatively short periods of time, following subjective advice from the person exposed on where to sample, and analysed by methods which are not fully automated. The result may be substantial error in the measurement of exposure.

The sensitivity of environmental measurements can be very high when modern methods are used and this is never a disadvantage. There is little point for epidemiological purposes, however, in pushing it to concentrations of the agent much below those likely to produce epidemiologically detectable effects. The specificity characteristics of an environmental measurement may be more difficult to determine. Where, for example, the biologically relevant exposure is a complex mixture, it may be more appropriate to base measurements on a biologically relevant characteristic of the whole mixture than to measure a specific chemical.

The measurement of present exposure and the reconstruction of past exposure require quite different approaches. Sampling strategies for current exposures have to take into account the nature of the exposure and its expected effect, whether immediate or delayed in time. The extent of sampling in space and time must also be determined and requires knowledge, not often available in adequate detail, of exposure variability, for example, between and within workers exposed to a pollutant in a working environment.

Actual measurements taken in the past may occasionally be available for measurement of past exposure. These measurements will usually have been taken for purposes other than an epidemiological study, typically environment control, and may not be representative of the actual distribution of the exposure. Most often, few or no past measurements will be available for the reconstruction of past exposure.

Substantial experience has been gained in recent years in the reconstruction of past occupational exposures. Job titles, as they appear in work histories, are broken down into elementary task components. An estimate is made, for each of these components, of exposure levels at appropriate times in the past, by use of whatever measurements are available, and knowledge of factors likely to have affected exposure such as the production processes in use, the physical characteristics of the agent, use of protective devices, etc.

When some past measurements are available, it may be necessary to convert measurements obtained by one method to estimates of those that would have been obtained by another usually more recent and more accurate method. The 'conversion factors' used may be subject to substantial uncertainty.

When no direct measurements are feasible for either past or present environments, an attempt may be made to measure exposure by use of conversion tables, such as job-exposure matrices and food tables linked to data derived from records or questionnaires. Additional error may be introduced, however, because of the error inherent in the conversion tables themselves.

REFERENCES

Cherrie, J., Dodgson, J., Groat, S., and McLaren, W. (1986). Environmental surveys in the European man-made fiber production industry. *Scandinavian Journal of Work Environment and Health*, **12**, (Suppl. 1), 18–25.

Cherrie, J., Krantz, S., Schneider, T., Öhbert, I., Kamstrup, O., and Linander, W.

(1987). An experimental simulation of an early rock wool/slag wool production process. *Annals of Occupational Hygiene*, **31**, 583–93.

Clayton, G. D. and Clayton, F. E. (ed.) (1978, 1979, 1981). *Patty's industrial hygiene and toxicology*, vols 1, 2, and 3 (3rd edn.) John Wiley and Sons, Chichester.

Corn, M. (1981). Strategies of air sampling. In *Recent advances in occupational health*, (ed. J. C. McDonald), **1**, pp. 199–210. Churchill Livingstone, Edinburgh.

Corn, M. (1985). Strategies of air sampling. *Scandinavian Journal of Work Environment and Health*, **11**, 173–80.

Corn, M. and Esmen, N. A. (1979). Workplace exposure zones for classification of employee exposures to physical and chemical agents. *American Industrial Hygiene Association Journal*, **40**, 47–57.

Dagbert, M. (1976). *Etudes de correlation de mesures d'empoussièrage dans l'industrie de l'amiante*, document 5 (Beaudry report). Québec comité d'étude sur la salubrité dans l'industrie de l'amiante, Montreal.

Dodgson, J., Cherrie, J., and Groat, S. (1987). Estimates of past exposure to respirable man-made mineral fibres in the European insulation wool industry. *Annals of Occupational Hygiene*, **31**, 567–82.

Doll, R. and Peto, J. (1985). *Asbestos: effects on health of exposure to asbestos*, pp. 19–22. Her Majesty's Stationery Office, London.

Dupré, J. G., Mustard, J. F., Uffen, R. J., Dewees, D. N., Laskin, J. I., and Kahn, L. B. (1984). *Report of the Royal Commission on matters of health and safety arising from the use of asbestos in Ontario*. Vol. 2, pp. 659–70. Ontario Ministry of the Attorney General, Toronto.

Esmen, N. (1979). Retrospective industrial hygiene surveys. *American Industrial Hygiene Association Journal*, **40**, 58–65.

Gérin, M., Siemiatycki, J., Kemper, H., and Bégin, D. (1985). Obtaining occupational exposure histories in epidemiological case-control studies. *Journal of Occupational Medicine*, **27**, 420–6.

Gilbert, R. O. (1987). *Statistical methods for environmental pollution monitoring*. Van Nostrand Reinhold, New York.

Hale, W. E. (1972). Sample size determination for the log-normal distribution. *Atmospheric Environment*, **6**, 419–22.

Horwitz, W. (1977). The variability of AOAC methods of analysis as used in analytical pharmaceutical chemistry. *Journal of the Association of Official Analytical Chemists*, **60**, 1355–63.

IARC (International Agency for Research on Cancer) (1978–88). *Environmental carcinogens. Selected methods of analysis*. Volumes 1–10. International Agency for Research on Cancer, Lyon.

Kaldor, J. M. (1991). Modeling complex exposure histories in epidemiological studies. In *Statistical models for longitudinal studies of health* (ed. J. H. Dwyer, M. Feinleib, P. Lippert, and H. Hoffmeister), pp. 332–48. Oxford University Press, New York.

Mace, A. E. (1964). *Sample-size determination*, pp. 35–37, 69–70. Reinhold Publishing Company, New York.

Nicholson, W. J. (1989). Airborne mineral fibre levels in the non-occupational environment. In *Non-occupational exposure to mineral fibres* (eds. J. Bignon, J. Peto, and R. Saracci), IARC Scientific Publications No. 90, pp. 239–61. International Agency for Research on Cancer, Lyon.

National Research Council (1985). *Epidemiology and air pollution.* National Academy Press, Washington.

Paul, A. A. and Southgate, D. A. T. (1978). *McCance and Widdowson's The composition of food,* 4th Edition. p. 31 Elsevier North-Holland, Amsterdam.

Preston, D. L. and Pierce, D. A. (1987). The effects of changes in dosimetry on cancer mortality risk estimates in the atomic bomb survivors. *Radiation Effects Research Foundation technical report 9–87.* Radiation Effects Research Foundation, Hiroshima.

Rajhans, G. S., and Sullivan, J. L. (1981). *Asbestos sampling and analysis.* Ann Arbor Science, Ann Arbor, Michigan.

Rappaport, S. (1991). Selection of the measures of exposure for epidemiology studies. *Applied occupational and environmental hygiene,* 6, 448–457.

Roach, S. A. (1966). A more rational basis for air sampling. *American Industrial Hygiene Association Journal,* 27, 1–12.

Saracci, R., Simonato, L., Acheson, E. D., Andersen, A., Bertazzi, P. A., Claude, J. *et al.* (1984). Mortality and cancer incidence of workers in the man-made vitreous fibres producing industry: an international investigation at thirteen European plants. *British Journal of Industrial Medicine,* 41, 425–36.

Simonato, L., Fletcher, A. C., Cherrie, J. W., Andersen, A., Bertazzi, P., Charnay, N. *et al.* (1987). The International Agency for Research on Cancer historical cohort study of MMMF production workers in seven European countries: extension of the follow-up. *Annals of Occupational Hygiene,* 31, 603–23.

Snedecor, G. W. and Cochran, W. G. (1980). *Statistical methods,* 7th edn, pp. 171–4. Iowa State University Press, Ames, Iowa.

Stewart, P. A., Blair, A., Cubit, D. A., Bales, R. E., Kaplan, S. A., Ward, J., *et al.* (1986). Estimating historical exposures to formaldehyde in a retrospective mortality study. *Applied Industrial Hygiene,* 1, 34–41.

Thain, W. (1980). *Monitoring toxic gases in the atmosphere for hygiene and pollution control,* pp. 91–8. Pergamon Press, Oxford.

Whitaker, T. B. and Dickens, J. W. (1974). Variability of aflatoxin test results. *Journal of the American Oil Chemists' Society,* 51, 214–218.

Woitowitz, H. J., Schake, G., and Woitowitz, R. (1970). Ranking estimation of the dust exposure and industrial-medical epidemiology. *Staub Reinhaltung der Luft,* 30, 15. (English translation).

11

Response rates and their maximization

The only correct method of handling persons lost to follow-up is not to have any. (Dorn 1950)

INTRODUCTION

In epidemiology and survey research in general, the word *response* has several meanings. Two of them are relevant to exposure measurement:

- the reply or 'response' that a research subject gives to a question put to him or her
- the participation (ability or willingness to 'respond') of the subject in an epidemiological or other study.

The emphasis of this book is on the first of these — obtaining responses with minimum error *at the level of the individual subject*. In epidemiology, however, we are concerned not just with individual subjects, but with the wider populations that they represent. Our inferences about population exposures may be affected by two sources of error additional to those that affect the data obtained from individual subjects: random sampling error and selection bias. Random sampling error occurs when statistics derived from the sample are not equal to the underlying population parameters because, *by chance*, members of the sample do not accurately represent the population as a whole. Selection bias occurs when statistics in the sample are not equal to the population parameters because the sample is not a true random sample of the population. Our attention in this chapter is directed to selection bias.

Selection bias may arise in several ways (Kalton 1983).

(a) The sample may not be a true random sample either because of errors in sample selection or because the sampling frame fails to include some units of the population (i.e. 'non-coverage' of the population).

(b) No information may be collected from some members of the sample, referred to as 'unit' or 'total' non-response, because of failure to locate or contact them, denial of access to them, their refusal to participate, their inability to co-operate (due to age, illness, language barrier, etc.) or other problems (distance, loss of questionnaires, etc.).

(c) The subject may participate but may not answer some questions, referred to as 'item' non-response, because he or she lacks the necessary information, does not make the effort necessary to retrieve it or refuses to give it, or the interviewer fails to record it, or the answer recorded is rejected in an edit check (perhaps because of error in recording, coding or data entry, or lack of consistency with other data provided by the respondent).

Attention in this chapter is directed mainly to the second of these sources of selection bias — non-response by subjects. It is considered relevant to exposure measurement because it can affect the measurement of the exposure of *populations* to agents of disease and, more important for the purpose of this book, because it can vary with the method of exposure measurement. In addition, the methods used to maximize response rates are at least partly method specific.

Item non-response too is clearly important to exposure measurement and may be method specific (e.g. it is more difficult to prevent when using a self-administered questionnaire than when using a personal interview approach). It is not dealt with here, however, because its prevention is largely a matter of quality control in the individual measurement procedure; a topic which has been dealt with both in Chapter 5 and in relation to the different measurement methods.

In this chapter, therefore, we define response rates, examine the way in which they vary according to the method of exposure measurement, describe the observed effects of non-response on measurements of exposure in populations, and give an account of strategies that can be used to maximize response rates.

RESPONSE RATES

Definition and calculation

There is no standard definition of the response rate, although the term is commonly used and response rates (actually response *proportions*) are often reported as essential inputs to the judgement of methodological adequacy of epidemiological studies. There are two proportions that should be distinguished: the completion rate and the response rate (Kviz 1977). The *completion rate* is the proportion of all persons selected for the study who are eligible and participate. The *response rate* is the proportion that eligible participants form of those selected for the study who were actually eligible to participate. The two commonly differ because sampling frames are often in error and not all those selected are truly eligible to participate — that is, some members of the sample are not actually members of the population from which the sample was supposedly drawn. For example, in a population-based case-control study, controls who were found, following attempted contact, to have been non-resident in the area of the study during the period in which the cases were diagnosed would be deemed ineligible and excluded from response rate calculations.

It is clear from the above that a response rate cannot be calculated unless the population being sampled is clearly defined. Without such a definition, there are no criteria by which eligibility can be determined. Similarly, a valid response rate cannot be calculated unless the eligibility of all members of the sample can be determined. The eligibility of *participants* will usually be known, but the eligibility of *non-participants* may not be. For example, in a mail survey the only information available about non-participants may be the initial data that allowed them to be selected, and the knowledge that they have failed to respond. Their non-response may be due to ineligibility or true non-response. Frequently the eligibility of non-respondents in face-to-face or telephone interview surveys will be known more completely than in mail surveys, thus giving rise to problems in the comparison of response rates among surveys conducted by different methods.

Eligibility of non-respondents may also be uncertain in surveys conducted by telephone when the sample has been selected by random digit dialling. Some of the telephone numbers dialled (about 5 per cent in the United States) are not answered after multiple calls, even though the line is apparently in working order. Whether or not these numbers represent eligible households that could contain eligible respondents is not known, and so an exact response rate cannot be calculated.

A further difficulty arises in selection of samples for interview by random digit dialling or any other method that involves an initial approach to randomly selected households. If the initial respondent refuses to provide any information about the composition of the household, it is not possible to determine whether the household contains an eligible respondent. In these surveys, the final 'response rate' is calculated as the product of the proportion of households that agrees to provide data for respondent selection and the proportion of respondents selected who participate fully. (For this to be a true response rate, it must be assumed, at least, that the proportion of refusing households that would have yielded an eligible respondent is the same as the proportion in non-refusing households.) Typically, both of these proportions lie between 80 per cent and 90 per cent in random digit dialling surveys (Hartge *et al.* 1984), so that the final response rate is not higher than about 75 per cent.

Where there are difficulties in determining the eligibility of non-respondents, it is usual to calculate a range of possible response rates by assuming, alternately, that all non-respondents of unknown eligibility were eligible and that all were not eligible. This approach is probably better than the calculation of a completion rate only, except when the response rates of different samples selected in the same way from the same population are being compared. When populations or methods of sampling differ, completion rates are likely to be too much affected by variation between samples in the proportion of eligible respondents to give a reliable guide to response rates.

A further difficulty in evaluating response rates arises in mail surveys when failure to mail a reply is taken as an indication of non-response. In an experiment in which letters were mailed to fictitious addresses and to fictitious persons at valid addresses (Sandler and Holland 1990), all those mailed to fictitious addresses were returned as undelivered by the US Mail Service while 13 per cent of those sent to fictitious persons were not returned. This finding suggests that a proportion of those who apparently fail to respond in a mail survey may have never received the questionnaire and are not truly non-respondents in that they never had the opportunity to respond. Their absence from the sample, however, could still bias the results. This ambiguity is best dealt with by trying to contact apparent non-respondents by telephone or home visit, with the added benefit of improvement in the final response rate.

Time trends

There is a widely held belief supported by evidence (Steeh 1981), particularly in the United States, that response rates for personal interview surveys have become increasingly poor with time. Analysis of rates of non-response in the National Election Studies and Surveys of Consumer Attitudes conducted by the Survey Research Center, University of Michigan, between 1952 and 1979 showed refusal proportions increasing from 6–8 per cent in the 1950s to 16–20 per cent in the 1970s. There was little net trend in the proportion of other reasons for non-response. The increase in the refusal proportion was greatest for large cities and least for small towns, and there was some increase in other reasons for non-response, probably mainly failure to make contact with the respondent, in large cities only.

The reasons for the fall in response rates during the 1960s and 1970s are poorly understood. They are probably not due, at least in the data from the Survey Research Center, to changes in survey methods. The possibility that they are due to fear, and a greater concern for personal safety of both the subject and the interviewer in urban areas, has led to the suggestion that the trend may be halted by a method that reduces fear of co-operation – the telephone survey (Groves and Kahn 1979). Initial data from the Survey Research Center, following a change to random digit dialling for the Survey of Consumer Attitudes, suggests that response rates may have stopped falling with the change. In addition, Schleifer (1986) found that response rates to public opinion surveys conducted by telephone were stable through the first half of the 1980s. However, an analysis of response rates in control subjects in case control studies of cancer conducted by the US National

Cancer Institute, selected by random digit dialling and interviewed by telephone, showed a fall in estimated overall response rate from 74 per cent in 1979 to 61 per cent in 1982–4 (Hartge *et al*. 1984). Thus it is not clear, on present evidence, that telephone interviewing has brought an end to falling response rates.

Other relevant variables that have varied with time and may affect the proportion of people likely to respond to surveys include:

- the frequency with which their participation has previously been sought (56 per cent of people interviewed in 1984 had been approached more than once in the past year)

- an increasing incidence of 'false surveys' (marketing campaigns disguised as opinion surveys)

- an increase in prevalence of the opinions that survey interviews were too long and that being interviewed was an unpleasant experience (Schleifer 1986).

EFFECT OF METHOD OF EXPOSURE MEASUREMENT ON RESPONSE RATES

A number of comparisons have been made, in epidemiological or health-related studies, of response rates achievable by the three main methods of obtaining data directly from respondents: face-to-face interview, telephone interview, and mailed, self-administered questionnaire (Hochstim 1967; Siemiatycki 1979; Battistutta *et al*. 1983; Weeks *et al*. 1983; Rolnick *et al*. 1989). All except one of these studies were conducted by assigning random samples of the study population, selected in the same way, to each method of data collection.

These studies were consistent in showing that response rates of over 80 per cent have been achieved for health-related surveys in a variety of populations as recently as 1981. They also showed that the highest response-rate is usually achieved through face-to-face interview and the lowest through mailed, self-administered questionnaire. The differences in response rates were greatest if only one survey method was employed, and were reduced substantially if additional methods were used to follow up those from whom a response was not obtained by the first method. For example, in methodological work in the Alameda County Human Population Laboratory, Hochstim (1967) observed that an initial home visit with callbacks as necessary gave a 90 per cent response rate, an initial telephone call with callbacks if necessary and mail to households without a telephone gave a response rate of 86 per cent, and an initial approach by mail with up to two additional mailings gave a response rate of 81 per cent. Follow-up of the home visit group by mail or telephone increased the response rate to 93 per cent, follow-up of the telephone group by mail increased the rate to 91 per cent, and follow-up of the mail group by telephone or home visit increased it to 88 per cent. Thus, use of the follow-up procedures substantially reduced the response-rate gap between the methods. Similar results were obtained by Siemiatycki (1979).

Use of multiple methods of approach may be useful in reducing differential non-response between different groups of subjects. In a case-control study of sexually transmitted disease, Rolnick *et al.* (1989) found a much larger difference between methods of approach in the response of cases (65 per cent responded to a mailed questionnaire and 79 per cent responded to a face-to-face interview) than in the response of controls (82 per cent and 84 per cent responded respectively). It is possible that the use of telephone or home visit follow-up could have eliminated this differential response to the mailed questionnaire.

The cost advantage of the cheaper methods of approach — telephone and mail — is not eliminated by the use of other methods of approach after initial failure to obtain a response. For example, Hochstim (1967) found the final cost per response, after use of multiple methods of follow-up, to be US$9.04 for a home visit, US$4.49 for telephone, and US$4.05 for mail. Similarly, Siemiatycki (1979) found it to be US$16.10 for a home visit, US$8.22 for telephone, and US$8.69 for mail.

Given the improvement in response rate that occurs with use of multiple methods of data collection, the question arises as to whether differences in quality of response by method should influence their combination in a single study. Evidence summarized in Chapter 2 suggests that any differences in response quality between the three methods are not large. The use of several of them to maximize response rates is unlikely, therefore, to bias estimates of exposure for the population away from what would have been obtained by use of only one method which obtained a high response rate.

SELECTION BIAS DUE TO NON-RESPONSE

Evidence of selection bias due to non-response

An early review of studies of the characteristics of respondents and non-respondents in medical surveys noted that non-response was consistently more common in the old and the less-well educated; it was unrelated to sex and inconsistently related to economic status. Whites were noted to have higher non-response rates than blacks, and housewives, self-employed, and unemployed people to have higher non-response rates than employed people (Cobb *et al.* 1957). The results of a number of more recent studies are summarized in Table 11.1. These results have been obtained in a number of different ways.

(a) There have been direct comparisons of those who respond with those who do not, either in cross-sectional surveys of newly recruited subjects or on follow-up of subjects who have been surveyed before.

(b) A number of comparisons have been made between early and late responders to surveys, or those who respond with little prompting and those who require much persuasion. The assumption here is that those who are persuaded to respond with difficulty are intermediate in their characteristics between those who respond readily and those who do not respond at all.

(c) Dropouts in long-term follow-up studies have been compared with continuing participants.

(d) In a few instances, comparisons have been made between characteristics of population samples that have a low response rate and characteristics of samples of the same population with a high response rate. This approach addresses more directly the extent of selection bias likely to be present as a result of a low response rate.

The results of these four approaches have generally been consistent in pointing to the same variables as being associated with non-response.

Table 11.1 shows that the correlates of non-response identified by Cobb *et al.* (1957) have generally been associated with non-response in more recent data. In addition, current smoking has emerged as a consistent and strong correlate of non-response. While Cobb *et al.* (1957) stated that blacks were better respondents than whites, four recent studies have observed the opposite. It would not be unreasonable to speculate that social changes of the past 30 years might have created this difference. Poor response was also observed by Cartwright (1986) among women in ethnic minority groups in the United Kingdom and particularly among those of Moslem religion. The recent studies show a more consistent pattern of association between the various indicators of low socioeconomic status and non-response than was observed by Cobb *et al.* (1957). A number of other variables have been associated with non-response, such as poor social support and low body weight (Iversen and Sabroe 1988; Benfante *et al.* 1989), but too infrequently to be certain of the consistency of the association.

A number of studies have examined the association of non-response with measures of health status (Loewenstein *et al.* 1969; Oakes *et al.* 1973; Wilhelmsen *et al.* 1976; Criqui *et al.* 1978; Greenlick *et al.* 1979; Vernon *et al.* 1984; Siemiatycki and Campbell 1984; Brambilla and McKinlay 1987; Cottler *et al.* 1987; Iversen and Sabroe 1988). Non-response was fairly consistently associated with poor current health status as measured, for example, by time away from work due to illness, presence of current symptoms of ill health, and alcohol problems, but not consistently with presence of chronic conditions or disabilities. This inconsistency may be explained by the evidence of higher response rates in people with recent medical care, which may

Table 11.1 Summary of results of studies comparing characteristics of respondents and non-respondents in medical surveys[a]

Characteristic	Association with non-response[b]
Greater age	Positive
Male sex	(Positive)[b]
Married	Inconsistent
Non-white race	Positive
Urban residence	Positive
Low educational status	Positive
Unemployed or low occupational status	Positive
Low family income	(Positive)[b]
Large household size	Inconsistent
Smoker	Positive
Recent illness or poor present health	Positive
Presence of chronic conditions or impairments	Inconsistent
High use of medical care	Negative

[a] Studies reviewed included Theodore *et al.* (1956), Cobb *et al.* (1957), Heath (1958), Hammond (1959), Robins (1963), Hochstim (1967), Loewenstein *et al.* (1969), Burgess and Tierney (1970), Kaplan and Cole (1970), Comstock and Helsing (1973), Oakes *et al.* (1973), Wilhelmsen *et al.* (1976), Criqui *et al.* (1978), Greenlick *et al.* (1979), Barton *et al.* (1980), De Maio (1980), Wu and Brown (1983), Weeks *et al.* (1983), Siemiatycki *et al.* (1984), Vernon *et al.* (1984), Brambilla and McKinlay (1987), Cottler *et al.* (1987), Walker *et al.* (1987), Bull *et al.* (1988), Iversen and Sabroe (1988), Wingo *et al.* (1988), Benfante *et al.* (1989).
[b] Pattern of association based on one or two significant associations.

indicate that contact with medical services encourages response in people whose probability of responding would otherwise be reduced by their poor health. Thus the pattern observed in people with chronic illness or disability could depend on their experience of medical care.

There is an apparent conflict between the study of Loewenstein *et al.* (1969) which showed an association between present good health and non-response, and the studies of Wilhelmsen *et al.* (1976) and Criqui *et al.* (1978) which showed the opposite. The former, however, was a survey of health and health care use while the latter two sought subjects for screening. It would be reasonable to postulate that healthy subjects might seek screening but avoid surveys of past illness and medical care. The study of Criqui *et al.* (1978) showed, in addition, that respondents were more likely than non-respondents to have a past history of hyperlipidaemia and a family history of heart disease. Thus it appears that the '*worried* well' may be the most likely to accept an invitation to be screened.

Evidence that those already ill fail to respond to invitations to be screened is also provided by studies in which mortality has been compared in participants and non-participants of screening studies. In the study of Wilhelmsen *et al.* (1976), the Framingham Study (Gordon *et al.* 1959), the Honolulu Heart Study (Benfante *et al.* 1989), and the British Regional Heart Study (Walker *et al.* 1987), those who were screened had lower subsequent mortality rates than those who were not. Similar differences were observed in the British Doctors Study (Doll and Hill 1964), a prospective cohort study that did not require initial health screening, thus suggesting that this effect is not confined to studies involving health screening. In one screening study, the Western Electric Company study, there was no difference in mortality between participants and non-participants (Paul *et al.* 1963). This study was based on men who were all working at the time of the invitation to be screened and were therefore unlikely to be ill. In this case, the 'healthy worker' bias appears to have protected against the 'healthy screenee' bias!

While there is clearly potential for selection bias due to non-response, the extent of this bias depends both on the prevalence of non-response in any study and the difference between respondents and non-respondents in the prevalence of the characteristics under consideration. The studies of Weeks *et al.* (1983) and Siemiatycki and Campbell (1984) addressed this question of net bias. In both, the differences in prevalence of characteristics between the low-response-rate sample and the final sample were very small. Criqui *et al.* (1978) also noted that respondents in their survey were 'generally representative' of the target population, and Loewenstein *et al.* (1969) reported that when the distributions of 200 variables were compared in samples with and without the late respondents only 15 variables had distributions that differed by as much as two to three percentage points in one or more categories. A more important issue, however, is the extent of bias in epidemiological measures of effect that might flow from these small effects of non-response on prevalence of exposure.

Effect of selection bias due to non-response

The effect of selection bias due to non-response on incidence rate ratios in epidemiological studies has been discussed by a number of authors (Greenland 1977; Criqui 1979; Criqui *et al.* 1979; Kleinbaum *et al.* 1981; Austin *et al.* 1981). Criqui (1979) showed that bias in the incidence rate ratio would be most likely to occur if there was 'combined risk factor and disease response bias'; i.e. response proportions differed both between those with and without the risk factor and those with and without the disease. In the following two by two table, the values P_a, P_b, P_c, and P_d represent, respectively, the response proportions in those with the risk factor and the disease, those with the risk factor but without the disease, those without the risk factor but with the disease, and those without the risk factor and without the disease.

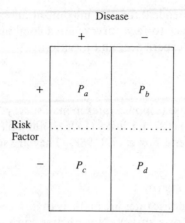

It may be shown quite simply (Austin *et al.* 1981) that the crude odds ratio for the association between risk factor and disease derived from the respondents (OR_R) is related to the crude odds ratio in the whole population (OR_P) as follows:

$$OR_R = \frac{P_a P_d}{P_b P_c} \times OR_P \qquad [11.1].$$

If the values of P_a, P_b, P_c, and P_d are known, the odds ratio in the population can be calculated from the odds ratio in the respondents and the extent of bias in the latter evaluated. Equation 11.1 also shows that provided the response proportion is the same in those with and without disease, given risk factor status, that is $P_a = P_b$ and $P_c = P_d$, variation in the response proportion by risk factor status will not bias OR_R. Similarly, if response proportions are the same, given disease status, in those with and without the risk factor, variation in the response proportion by disease status will not bias OR_R.

In the study of Criqui *et al.* (1978), data on six risk factors for cardiovascular disease (family history of heart attack, stroke and diabetes, past history of hyperlipidaemia and hypertension, and present cigarette use) and history of four diseases (past hospitalization for heart attack, heart failure, stroke, and history of diabetes) were obtained by telephone from a sample of 60 per cent of the non-respondents. This permitted estimation of P_a, P_b, P_c, and P_d and, therefore, calculation of OR_P from OR_R for each of the risk factor–disease combinations from Equation 11.1. Values of $P_a P_d / P_b P_c$ varied from 0.83 to 1.63; that is, the bias in OR_R varied from −17 per cent to +63 per cent. Thus appreciable bias was observed in some odds ratios even though the overall response rate was high (82.1 per cent).

MAXIMIZATION OF RESPONSE RATES

The strategies recommended for the maximization of response rates in mail, telephone, and face-to-face surveys are a combination of empirically supported techniques, experience, and intuition.

Mail surveys

Factors that may increase response rates in mail surveys have been reviewed by Kanuk and Berenson (1975), Linsky (1975), Dillman (1978), Baumgartner and Heberlein (1984), and Fox *et al.* (1988). They are summarized in Table 11.2.

Topic and sponsor of survey

Potential effects on response rates are unlikely to influence greatly the choice of a topic or sponsor for a survey. Nonetheless some choices can be exercised, and may influence response. Surveys on highly salient topics can achieve response rates some 30 percentage points higher than those on non-salient topics (Baumgartner and Heberlein 1984). It is clearly important, therefore, to bring out the salience of the survey as strongly as possible in the introductory letter. For example, Walter *et al.* (1988) found that response

Table 11.2   Factors that may increase response rates in mail surveys

---

Empirically supported
  A salient topic
  Advance notice that a questionnaire will be sent
  Government or University sponsorship
  A handwritten address
  Special class (e.g., certified) mailings
  Letter signed by patient's usual medical practitioner rather then research
    doctor
  An incentive included with the questionnaire
  A coloured questionnaire
  Stamped return envelope
  Multiple mailings
  Inclusion of a questionnaire with later mailings
  Follow-up and interview by telephone or home visit

Recommended
  Blanket publicity
  Personalization of correspondence
  Introductory letter explaining importance of respondent to the survey
  Small format questionnaire
  Commemorative stamps on outward mailing

---

to a letter seeking participation of controls in a case-control study increased from 74 per cent to 85 per cent when the letter, which initially referred to a 'study of health and environmental/lifestyle risk factors', was changed to refer to a 'study of cancer and the environment' and indicated that it involved 'questions about the relationship between environmental factors and cancer'. This increased response can presumably be attributed to the increased salience of cancer, and, perhaps, 'the environment' to the subjects.

There is consistent evidence that surveys conducted under the auspices of government departments or universities (especially government census bureaus) achieve higher response rates than those conducted by commercial survey organizations (Baumgartner and Heberlein 1984; Fox *et al.* 1988). Hammond (1959) found that the response to a questionnaire on smoking habits was consistently higher when the covering letter was from the Yale Statistical Laboratory than when it was from the American Cancer Society (both organizations were associated with the survey). Thus where several organizations are involved in a survey, the stationery used for the covering letter should be that of the organization thought likely to bring the greatest response.

Blanket publicity

'Blanket publicity', by way of newspapers and other news media, has been shown to be effective in increasing response rates in the US Health Examination Survey to a request for a personal interview followed by appointment for an examination (Schaible 1972). While similar data are not available for mail or telephone surveys, it seems reasonable to believe that advance publicity would have a beneficial effect on their response rates also. The publicity probably helps to establish the reputability of the investigators and the importance of their work in the eyes of potential respondents.

Advance notice

Advance notice, by mail or telephone, that a questionnaire will be sent does increase response rates (Linsky 1975; Spry *et al.* 1989), although not necessarily in all populations (Shiono and Klebanoff 1991). The advance letter generally identifies the researchers, states the study's purpose, and requests co-operation. It is doubtful, however, whether this approach achieves any more than can be achieved by an appropriate programme of follow-up mailing after the questionnaire has been sent. Because follow-up mailings need be sent only to those who do not respond, they are cheaper per unit of additional response than an advance mailing; they are therefore preferred.

Personalization of correspondence

Personalization of correspondence is commonly recommended, but has not been shown to either increase or decrease response rates in most studies (Baumgartner and Heberlein 1984). Its rationale is to distinguish the questionnaire from 'junk mail', and it may become effective in increasing response rates as the prevalence of 'junk mail' increases. Dillman (1978) recommends that the letter be dated as near as possible to the real date of mailing, and that the name, address, and salutation be individually typed on each letter in the normal business letter position. The sponsoring organization's normal business stationery should be used, and the letter should be signed personally by the study director using a blue pen. There is evidence that a handwritten address will increase response significantly over that obtained with a typed address (Rimm *et al*. 1990). The latter obtained a response rate no better than a computer-printed address in a window envelope.

Introductory letter
While common sense dictates that the introductory letter must be important in securing responses, there are few empirical data available to guide its construction. There are some suggestions from data that an appeal to ego ('you are important') gives higher response rates than an appeal to altruism ('your response will benefit the community'; Marshall and Gee 1976). Hammond (1959) found that a simple request for information appeared to be more effective than a 'hard sell' letter. Dillman (1978) recommends that the letter should include the following components:

- a statement of what the study is about and its usefulness (see section on 'topic and sponsor of survey' above)
- a statement of why the subject is important to the study
- a promise of confidentiality (including an explanation of the identifying number on the questionnaire)
- reference to the incentive (if any)
- a statement of what to do if questions arise (including direct access to the signatory)
- an expression of appreciation.

Additional components of the introduction to any questionnaire have already been discussed in Chapter 6. The letter should be no more than a single page, and there is some evidence that response rates are improved if the signatory has a title (Kanuk and Berenson 1975). Response rates have been shown to be better if, when possible and relevant, the letter is signed by the subject's usual medical practitioner rather than by the research worker (Smith *et al*. 1985).

A postscript reinforcing the request for co-operation has not been found to increase response rates (Fox *et al*. 1988). A promise of complete anonymity produced no greater initial response, and ultimately a poorer response because of inability to follow-up non-responders, than an explanation that the questionnaire was numbered and a follow-up letter would be sent if no reply was received (Campbell and Waters 1990).

Questionnaire size

Response rates appear to be comparatively insensitive to length of the questionnaire, up to about 12 pages (see Chapter 6). Dillman (1978), however, recommends that it be printed with reduction to 20 cm by 15 cm ($8\frac{1}{4} \times 6\frac{1}{8}$ in)) so that it looks quite small. For similar reasons it should be printed on both sides of the paper, and in booklet form for ease of use.

Special class mailings

A number of studies have shown that first-class mail, as compared with lower class or bulk rate mail, and special class mailings, such as air mail, where air mail is not routine, and certified or recorded delivery mail, as compared with first-class mail, increase response rates (Baumgartner and Heberlein 1984; Fox *et al*. 1988). There is evidence to suggest that initial use of certified mail can get a better overall response rate even when certified mail is used for all non-respondents, whether contacted initially by certified mail or by regular first-class mail (Rimm *et al*. 1990). Thus the full effect of certified mailings may not be achievable if they are restricted to follow-up mailings. It is also the practice of some to use commemorative or multiple small denomination stamps on outward mailings to increase the respondent's initial interest in the letter. The effectiveness of these practices has not been established.

Incentives

The most effective incentive appears to be something enclosed with the original or a follow-up letter, usually cash (Linsky 1975; Baumgartner and Heberlein 1984; Berry and Kanouse 1987). Other incentives that are used include an offer of a report of the results of the survey, lottery tickets, or participation by respondents in some other kind of prize draw, pens, etc. Of these, participation in a prize draw (US$200) has been shown to be effective but not apparently as effective as a US$1 cash incentive (Hubbard and Little 1988; Spry *et al*. 1989). A promise of a donation to charity was not effective (Hubbard and Little 1988).

The monetary incentive need not be large. Most of the original research, done some years ago, used a 25 cent coin. A dollar, or its approximate equivalent in another currency, is now more effective (Hubbard and Little 1988). Larger sums (up to US$20) have been used, but there are some indications that the use of too large a sum may be counterproductive. It appears that the incentive, given unconditionally (i.e. included with the initial mailing), acts as a token of good faith between the investigator and the subject. A large sum may appear to be less of a token and more like compensation which will almost inevitably be insufficient. There is evidence that final response rates may be just as high if the incentive is enclosed only with later mailings to non-respondents. This approach will lead to financial savings.

A coloured questionnaire

In a meta-analysis covering three studies, it was found that a green question-naire obtained a better response rate than a white questionnaire (Fox *et al.* 1988).

Stamped return envelope

A stamped return envelope is effective in increasing response rates when used as an alternative to a 'business reply paid' or franked envelope (Fox *et al.* 1988; Shiono and Klebanoff 1991). The stamp may have a token value like that of a small monetary incentive.

Multiple mailings

A programme of multiple mailings is probably the single most important strategy for increasing response rates in mail surveys. Dillman (1978) recommends the following programme as part of his 'total design method'.

1. Exactly 1 week after the questionnaire is first mailed, a postcard (a sealed letter is likely to be preferable for most epidemiological purposes) is sent to all subjects to thank those who have responded already and to remind those who have not.
2. A follow-up letter is mailed to non-respondents exactly 3 weeks after the first mailing. This letter informs them that their questionnaire has not been received and restates the importance of their response.
3. A further follow-up letter is sent to non-respondents, by certified mail, 7 weeks after the first mailing. This mailing includes a copy of the questionnaire—a strategy that has been shown to be effective in increasing response (Baumgartner and Heberlein 1984).

Follow-up and interview by telephone or home visit

The value of follow-up by different survey modes is well established (see p. 298). In follow-up in a mail survey, it is usual to begin first with an attempted contact by telephone, and then by home visit if there is no telephone available or telephone contact is not achieved. The study by Battistutta *et al.* (1983) suggests that telephone or home visit *reminders* are unlikely to be effective in obtaining responses and so, when contact is made, the questionnaire should be completed by interview if at all possible.

Telephone interview surveys

The factors that increase response in telephone and face-to-face interview surveys have received a great deal less attention than those influencing response to mail surveys—probably because of a perception that mail surveys are more in need of response-maximization strategies. However, many

Table 11.3 Factors that may increase response rates in telephone surveys

---

Empirically supported
  Advance letter
  Experienced interviewers
  Interviewers perceived as sounding confident and competent
  Personalized approach on telephone contact
  Delay in household screening
  Brief household screening procedures with immediate approach to
    selected respondent (random digit dialling)
  Callbacks to households that initially fail to participate (random digit
    dialling)
  Multiple attempts at contact
  Follow-up by mail questionnaire or home visit and face-to-face interview

Recommended
  Blanket publicity
  Carefully constructed introduction
  Availability of verification of interview's credentials
  Elimination of interviewers with high refusal rates
  Use of particularly experienced interviewers to follow-up near refusals

---

of the principles outlined above for mail surveys can be applied to telephone and face-to-face surveys. Factors that may increase response rates in telephone surveys have been reviewed by Dillman (1978) and Groves and Lyberg (1988) and are summarized in Table 11.3. Many of these factors also apply to the recruitment of subjects for a survey by telephone (e.g. by random digit dialling).

Advance letter

An advance letter does increase the response in telephone surveys in which the name and address of the subject is known (Dillman *et al.* 1976; Cannell and Fowler 1977). An initial, purely introductory telephone call may have similar effects (Groves and Kahn 1979). According to Dillman (1978), an advance letter '. . . eliminates the element of surprise . . . [and] provides tangible evidence that the interviewer is legitimate and that the telephone call is neither a sales gimmick nor a practical joke'. The letter should advise that the subject will be called soon, provide a brief description of the study topic and its importance, give an indication of how long the interview will take, offer the possibility of requesting callback at a later time if the call comes at an inconvenient time, and, finally, express appreciation to the subjects and give them the option of calling the study director for more information (Dillman 1978). The letter should not ask the subjects whether they are willing to be interviewed, or ask them to indicate their willingness to participate prior to the telephone call. The seeking of consent to interview prior to the first telephone contact reduces participation rates (Mueller *et al.* 1986).

Blanket publicity

Blanket publicity in the news media has been recommended by Gorden (1975), and probably has the same effect as an advance letter. The subject is more likely to accept the interviewer's credentials when he or she calls.

Interviewers

Hartge *et al.* (1984) noted that the highest response rates in their experience of random digit dialling surveys were obtained by experienced interviewers. Response rates do appear to vary among interviewers, and response rates have been increased by 'weeding out' interviewers with consistently high refusal rates (Dillman *et al.* 1976). Male and female interviewers do not differ in response rates when level of experience is controlled (Groves and Lyberg 1988). There is evidence that interviewers who are perceived as sounding confident and competent obtain better response rates than those who do not (Oksenberg and Cannell 1988). These perceptions are contributed to by the interviewer speaking rapidly (at least in the introduction), loudly, with standard pronunciation, and with a falling rather than a rising tone on key words.

Personalized approach

Dillman *et al.* (1976) found that when approaching a named respondent, response rates were higher when the opening introduction was personalized ('Hello. Is this Mr/Mrs *(first and last name)*?') than when an impersonal opening introduction was given ('This is *(interviewer's name)* at Washington State University in Pullman and I'm calling for our Social Research Center.'). The respondent's name will be known in most epidemiological studies, although not when subjects are being obtained by random digit dialling.

Carefully constructed introduction

Most refusals occur at the end of the introduction. While there are no empirical data to guide the construction of the introduction, clearly great care should be taken. Dillman (1978) recommends that the introduction should begin by ascertaining that the correct number and correct person (if relevant) have been reached. The interviewer should then introduce himself or herself and the sponsoring organization. A statement of the purpose of the call should be made, the respondent's selection explained, and the expected duration of the interview given. Finally the interviewer should offer to answer any questions that the subject may have and solicit participation by saying: 'Okay?'

Verification of the interviewer's credentials

Because the interviewer is unable in a telephone interview to offer visible proof of his or her identity and association with the sponsoring organization, he or she should, if challenged, offer the respondent the option of calling a number to verify the credentials and then come back to the interviewer.

Incentives

In the one study in which it has been tested, the offer of a monetary incentive (US$10) decreased rather than increased response rates in a telephone survey by random digit dialling (Ward *et al.* 1984).

Delay in household screening

A better response rate has been reported when personal information was first sought from the telephone answerer, and then information about other household members obtained, than when information about the whole household was sought first (Groves and Lyberg 1988). This result is consistent with the views of many interviewers that the household roster (the information needed for random selection of an appropriate respondent from the household) is one of the most difficult sets of information to obtain early in the interview.

Immediate interview of selected subject on random digit dialling

Harlow and Hartge (1983) reported a very high response rate (91 per cent) in a random digit dialling survey seeking an age-stratified sample of women 30–69 years of age when the selected woman was asked for an interview by telephone immediately after the household had been screened for eligible respondents. In a small experiment comparing this approach with the more usual approach of obtaining full names and addresses on screening and sending a preliminary letter to the selected subject, the direct approach achieved a 16 per cent higher response rate. In random digit dialling, refusal to co-operate occurs most commonly at the stage of household screening, and it was thought that elimination of the need to ask for full name and address contributed to the high response rate of the direct approach. Respondent selection rules must be simple enough for immediate application by the interviewer in this approach. The loss in sampling efficiency that results from immediate selection of respondents may be a small price to pay for a substantially increased response rate.

Callbacks to initial or impending refusals

Callbacks by another, usually more experienced, interviewer to households that initially failed to co-operate can result in interviews in 25–40 per cent of cases (Groves and Lyberg 1988). This second-round success probably results from a different person answering the telephone, the call coming at a more convenient time for the respondent, or the superior skills of the second interviewer. A policy of calling back to households where initial refusal has occurred, however, may be viewed as unethical by some ethical review committees.

Multiple attempts at contact

About a third of possible interviews can be completed after three calls. In the USA at least, it takes 12 calls to complete 75 per cent of interviews and 24 calls to complete 90 per cent (Sebold 1988). Attempts should be made both in the evening and at weekends. Extension of the period over which calls are made will reduce the proportion of telephones that are unanswered at the end of a study. A careful record should be kept of calls made so that the call strategy can be carefully planned.

Follow-up mail questionnaire or home visit

Response rates to telephone surveys can be increased by mail or home visit follow-up, if contact is not established by telephone. The mail may catch an elusive but otherwise willing respondent, and a home visit may provide information about the reasons for non-contact (e.g. by asking the neighbours) that will lead to later contact. If the sample has been selected by random digit dialling, only the proportion of selected respondents who participate can be increased by such follow-up methods, as refusal at the household level usually occurs before the name and address of any member of the household has been obtained (Ward *et al.* 1984).

Face-to-face interview surveys

Factors that may increase response rates in face-to-face interview surveys are summarized in Table 11.4.

Blanket publicity

Blanket publicity in the news media has been shown to increase participation in the US Health Examination Survey (Schaible 1972).

Advance contact

Several studies have shown that advance contact by mail or telephone has decreased rather than increased response rates — possibly because the subject was given the opportunity to refuse (easily) by mail or telephone (Cartwright and Tucker 1967; Brunner and Carroll 1968). On the other hand, Bergsten *et al.* (1984) found that an advance letter and telephone call gave a 20 per cent saving in data collection costs (because of the greater efficiency of arranged home visits) with only a 1 per cent reduction in response rate. A very high response rate was reported for a face-to-face interview survey in which subjects were mailed a copy of a news story about the survey with a photograph

Table 11.4 Factors that may increase response rates in face-to-face interview surveys

---

Empirically supported
  Blanket publicity
  Prior mailing of copy of news story about survey including photograph of
    interviewer
  Experienced interviewers
  Avoidance of signed consent procedures
  Multiple attempts at contact
  Follow-up by mail questionnaire or telephone contact and interview

Recommended
  Careful selection and training of interviewers
  Carefully constructed introduction
  Well-planned callbacks
  Use of particularly experienced interviewers to follow-up near refusals

---

of the interviewer (Gorden 1975). On balance, it seems likely that some form of advance contact will, at least, increase efficiency without reducing response rates provided that it does not give the subject the opportunity to refuse. It has been the practice of one of the authors (B.K.A.), when conducting case-control studies by personal interview, to write giving a time at which the interviewer will call and asking for a response only if the proposed time is inconvenient to the respondent. While this does provoke a few refusals, it is often possible to encourage the subject to participate when he or she calls.

Interviewers

Experienced interviewers have the lowest refusal rates (US Bureau of the Census 1972). It is probably a good strategy for an interviewer to withdraw when refusal appears imminent but has not been made explicit, so that a more experienced interviewer can attempt to obtain the interview.

Signed consent

A request for signed consent at the beginning of an interview has been shown to reduce response rates (Bradburn and Sudman 1979). If necessary at all, the request should be made at the end of the interview provided, of course, that this approach is approved by the relevant ethical review committee (see Chapter 12). This approach may be particularly useful when the study involves both an interview and the collection of a blood sample, but signed consent is required only for the blood sample.

Incentives

Incentives are not generally recommended for face-to-face interview surveys except when something additional is being asked of the subject (e.g. completion of a diary or submission to some form of physical examination or test; Cannell and Fowler 1977). A US$10 honorarium was found to increase response to requests for examination in the US Health Examination Survey (Bryant *et al.* 1975).

Multiple attempts at contact

A minimum of four calls should be made to a house when trying to obtain a face-to-face interview. It is usual, after the first or second contact failure, to attempt to find out the subject's movements or whereabouts from neighbours so that subsequent calls can be more strategically planned.

Follow-up by mail or telephone contact

It may be possible to contact a subject by mail or telephone when contact in person at home has not been achieved.

Tracing subjects who are hard to find

When the subjects of a study have been individually identified before measurement of exposure begins (e.g. in a disease register, in a population register, among the members of a cohort with a particular exposure experience), one element of maximization of response rates is the successful initial tracing of subjects so that their present vital status can be determined and exposure data collected, when that is appropriate. There is evidence to suggest that subjects who cannot be found may differ more from subjects who respond than do subjects who can be found but refuse to respond (Decouflé *et al.* 1991). Thus, finding subjects who are hard to find may be as or more important in minimizing bias as obtaining a high response rate in those who are easily found.

Maintaining contact with and finding the whereabouts of subjects of cohort studies and clinical trials has been reviewed in detail elsewhere (Kelsey *et al.* 1986; Meinert and Tonascia 1986; Checkoway *et al.* 1989). Most of the strategies used in these circumstances are also appropriate when subjects must be found for exposure mesurement. Those that are particularly relevant to this purpose are summarized in Table 11.5; they are largely self-explanatory. They have been listed in order of perceived degree of difficulty and/or cost. It is usual to pursue the simpler approaches first, and resort to the more difficult approaches only when simpler ones fail and the additional effort and cost is considered to be justified by the likely reduction in bias that might result.

Not all the approaches listed in Table 11.5 are available in all study areas.

Table 11.5 Strategies for locating subjects who are hard to find

- Check telephone books and/or directory assistance for new telephone numbers and addresses.
- Check town or city residents' directories if they exist.
- Seek new address information through whatever facilities may exist for this in the local postal service.
- Contact physicians or hospitals who provided original identification of cases or controls.
- Check with personal contacts or relatives of subjects if any are known.
- For someone with an unusual last name, call others with the same name listed in the telephone book for the same area.
- Use reverse directories (telephone number by address), if they exist, to telephone new residents of old addresses or old neighbours.
- Write to or visit new residents of old addresses or old neighbours.
- If home has been sold, see if real estate agency has new address.
- Check national registers (e.g. electoral records, social security records, driver's licence records, public utility subscribers, taxation records, health insurance records, death index) for new address or vital status information.
- Check with marriage registers for changes of last names.
- Use credit bureau or other private agency that specializes in locating people.

Some (e.g. checking national registers) will depend on the existence of a good working relationship between the investigators and the relevant authorities and the absence of legal restrictions to access. In some situations, custodians of national registers may be willing to forward correspondence to a new address without making that new address available to the investigator; while not optimal, this approach will sometimes have the desired result. Some of the strategies may be possible only when special provision has been made for follow-up in an earlier phase of the study. For example, the data initially collected in a well-conducted cohort study may include names of relatives or other personal contacts. These contacts may be able to provide tracing information when subjects must be contacted again to provide exposure data for a case-control study being conducted within the cohort study, or for other reasons.

SUMMARY

The determinants of the probability that a subject will participate (respond) in an epidemiological study, the effects of low response rates, and techniques for increasing response rates have been dealt with in this chapter because of their importance to the measurement of exposure in whole populations and because they may vary between methods of measurement of exposure.

There is evidence that the response rates in population surveys in the United States has fallen over the past 40 years, with the change being most evident in large cities. This trend may have been halted by the introduction of telephone survey techniques.

Response rates tend to be highest for face-to-face interviews, intermediate for telephone interviews, and least for mailed questionnaires. The use of multiple methods of approach after initial non-response, however, can narrow the response gap between methods while not reducing the cost advantage of telephone and mail approaches.

Failure to participate in surveys is not a random phenomenon; it correlates with a variety of characteristics of individuals, particularly greater age, less education, lower socioeconomic status, current smoking, and poor present health. Thus, in theory at least, non-response can lead to appreciable bias in some characteristics of the sample of subjects although, when samples of the same population with low and high response rates have been compared, the differences in prevalence proportions of relevant characteristics have been small.

The effect of selection bias due to non-response on the odds ratio of disease in a population can be simply estimated from Equation 11.1:

$$OR_R = \frac{P_a P_d}{P_b P_c} \times OR_P$$

where OR_R is the odds ratio in the respondents, OR_P is the odds ratio in the population, and $P_a, P_b, P_c,$ and P_d are respectively the response proportions in those with the risk factor and the disease, those with the risk factor but without the disease, those without the risk factor but with the disease, and those without the risk factor and without the disease. In a study in which these proportions were estimated, OR_R varied from 0.83 to 1.63 times OR_P depending on the risk factor and disease combination being studied.

A variety of techniques can be used to maximize response rates in different kinds of epidemiological studies. They include:

- Blanket publicity before the survey
- appropriate advance notice of contact
- personalization of correspondence and approaches by telephone
- use of special class mailings (e.g. certified mail)
- a carefully constructed introductory letter or statement signed, if possible, by someone salient to the subject
- telephone interviewers perceived as sounding confident and competent
- availability of checking of telephone interviewers credentials
- an immediate approach to subjects identified through random digit dialling
- the offer of a monetary incentive
- *stamped* return envelopes
- avoidance of signed consent procedures at the beginning of interviews
- use of experienced interviewers
- multiple approaches to subjects

- a further approach by especially experienced interviewers to subjects who refuse initially.

Strategies should also be adopted to locate study subjects who are initially hard to find.

REFERENCES

Austin, M. A., Criqui, M. H., Barrett-Connor, E., and Holdbrook, M. J. (1981). The effect of response bias on the odds ratio. *American Journal of Epidemiology*, **114**, 137-43.

Barton, J., Bain, C., Hennekens, C. H., Rosner, B., Belanger, C., Roth, A., and Speizer, F. (1980). Characteristics of respondents and non-respondents to a mailed questionnaire. *American Journal of Public Health*, **70**, 823-5.

Battistutta, D., Byth, K., Norton, R., and Rose, G. (1983). Response rates: a comparison of mail, telephone and personal interview strategies for an Australian population. *Community Health Studies*, **7**, 309-13.

Baumgartner, R. M. and Heberlein, T. A. (1984). Recent research on mailed questionnaire response rates. In *Making effective use of mailed questionnaires*, (ed. D. C. Lockhart), pp. 65-76. Jossey-Bass, San Francisco, California.

Benfante, R., Reed, D., MacLean, C., and Kagan, A. (1989). Response bias in the Honolulu Heart Program. *American Journal of Epidemiology*, **130**, 1088-100.

Bergsten, J. W., Weeks, M. F., and Bryan, F. A. (1984). Effects of an advance telephone call in a personal interview survey. *Public Opinion Quarterly*, **48**, 650-7.

Berry, S. H. and Kanouse, D. E. (1987). Physician responses to a mailed survey, an experiment in timing of payment. *Public Opinion Quarterly*, **51**, 102-14.

Bradburn, N. M. and Sudman, S. (1979). *Improving interview method and questionnaire design*. Jossey-Bass, San Francisco.

Brambilla, D. J. and McKinlay, S. M. (1987). A comparison of responses to mailed questionnaires and telephone interviews in a mixed mode health survey. *American Journal of Epidemiology*, **126**, 962-71.

Brunner, G. A. and Carroll, S. J. (1968). The effect of prior telephone appointments on completion rates and response content. *Public Opinion Quarterly*, **31**, 652-4.

Bryant, E. E., Kovar, M. G., and Miller, H. (1975). A study of the effect of remuneration upon responses in the health and nutrition examination survey. *Vital and Health Statistics*, Series 2, No. 67. Department of Health, Education, and Welfare, Washington. (DHEW Publication No. (HRA) 76-1341).

Bull, S. B., Pederson, L. L., Ashley, M. J., and Lefcoe, N. M. (1988). Intensity of follow-up. Effects on estimates in a population telephone survey with an extension of Kish's (1965) approach. *American Journal of Epidemiology*, **127**, 552-61.

Burgess, A. M. and Tierney, J. T. (1970). Bias due to non-response in a mail survey of Rhode Island physicians' smoking habits – 1968. *New England Journal of Medicine*, **282**, 908.

Campbell, M. J. and Waters, W. E. (1990). Does anonymity increase response rate in postal questionnaire surveys about sensitive subjects? A randomised trial. *Journal of Epidemiology and Community Health*, **44**, 75-6.

Cannell, C. F. and Fowler, F. J. (1977). Interviewers and interviewing techniques. In

Advances in health survey research methods: Proceedings of a National Invitational Conference, National Center for Health Services Research Proceedings Series, (ed. L.G. Reeder), pp. 13–23. Department of Health, Education, and Welfare, Washington. (DHEW Publication No. (HRA) 77–3154).

Cartwright, A. (1986). Who responds to postal questionnaires? *Journal of Epidemiology and Community Health*, **40**, 267–73.

Cartwright, A. and Tucker, W. (1967). An attempt to reduce the number of calls in an interview inquiry. *Public Opinion Quarterly*, **31**, 652–4.

Checkoway, H., Pearce, N., and Crawford-Brown, D. J. (1989). *Research methods in occupational epidemiology*. Oxford University Press, New York.

Cobb, S., King, S., and Chen, E. (1957). Differences between respondents and non-respondents in a morbidity survey involving clinical examination. *Journal of Chronic Diseases*, **6**, 95–108.

Comstock, G.W. and Helsing, K. (1973). Characteristics of respondents and non-respondents to a questionnaire for estimating community mood. *American Journal of Epidemiology*, **97**, 233–9.

Cottler, L.B., Zipp, J.F., Robins, L.N., and Spitznagel, E.L. (1987). Difficult-to-recruit respondents and their effect on prevalence estimates in an epidemiologic survey. *American Journal of Epidemiology*, **125**, 329–39.

Criqui, M.H. (1979). Response bias and risk ratios in epidemiologic studies. *American Journal of Epidemiology*, **109**, 394–9.

Criqui, M.H., Austin, M., and Barrett-Connor, E., (1979). The effects of non-response on risk ratios in a cardiovascular disease study. *Journal of Chronic Diseases*, **32**, 633–8.

Criqui, M.H., Barrett-Connor, E., and Austin, M. (1978). Differences between respondents and non-respondents in a population-based cardiovascular disease study. *American Journal of Epidemiology*, **108**, 367–72.

Decoufflé, P., Holmgreen, P., Calle, E.E., and Weeks, M.F. (1991). Nonresponse and intensity of follow-up in an epidemiologic study of Vietnam-era veterans. *American Journal of Epidemiology*, **133**, 83–95.

De Maio, T.J. (1980). Refusals: who, where and why. *Public Opinion Quarterly*, **44**, 223–33.

Dillman, D.A., (1978). *Mail and telephone surveys*. John Wiley and Sons, New York.

Dillman, D.A. Gallegos, J.G., and Frey, J.H. (1976). Reducing refusal rates for telephone interviews. *Public Opinion Quarterly*, **40**, 66–78.

Doll, R. and Hill, A.B. (1964). Mortality in relation to smoking: ten years' observations of British doctors. *British Medical Journal*, **1**, 1399–410.

Dorn, H.F. (1950). Methods of analysis for follow-up studies. *Human Biology*, **22**, 238–48.

Fox, R.J., Crask, M.R., and Jonghoon, K. (1988). Mail survey response rate. A meta-analysis of selected techniques for inducing response. *Public Opinion Quarterly*, **52**, 467–91.

Gorden, R.L. (1975). *Interviewing: strategy, techniques and tactics*. Dorsey Press, Homewood, Illinois.

Gordon, T., Moore, F.E., Shurtleff, D., and Dawber, T.R. (1959). Some methodological problems in the long-term study of cardiovascular disease: observations on the Framingham Study. *Journal of Chronic Diseases*, **10**, 186–206.

Greenland, S. (1977). Response and follow-up bias in cohort studies. *American Journal of Epidemiology*, **106**, 184–7.

Greenlick, M.R., Bailey, J.W., Wild, J., and Grover, J. (1979). Characteristics of men most likely to respond to an invitation to be screened. *American Journal of Public Health*, **69**, 1011–5.

Groves, R.M. and Kahn, R.L. (1979). *Surveys by telephone. A national comparison with personal interviews*. Academic Press, New York.

Groves, R.M. and Lyberg, L.E. (1988). An overview of non-response issues in telephone surveys. In *Telephone survey methodology*, (ed. R.M. Groves, P.P. Biemer, L.E. Lyberg, J.T. Massey, W.L. Nicholls, and J. Waksberg), pp. 191–211. John Wiley and Sons, New York.

Hammond, E.C. (1959). Inhalation in relation to type and amount of smoking. *Journal of American Statistical Association*, **54**, 35–51.

Harlow, B.L. and Hartge, P. (1983). Telephone household screening and interviewing. *American Journal of Epidemiology*, **117**, 632–3.

Hartge, P., Brinton, L.A., Rosenthal, J.F., Cahill, J.I., Hoover, R.N., and Waksberg, J. (1984). Random digit dialling in selecting a population-based control group. *American Journal of Epidemiology*, **120**, 825–33.

Heath, C.W. (1958). Differences between smokers and non-smokers. *Archives of Internal Medicine*, **101**, 377–88.

Hochstim, J.R. (1967). A critical comparison of three strategies of collecting data from households. *Journal of American Statistical Association*, **62**, 976–82.

Hubbard, R. and Little, E.L. (1988). Promised contributions to charity and mail survey responses. Replication with extension. *Public Opinion Quarterly*, **52**, 223–30.

Iversen, L. and Sabroe, S.(1988). Participation in a follow-up study of health among unemployed and employed people after a company closedown: drop outs and selection bias. *Journal of Epidemiology and Commununity Health*, **42**, 396–401.

Kalton, G. (1983). *Compensating for missing survey data*. Institute of Social Research, University of Michigan, Ann Arbor, Michigan.

Kanuk, L. and Berenson, C. (1975). Mail surveys and response rates: A literature review. *Journal of Marketing Research*, **12**, 440–53.

Kaplan, S. and Cole, P. (1970). Factors affecting response to postal questionnaires. *British Journal of Preventive and Social Medicine*, **24**, 245–7.

Kelsey, J.L., Thompson, W.D., and Evans, A.S. (1986). *Methods in observational epidemiology*. Oxford University Press, New York.

Kleinbaum, D.G., Morgernstern, H., and Kupper, L.L. (1981). Selection bias in epidemiologic studies. *American Journal of Epidemiology*, **113**, 452–63.

Kviz, F. (1977). Towards a standard definition of response rate. *Public Opinion Quarterly*, **41**, 265–7.

Linsky, A.S. (1975). Stimulating responses to mailed questionnaires: A review. *Public Opinion Quarterly*, **39**, 82–101.

Loewenstein, R., Colombotos, J., and Elinson, J. (1969). Interviews hardest-to-obtain in an urban health survey. *Milbank Memorial Fund Quarterly*, **47**, 195–200.

Marshall, B.G. and Gee, C.A. (1976). *Mail questionnaire research: a selected bibliography with selected annotations*. Council of Planning Librarians, Exchange Bibliography No. 994, March 1976.

Meinert, C. L., and Tonascia, S. (1986). *Clinical trials. Design, conduct and analysis.* Oxford University Press, New York.

Mueller, B. A., McTiernan, A., and Daling, J. R. (1986). Level of response in epidemiologic studies using the card-back system to contact subjects. *American Journal of Public Health*, **76**, 1331–2.

Oakes, T. W., Friedman, G. D., and Seltzer, C. C. (1973). Mail survey response by health status of smokers, non-smokers, and ex-smokers. *American Journal of Epidemiology*, **98**, 50–5.

Oksenberg, L. and Cannell, C. (1988). Effects of interviewer vocal characteristics on non-response. In *Telephone survey methodology*, (ed. R. M. Groves, P. P. Biemer, L. E. Lyberg, J. T. Massey, W. L. Nicholls, and J. Waksberg), pp. 257–69. John Wiley and Sons, New York.

Paul, O., Lepper, M. H., Phelan, W. H., Dupertuis, G. W., MacMillan, A., McKean, H., and Park, H. (1963). A longitudinal study of coronary heart disease. *Circulation*, **28**, 20–31.

Rimm, E. B., Stampfer, M. J., Colditz, G. A., Giovannucci, E., and Willett, W. C. (1990). Effectiveness of various mailing strategies among non-respondents in a prospective cohort study. *American Journal of Epidemiology*, **131**, 1068–71.

Robins, L. N. (1963). The reluctant respondent. *Public Opinion Quarterly*, **27**, 276–86.

Rolnick, S. J., Gross, C. J., Garrard, J., and Gibson, R. W. (1989). A comparison of response rate, data quality, and cost in the collection of data on sexual history and personal behaviours. Mail survey approaches and in-person interviews. *American Journal of Epidemiology*, **129**, 1052–61.

Sandler, R. S. and Holland, K. L. (1990). Fate of incorrectly addressed mailed questionnaires. *Journal of Clinical Epidemiology*, **43**, 45–7.

Schaible, W. L. (1972). Quality control in a National Health Examination Survey. *Vital and Health Statistics*, Series 2, No. 34. Department of Health, Education, and Welfare, Washington. (DHEW Publication No. (HSM) 72–1023.)

Schleifer, S. (1986). Trends in attitudes toward participation in survey research. *Public Opinion Quarterly*, **50**, 17–26.

Sebold, J. (1988). Survey period length, unanswered numbers, and non-response in telephone surveys. In *Telephone survey methodology*, (R. M. Groves, P. P. Biemer, L. E. Lyberg, J. T. Massey, W. L. Nicholls, and J. Waksberg) pp. 247–56. John Wiley and Sons, New York.

Shiono, P. H. and Klebanoff, M. A. (1991). The effect of two mailing strategies on the response to a survey of physicians. *American Journal of Epidemiology*, **134**, 539–42.

Siemiatycki, J. (1979). A comparison of mail, telephone, and home interview strategies for household health surveys. *American Journal of Public Health*, **69**, 238–45.

Siemiatycki, J. and Campbell, S. (1984). Non-response bias and early versus all responders in mail and telephone surveys. *American Journal of Epidemiology*, **120**, 291–301.

Smith, W. C. S., Crombie, I. K., Campion, P. D., and Knox, J. D. E. (1985). Comparison of response rates to a postal questionnaire from a general practice research unit. *British Medical Journal*, **291**, 1483–5.

Spry, V. M., Hovell, M. F., Sallis, J. G., Hofstetter, C. R., Elder, J. P., and Molgaard,

C. A. (1989). Recruiting survey respondents to mailed surveys: Controlled trials of incentives and prompts. *American Journal of Epidemiology*, **130**, 166–72.

Steeh, C. G. (1981). Trends in non-response rates, 1952–1979. *Public Opinion Quarterly*, **45**, 40–57.

Theodore, A., Berger, A. G., and Palmer, C. E. (1956). A follow-up study of tuberculosis in former student nurses I. Methods of locating and obtaining information from a study population of 25,752. *Journal of Chronic Diseases*, **3**, 499–520.

US Bureau of the Census (1972). *Investigation of census bureau interviewer characteristics, performance and attitudes: a summary*, Working Paper No. 34. US Government Printing Office, Washington.

Vernon, S. W., Roberts, R. E., and Lee, E. S. (1984). Ethnic status and participation in longitudinal health surveys. *American Journal of Epidemiology*, **119**, 99–113.

Walker, M., Shaper, A. G., and Cook, D. G. (1987). Non-participation and mortality in a prospective study of cardiovascular disease. *Journal of Epidemiology and Community Health*, **41**, 295–9.

Walter, S. D., Marrett, L. D., and Mishkel, N. (1988). Effect of contact letter on control response rates in cancer studies. *American Journal of Epidemiology*, **127**, 691–4.

Ward, E. M., Kramer, S., and Meadows, A. T. (1984). The efficacy of random digit dialling in selecting matched controls for a case-control study of pediatric cancer. *American Journal of Epidemiology*, **120**, 582–91.

Weeks, M. F., Kulka, R. A., Lessler, J. T., and Whitmore, R. W. (1983). Personal versus telephone surveys for collecting household health data at the local level. *American Journal of Public Health*, **73**, 1389–94.

Wilhelmsen, L., Ljunberg, S., Wedel, H., and Werko, L. (1976). A comparison between participants and non-participants in a primary preventive trial. *Journal of Chronic Diseases*, **29**, 331–9.

Wingo, P. A., Ory, H. W., Layde, P. M., and Lee, N. C. (1988). The Cancer and Steroid Hormone Study Group: The evaluation of the data collection process for a multicenter, population-based, case-control design. *American Journal of Epidemiology*, **128**, 206–17.

Wu, M. and Brown, B. W. (1983). Detection and evaluation of bias in a postal survey of the health of dental personnel. In *Methods and issues in occupational and environmental epidemiology*, (ed. L. Chiazze, F. E. Lundin, and D. Watkins), pp. 133–42. Ann Arbor Science, Ann Arbor, Michigan.

12

Ethical issues

It may be accepted as a maxim that a poorly or improperly designed study involving human subjects . . . is by definition unethical. Moreover, when a study is in itself scientifically invalid, all other ethical considerations become irrelevant. There is no point in obtaining 'informed consent' to perform a useless study. (Attributed to David Rutstein by Silverman 1986)

INTRODUCTION

Ethics are rules or principles that govern right conduct. In the research context, 'right conduct' may be defined in terms of what is right for science, what is right for the subjects of the research, or what is right for society at large. Ethics based on social benefit and scientific merit are potentially in conflict with ethics that protect the rights of research subjects. A highly informative and therefore socially valuable investigation which is conducted according to sound scientific principles may carry unacceptable hazards to the subjects. Removal of the hazards may render the investigation less satisfactory, or even worthless scientifically, and therefore less useful, or even useless, socially. Resolution of this conflict between ehtics will almost always involve compromise and lead to a result which is less than wholly desirable when measured against some scale of values.

The atrocities committed in the name of medical science during World War II, the resulting Nuremberg trials, the Nuremberg Code which arose from them, and the Declaration of Helsinki, adopted by the World Medical Association in 1964 and revised in 1975, 1983, and 1989, have placed the ethical emphasis in biomedical research on protection of the rights of individual subjects (Bower and De Gasparis 1978). This chapter aims to outline the ethical principles involved in research on human subjects as they relate to the rights of those subjects, and how they might be applied in exposure measurement in epidemiology. A discussion of broader ethical issues in epidemiological research can be found in Soskolne (1989).

HUMAN RIGHTS AND EPIDEMIOLOGICAL RESEARCH

The United Nations Universal Declaration of Basic Human Rights is probably the most widely accepted statement of its kind. Those articles of it which are relevant to the participation of human subjects in epidemiological research are listed in Table 12.1. Articles 1 and 3 declare the right of freedom of the individual to decide whether or not to participate in research, Articles 3 and 5 declare the right of freedom from harm during the course of experimentation, and Article 12 declares the right of personal privacy.

The Nuremberg Code and the Declaration of Helsinki (Reynolds 1979) were aimed at protecting these rights by establishing a code of practice to be followed in biomedical research. They dealt mainly with the provision of informed consent, protection of the subject against physical injury, and the freedom of the subject to withdraw from the research at any time. The Nuremberg Code also made some cogent points about the quality of the research that might justify limitation of the rights of human subjects (Table 12.2). It is clear from these statements that the justification of the research in social terms and the quality of the methods whereby it is to be conducted must form part of the judgement as to whether or not it is ethical. Poor-quality research is unethical if it presents any threat at all to human rights and, perhaps, even if it presents no such threat because it wastes resources. This concept is also embodied in paragraph 20 of the 'Proposed International Guidelines for Biomedical Research Involving Human Subjects' published by the World Health Organization and the Council for International Organizations in Medical Sciences (CIOMS 1982): '. . . an experiment on human subjects that is scientifically unsound is *ipso facto* unethical, in that it may expose the subjects to risk of inconvenience to no purpose.'

Table 12.1 Articles of the United Nations Universal Declaration of Basic Human Rights that are relevant to the participation of human subjects in epidemiological research (see Reynolds 1979)

Article 1
All human beings are born free and equal in dignity and rights. They are endowed with reason and conscience and should act towards one another in a spirit of brotherhood.

Article 3
Everyone has the right to life, liberty and security of person.

Article 5
No one shall be subjected to torture or to cruel, inhuman or degrading treatment or punishment.

Article 12
No one shall be subjected to arbitrary interference with his privacy, family, home or correspondence, nor to attacks upon his honour and reputation. Everyone has the right to the protection of the law against such interference or attacks.

Table 12.2   Elements of the Nuremberg Code that deal with the quality of research in balance with the rights of human subjects

---

Article 2
The experiment should be such as to yield fruitful results for the good of society, unprocurable by other methods or means of study, and not random and unnecessary in nature.

Article 3
The experiment should be so designed and based on the results of animal experimentation and a knowledge of the natural history of disease or other problem under study that the anticipated results will justify the performance of the experiment.

These statements imply that judgements of the scientific quality and ethical acceptability of research should go hand in hand. This conjunction may be difficult to achieve in practice, at least by means of one committee, because of the different types of people required for each judgement (May 1975; Denham *et al.* 1979). For the research practitioner, they imply an ethical obligation to pursue excellence in research and thus, for example, to seek peer review of the objectives and methods of the research, in addition to seeking ethical review of the safeguards provided for human rights. They lead to the almost absolute requirement that all research on humans be conducted according to written protocols; without a written protocol the quality and ethical nature of the research cannot be assured nor judged by persons other than the investigators.

An ethical duty also logically arises, although it is not often clearly recognized, to publish the results of all research carried out on human subjects, whatever the results may be. If research is conducted which potentially impinges on the rights of human subjects, then the counterbalancing 'greater good' to society will not be realized unless the data are published. Also, it may be argued, given the application-oriented rather than purely biological character of most epidemiological research, that the epidemiologist has an ethical duty not to regard the publication of results as an end in itself, with no concern for any action that may appear to be needed in their light. This is of crucial importance in developing countries where the research epidemiologist also often has wider public health responsibilities. But even in developed countries the duty can be considered to arise ' . . . to speak as experts on behalf of the public health' (Rose 1989).

The conduct of epidemiological research, and specifically the measurement of exposure, may raise a number of problems relevant to the rights of research subjects. The three areas in which problems are most likely to arise are:

• free and informed consent to participate in research

- protection of personal privacy and confidentiality of personal data
- risk of physical or psychological harm.

Free and informed consent

The use of unreasonable pressure to elicit the co-operation of research subjects may violate Articles 1 and 3 of the United Nations Declaration (Table 12.1). High response rates are necessary if unbiased data are to be obtained. However, the use of multiple methods of approach to subjects, as recommended in Chapter 11, may be considered by some to be unreasonable pressure. At least one ethics committee has ruled that more than one postal reminder or a follow-up home visit were ethically unacceptable in a survey conducted initially by mail (Allen and Waters 1982). The use of financial incentives to obtain co-operation may also be considered by some to represent unreasonable pressure, although it is an effective way of increasing response (Chapter 11) and thus increasing the validity of the study.

There is a clear conflict between the ethical principle that subjects should be completely free to choose to participate or not in research and the ethical need, in most epidemiological studies, to ensure that a high participation rate is obtained for the sake of scientific validity. Where participation in the research presents minimal risk of harm to subjects, it seems reasonable to permit the use of methods of recruitment that maximize response. The issue of 'minimal risk' is dealt with in greater detail below.

Subjects may also be given incomplete information about the research. However, what constitutes 'incomplete' information may not be clear-cut or absolute and, like what constitutes 'unreasonable pressure', may be influenced by other ethical considerations. For example, it is common in case-control studies that the research hypotheses are not outlined in detail so as to avoid bias in the recall of exposures. In a case-control study of malignant melanoma, both cases and controls were told only that they were participating in a study of 'environment, lifestyle and health' (Holman and Armstrong 1984). It was hoped, thereby, to make the study equally salient to cases and controls. In a randomized-controlled trial of a vegetarian diet in the control of mild hypertension, subjects were all given 50 mg of vitamin C daily and told that the aim of the study was to determine the effect of vitamin C on blood pressure in interaction with dietary change (Margetts *et al*. 1985). This was intended to create a uniform placebo response across the experimental and control diets because of the impossibility of keeping the subjects blind to the dietary change. It is doubtful whether, in either of these examples, it would have been ethically more appropriate to inform the subjects of all details of the research at the risk of prejudicing the scientific validity of the studies, itself a prerequisite for an ethically acceptable investigation.

Privacy and confidentiality

Privacy has been defined, with survey research in mind, as 'the freedom of the individual to choose for himself the time and circumstances under which and the extent to which his attitudes, beliefs, behaviour and opinions are to be shared or withheld from others' (Rubehausen and Brim 1966). Invasion of privacy may violate Article 12 of the United Nations Declaration. In exposure measurement, privacy is fully preserved only if subjects interviewed by telephone or in person by an interviewer are contacted in advance by letter to obtain consent. Such an approach, however, may substantially reduce participation rates and so threaten the validity of the research.

Confidentiality is automatically preserved if epidemiological studies are restricted to the use of data which cannot be identified with the individuals to whom it relates. Such a restriction, however, greatly limits the capacity of epidemiology to provide answers to socially important questions (Gordis *et al.* 1977). When personal data provided by the subject within a confidential relationship are passed to a third party for research purposes, confidentiality can be protected by obtaining the subject's consent. Obtaining consent may be logistically difficult, however, particularly in large studies. It may indeed be impossible if, for example, the subjects must be identified first to be traced or if they are already dead. Thus, again, it can be seen that the epidemiologist's ethical duty to individual subjects is in conflict with his or her ethical duty to the wider community to conduct valid research.

Physical or psychological damage

The occurrence of injury in the course of research potentially violates Articles 1, 3 and 5 of the United Nations Declaration. The possibility of physical injury is much less common in epidemiology than in most areas of biomedical research. Physically invasive procedures are, however, used for the measurement of exposure to agents of disease – for example, the sampling of blood or tissue for measurement of the concentration of chemicals or detection of the results of chemical exposure. Psychological injury is also a possibility, especially when subjects are required to recall events that are embarrassing (e.g. details of sexual history or of socially undesirable behaviours) or that they would prefer to suppress. The sharing of this information with the investigator may also lead to anxiety about the potential effects of any subsequent breach of confidentiality. Occasionally too, research brings to light information about subjects that they might prefer not to know and prefer others not to know (e.g. presence of antibodies to the human immunodeficiency virus) and thus may cause them substantial distress.

In a mail survey of 128 participants in a case-control study of cervical neoplasia, conducted up to 12 months after interview, Savitz *et al.* (1986) found that 24 per cent of subjects were 'bothered' in some way by the interview questions. Of these, 30 per cent were bothered by questions on sexual partners, 6 per cent by questions on sexually transmitted disease, and 5 per cent by questions on pregnancies. Fifteen per cent recalled a desire to stop the interview during its course and, in retrospect, 3 per cent regretted their participation. On the positive side, 90 per cent were very or somewhat happy about their participation. Similar results were obtained in a survey of patients who had been followed up after mastectomy (Funch and Marshall 1981). While the topics of both these research projects were sensitive ones to women and might, perhaps, have generated more than average numbers of adverse feelings, they do indicate the potential of epidemiological research to cause some psychological distress.

ETHICAL PRACTICE IN EPIDEMIOLOGICAL RESEARCH

It is not uncommon for particular professional groups to establish an ethical code of their own (see, for example, the American Psychological Association's 'Ethical Principles in the Conduct of Research with Human Participants', CPHPR 1982). In the medical field, the basic document is the Declaration of Helsinki as revised in 1975 (CIOMS 1982). Specific guidelines exist for epidemiologists in a number of countries (Fluss *et al.* 1990), and guidelines for epidemiologists have recently been proposed for discussion at the international level (Last 1990).

Biomedical research workers, including epidemiologists, are also coming more and more to be judged by ethical codes laid down by governments, research funding bodies, or both. Probably the most influential of these codes is that mandated by the US Department of Health and Human Services for research that it funds (USDHHS 1981). Institutions in which such research is conducted are required to have an Institutional Review Board which operates according to the principles laid down by the Department. This board reviews and approves or disapproves, on ethical grounds, all research proposing the use of human subjects. The US Department of Health and Human Services exempts certain types of research from its requirements, but it is doubtful whether much aetiological research in epidemiology would be covered by these exemptions (except for research based solely on analysis of publicly available data) and the wisest course for epidemiologists is to seek Institutional Review Board approval for most if not all of their research.

In Australia, guidance on ethical principles in the conduct of medical and health research is provided by the National Health and Medical Research Council through its Health Ethics Committee. This guidance has been published in a Council Statement on Human Experimentation and a series of Supplementary Notes dealing with particular ethical issues (NHMRC 1988).

One of these supplementary Notes deals specifically with epidemiological research. The Council has also issued Guidelines for the Protection of Privacy in the Conduct of Medical Research (NHMRC 1990) which are approved by the Australian Privacy Commissioner under the Privacy Act of 1988 and, if followed, can permit the use of personal records in medical research without the consent of the record subjects having been sought. The Council will not fund a research project unless its protocol has been passed by an institutional ethics committee (the Australian equivalent of the US Institutional Review Boards) operating in accordance with Council guidelines. Similar procedures are in operation in a number of other countries, and ethical guidelines for multinational epidemiological studies within the European Community are currently under discussion.

Internationally the best established set of guidelines is the 'Proposed International Guidelines for Biomedical Research Involving Human Subjects' prepared by the World Health Organization and the Council for International Organizations of Medical Sciences (CIOMS 1982). As well as covering the general principles enunciated in Helsinki II, these guidelines give special attention to ethical problems that may arise in the conduct of research in developing countries under sponsorship from international agencies or developed countries.

Based on the documents just cited and our personal experience and subjective values we have summarized below, under eight headings, our advice on how an ethically acceptable balance may be achieved between the rights of individuals and the wider good of society as pursued through epidemiological research.

Written protocols

All epidemiological research should be conducted according to written protocols that specifically address ethical issues.

The basis for this recommendation has already been outlined. In summary, neither the investigator nor anyone else can be assured of the justification, scientific quality, or ethical propriety of a proposed research programme unless it has been thought through sufficiently to be put down on paper.

Ethics committees

All protocols for epidemiological research involving human subjects should be passed by a properly constituted institutional review board or ethics committee.

This practice provides protection from the natural tendency of investigators to view their research in a more favourable light than others might view it. Pragmatically, it is no longer possible in many countries to obtain funds for research from most funding bodies unless the protocol has been approved by an ethics committee.

The submission to the ethics committee should:

- state the aims of the research and whether or not the protocol has passed scientific peer review (for an optimal assessment this should be the case)
- clearly identify the subjects in terms of their numbers, age, sex, state of health, other demographic characteristics, if different from the general population, etc.
- describe the research procedures with details of any intervention proposed and emphasis on anything likely to have adverse consequences, such as physically or psychologically invasive procedures or administration of a drug or other potentially harmful substance
- list any potential benefits of the research to the subjects and to society
- describe in detail the information about the research that will be given to participants and how consent will be obtained
- state whether or not subjects will be remunerated and to what extent
- describe how the confidentiality of information about the subjects will be preserved.

Investigators' ethical responsibility

The investigators should in any case assure themselves that a particular research programme involving human subjects contains adequate safeguards for the rights of those subjects and that these are put into effect throughout all stages of the investigation.

Ultimately, the investigators themselves have responsibility for ethical aspects of their research. They do not absolve themselves of this responsibility when they have a protocol passed by an institutional review board or ethics committee.

Subject's consent

Consent must be obtained from each research subject for their direct participation in epidemiological research.

In giving information prior to obtaining consent, all information that may be material to a subject's decision to participate should be given. It should include:

- a clear explanation, in terms that the subject can understand, of the purposes of the study and the procedures to be followed
- a description of any discomfort and possible hazards involved
- an accurate statement of how much of the subject's time will be needed
- a description of the potential benefits to them and to society

- a statement that they are free to withdraw their participation at any time
- a statement, when relevant, that their future interests will not be prejudiced in any way by refusal to participate
- an offer to answer any questions that they may have.

For 'minimal risk research' the requirement for both complete information and written consent may be waived provided that any information important to the subjects is given to them after their participation has ended. The US Department of Health and Human Services (USDHHS 1981) defined 'minimal risk research' as research that offers anticipated risks of harm that are not greater, considering probability and magnitude, than those ordinarily encountered in daily life or during the performance of routine physical or psychological examinations or tests. The US code (USDHHS 1981) permits both 'fully informed' and 'written' consent provisions to be waived for minimal risk research, and this approach seems reasonable. Most epidemiological research probably qualifies as minimal risk research, although what 'risks ordinarily encountered in daily life' means in practice is open to wide subjective interpretation. It seems reasonable to hold, however, that participation in an interview or completion of a self-administered questionnaire carries minimal risk, and that if a subject so participates they have consented to the procedure.

As noted above, it may be important to the scientific validity of an investigation that the subjects not be provided with complete information about the purposes of the study at the time of their participation. If no alternatives to this choice exist, the attention of the ethics committee that reviews the protocol should be drawn to it and to the reasons for it. For example, in a case-control study of the relationship between birth defects and prenatal use of a particular drug, it would be wrong to give the name of the drug in question when explaining the purpose of the study to the participating mothers. Disclosure of the name of the drug would be likely both to lead to recruitment into the study of a higher proportion of mothers exposed to the drug than mothers not exposed, and to lead to more assiduous recall of exposure to the drug by mothers of malformed children than mothers of healthy children. These effects could produce a positive and potentially spurious association between the drug and birth defects (NHMRC 1985). It is doubtful whether in this case it would be necessary to go back to the subjects after the study is terminated and explain the true purpose. In other situations, however, it may be important to go back to the subjects after their participation has ended and disclose the previously hidden information (CPHPR 1982). For example, participants in a randomized-controlled trial should be advised, after the code has been broken, of what treatment they received.

Waiver of the requirement to obtain written consent is important to some epidemiological research. There are logistic problems, for example, in obtaining written consent to a telephone interview, especially if the subject has been selected by a process such as random digit dialling. In addition, a requirement for signed consent does reduce the participation rate in otherwise apparently harmless research (Chapter 11). Lack of a requirement for written documentation of consent, however, does not absolve the investigator from providing the subject with information about the research. Thus the protocol should still specify what information will be provided and how it will be given when written consent is not going to be obtained.

In some studies, information may be provided and consent obtained in two steps: initially, say, for interview and, subsequently, for the taking of a blood sample. This procedure may be justified to obtain the highest possible rate of participation in the interview, unimpeded by subjects' disinclination to have a blood sample taken. Special care should be taken, if this approach is adopted, to explain to the subjects that they are at liberty to refuse to participate in the second or any subsequent phase of the study.

It is usually not feasible in community-based intervention trials to obtain consent to the intervention from each individual member of the community. The decision whether or not to permit or undertake the research will, in these circumstances, usually lie with the responsible public health authority. However, all possible means should be used to inform the community concerned of the aims and nature of the research, and any possible hazards or inconvenience. If feasible, dissenting individuals should have the option of not participating (CIOMS 1982).

The obtaining of consent for research on children requires special attention. It is axiomatic that children should never be the subjects of research that could equally well be done in adults (CIOMS 1982). When children are the subjects of research, both their own consent and the consent of a parent or other legal guardian should be obtained. While the capacity of children to consent will be influenced by age and understanding, their willing co-operation should be sought, after they have been informed of the purposes and nature of the research and any possible discomfort or inconvenience. The amount of information given, and whether or not written consent will be sought from the parent or guardian, will be determined by the considerations outlined above.

Special considerations regarding consent are also necessary for research involving people with impaired mental capacity. It has been argued for such persons that '. . . it is extremely unlikely whether valid third party consent can be given for procedures which are not essential for the preservation of life or health, such as . . . participation in medical research projects of no direct benefit to the patient.' (Hayes and Hayes 1983). A similar argument might be made with respect to research involving highly unsophisticated, 'third world' populations, individuals from which may have little prospect of understanding any explanation of a research project (Jamrozik 1984).

Access to personal data sources

Access to medical or other records, or biological specimens carrying the identification of the subjects of epidemiological research, may be obtained without the prior consent of the subjects provided a number of conditions are met.
The conditions that should be met include:

- the access is essential to achievement of the objectives of the research
- a requirement for consent would render the research logistically or economically impracticable or would prejudice its scientific value
- the consent of the custodian of the records or specimens is obtained
- the data obtained from record abstraction or analyses on biological specimens are the minimum necessary to achievement of the objectives of the research
- the data are protected against disclosure to persons not immediately involved in the research
- they are not used for new research without the further consent of the custodian of the records and further ethical review.

Access to confidential data is essential to the conduct of much epidemiological research (Gordis and Gold 1980; MRC 1985). Accepting that, the issue becomes whether or not such access should be permitted without the knowledge and consent of the record subject. Obtaining consent would be impracticable in many situations (Gordis and Gold 1980), and a requirement to obtain it would prevent much potentially important research.

The view of most legal authorities and government commissions that have considered the matter has been that the consent of the record subjects to the disclosure of information about them for research purposes need not be obtained provided that certain conditions are met (Armstrong 1984). (It should be noted, however, that legal and ethical requirements do not necessarily coincide.) For example, the conditions set down by the US Privacy Protection Commission were as follows:

- that the discloser [record owner or custodian] cannot violate any limitations under which the information was collected
- that the disclosure in individually identifiable form must be necessary to the research [disclosure in non-identifiable form does not represent a breach of confidentiality]
- that the institution or practitioner [discloser] must be satisfied that the importance of the research is such that it warrants the risk to the individual in the exposure of the information to the researcher
- that the institution or practitioner must be satisfied that the researcher has established adequate safeguards to protect the disclosed information from unauthorised use

- that the institution or practitioner must retain the authority to consent in writing to any further use or re-disclosure of the information in individually identifiable form (Curran 1978).

The implied requirement, that the consent of subjects be obtained for access to records when this course is practicable and does not threaten the success of the research, may be disputed. In some cases the correctness of this approach is obvious. For example, in a survey of skin cancer prevalence, subjects were asked about their recent past history of skin cancer (Kricker *et al.* 1990). Those who gave a positive history were asked to consent to the investigators obtaining access to their medical records to confirm the diagnosis and to obtain histopathological detail. It was an appropriate courtesy to seek consent, even though access to records could have been obtained without it, and, as it happens, consent was given by all subjects. At the other extreme, for example in the case of subjects who are dead or whose current whereabouts is not known or could be discovered only with great difficulty, the futility of requiring that consent be obtained is equally obvious. The grey areas between these extremes are those most likely to cause trouble, and it is in these areas that investigators, record custodians, and ethics committees must work together to reach mutually acceptable decisions.

Confidentiality of personal data

The confidentiality of personally identifiable data obtained in the course of epidemiological research should be protected in such a way as to render its disclosure to the detriment of the subject an extremely remote possibility.

If confidential data are to be adequately protected, it is important that investigators think through the safeguards required and prepare a written code of practice for the protection of confidential data. Briefly, such a code might include the following provisions:

(a) All persons who have access to name-identified research data during the course of their work sign a declaration that they will respect the confidentiality of the data with which they work.

(b) As far as possible, the records containing research information (whether on paper or in computer storage media) and the corresponding personal identifiers are kept physically and logically separate and are linkable only by means of a common non-personal identifier (e.g. record number.)

(c) Records containing personal identifiers are kept under lock and key when not being worked on or, in the case of computer records, under an equivalent level of security.

(d) The personal identifiers are retained only as long as is necessary to achieve the objectives of the research.

(e) Disposal of identified records is carried out with strict attention to security.

(f) Research results are never published in a form that would permit the identification of any individual subject.

While the destruction of personal identifiers as soon as the objectives of the research have been achieved obviously protects confidentiality it may often lead to the loss of future opportunities for the efficient conduct of worthwhile research. Many epidemiological studies have as their starting point data obtained in an earlier study to which the original personal identifiers can still be linked. For example, Newman *et al.* (1986) reported on the relationship between body weight and dietary fat intake and survival after diagnosis of breast cancer by follow-up of patients with breast cancer interviewed 5–7 years earlier in a case-control study of aetiology. Such follow-up studies are frequently not envisaged when the original data are being collected, and would not be possible if the personal identifying data were to be destroyed when no longer needed for the original study. However, if identified records are to be retained beyond their period of immediate usefulness, their retention should be justified specifically in the protocol, the manner in which they are to be stored should be stated, and both should be approved (or otherwise) by the ethics committee.

It may not be possible in all jurisdictions for epidemiologists to guarantee that personal data in their care can be protected against disclosure in court, a circumstance highlighting a potential conflict between ethical and legal obligations. Recently, however, the US Court of Appeals protected women in a study of the toxic shock syndrome from the disclosure of their identities to another party to the court proceedings, the manufacturers of one of the allegedly offending tampons (Curran 1986). In some states of Australia there exist amendments to the Health Acts that provide protection against use in court of data about identifiable individuals collected in the course of an approved research project. This kind of protection for research data should be sought whenever possible.

Consent to approach subjects

An approach to subjects identified through non-public records should only be made with the consent of the record custodian or whomever else the custodian should nominate.

An approach to patients with a particular disease identified through medical records is probably the commonest circumstance in which epidemiological research involves an approach to subjects identified through non-public records. In this situation, consent to the approach should be obtained from the doctor responsible for the patient's care at the time the record was made, an appropriate successor to that doctor, or the medical superintendent or other appropriate authority in the hospital in which the record is held. This consent is necessary for a number of reasons:

(a) It is a matter of common courtesy.

(b) It is the doctor responsible for care of the patient who is most likely to know whether an approach to the patient will cause emotional distress or other harm.

(c) Pragmatically, if this consent is not obtained it is likely that future access to the records in which the subjects were identified will be denied.

Objections may be raised that doctors do not 'own' their patients and should not be allowed to deny patients their right to participate in worthwhile research. In practice, doctors rarely deny access to their patients. Moreover, a recent study of women involved in a study of the causes of breast, ovarian, and endometrial cancers showed that 50 per cent considered that requesting their doctor's permission for access had been a necessary step (Boring *et al.* 1984).

Communication of research results

If, in the course of epidemiological research, information is obtained about a subject that necessitates some courses of action in the subject's interests, that course should be taken after due consultation with the subject.

This recommendation is usually applied when a previously unsuspected disease or physiological or biochemical risk factor for disease is discovered during the course of, for example, a prevalence survey or the collection of data on risk factors for an aetiological study. The investigator has an obligation to inform the subject of the finding, to explain its significance to him or her, to recommend an appropriate course of action, and to make reasonable efforts to ensure that this course is followed, provided that the subject consents. A common approach, when a risk factor such as high blood pressure or hypercholesterolaemia is found, would be to refer the subject to his or her usual medical practitioner.

This type of communication concerning medically controllable factors may be regarded only as a minimum, and the question might also be raised whether epidemiologists have an ethical duty to advise subjects regarding known hazardous or behavioural exposures that may be ascertained during data collection. For example, should smokers who participate in epidemiological research be advised, as part of the research programme, to give up smoking? What responsibility does an epidemiologist have towards a person who drinks in excess of, say, 40 g of alcohol a day? In these situations the subject himself or herself may be seen as responsible for the exposure, and the risk associated with it is already known rather than uncovered by the study. The ethical questions that they raise have not been discussed to any substantial extent in epidemiology, although the duty to notify the subjects has been considered to exist in some cases. For example, in a recent survey of non-melanocytic skin cancer (Kricker *et al.* 1990), an attempt was made to do this by providing all subjects, regardless of their exposure, with an educational leaflet on exposure to the sun. The efficiency of this indiscriminate approach to providing information would need to be compared, in each specific instance, with a more selective approach that entails the added cost of identifying and targeting subjects with particular levels of the exposure.

Taking the obligation to inform one step further, it may be argued that members of an exposed population, be it an occupational group (Schulte 1985) or a town's population, have, not only as individuals but as members of the group, the right to be informed about hazardous exposures uncovered during a research project so that they are in a position to take whatever protective action they deem appropriate. This duty towards the community in which a study is conducted, as well as the duty towards study subjects, is being considered in the ethical guidelines for epidemiology currently under discussion (Last 1990; Steering Committee 1990).

Clearly there are problems in deciding whether to notify or not, the most important of which is the need to be confident that the risk is real and that notification does not lead to anxiety which is out of proportion to the size of the risk.

In a cohort study of miners and millers of crocidolite (blue asbestos), recent results of which have been described in Armstrong *et al.* (1988), subjects who had been traced and were known to be cigarette smokers were notified of their increase in absolute risk of lung cancer as a consequence of exposure to both crocidolite and tobacco smoke. They were offered advice about giving up smoking, and access to assistance with it. It was assumed that the risks associated with exposure to asbestos only were already well known to the subjects as a consequence of media publicity and were, in any case, now irremediable since exposure had ended some 8 years before the study began. It could be argued, however, that this assumption was unjustified.

Finally, to what extent does an obligation exist to inform when the study has disclosed a hazard to others rather than to the subject? This is a highly controversial issue which may give rise to dilemmas that are not soluble in any way without serious infringement of somebody's rights. This dilemma is exemplified by the person at high risk of human immunodeficiency virus infection who does not want to know whether he or she is seropositive for the virus and thus poses a potential serious hazard to his or her sexual partners. A simpler case, perhaps, is that of smokers who are informed of the risk to others from passive exposure to their tobacco smoke. In this case, protecting others by refraining from smoking in their presence can protect the subjects themselves from tobacco-related disease.

SUMMARY

The overriding ethical principle in the conduct of research on human subjects is that the rights of individual subjects should take precedence over the expected benefits to human knowledge or the community. This principle does not preclude research that may lead to actual harm to subjects, provided that the subjects accept voluntarily, and with complete information, the possibility of harm. In addition, it can be modified when it may reasonably be judged that the probability of harm from the research is no greater than individuals assume daily as a part of the normal activities of life.

The disclosure of confidential information about research subjects has the potential for harm. This is the main ethical risk that most epidemiological research carries and should be treated with the same seriousness as would any more direct threat of harm.

The epidemiologist's ethical duty to the subjects of research is in potential conflict with his or her wider duty to society to conduct research that is scientifically valid and has the potential to improve the health of the community. This conflict can be resolved by the investigator's accepting personal responsibility for ensuring ethical practice in epidemiological research and adopting appropriate policies for this practice. These policies should include:

- working only from written research protocols that specifically address ethical issues
- ensuring that all research protocols have been passed by an appropriate ethical review committee
- obtaining fully informed consent from subjects to their participation in research except where the research is judged to present minimal risk to the subject
- obtaining access to personal data sources without the subjects' consent only under carefully defined conditions
- making express and adequate provision for maintenance of the confidentiality of personally identifiable data
- obtaining the consent of the custodian of the records for an approach to subjects identified through non-public records
- ensuring that results obtained during the course of research that may have a bearing on the health or welfare of subjects are communicated to them.

It is important for investigators to appreciate that scientifically poor research may be considered to be unethical because it can justify no risk to human subjects and because it wastes resources. Failure to publish the results of research in a readily accessible form is unethical for similar reasons.

REFERENCES

Allen, P. A. and Waters, W. E. (1982). Development of an ethical committee and its effects on research design. *Lancet*, **i**, 1233–6.

Armstrong, B. K. (1984). Privacy and medical research. *Medical Journal of Australia*, **141**, 620–1.

Armstrong, B. K., deKlerk, N. H., Musk, A. W., and Hobbs, M. S. T. (1988). Mortality in miners and millers of crocidolite in Western Australia. *British Journal of Industrial Medicine*, **45**, 5–13.

Boring, C. C., Brockman, E., Causey, N., Gregory, H. R., and Greenberg, R. S. (1984). Patient attitudes toward physician consent in epidemiologic research. *American Journal of Public Health*, **74**, 1406–8.

Bower, R. T. and de Gasparis, P. (1978). *Ethics in social research: protecting the interests of human subjects*. Praeger Publishers, New York.

CIOMS (Council for International Organizations of Medical Sciences) (1982). *Proposed international guidelines for biomedical research involving human subjects.* Council for International Organizations of Medical Sciences, Geneva.

CPHPR (Committee for the Protection of Human Participants in Research) (1982). *Ethical principles in the conduct of research with human participants.* American Psychological Association, Washington.

Curran, W. J. (1978). The privacy protection report and epidemiological research. *American Journal of Public Health*, **68**, 173.

Curran, W. J. (1986). Protecting confidentiality in epidemiologic investigations by the Centers for Disease Control. *New England Journal of Medicine*, **314**, 1027–8.

Denham, M. J., Foster, A., and Tyrrell, D. A. J. (1979). Work of a district ethical committee. *British Medical Journal*, **2**, 1042–5.

Fluss, S., Simon, F., and Gutteridge, F. (1990). A survey of policies and laws, pp. 7–9. Presented at the Conference on Development of International Ethical Guidelines for Epidemiological Research and Practice held by the Council for International Organizations of Medical Sciences, Geneva, November 1990.

Funch, D. O. and Marshall, J. R. (1981). Patients' atttiudes following participation in a health outcome survey. *American Journal of Public Health*, **71**, 1396–8.

Gordis, L. and Gold, E. (1980). Privacy, confidentiality, and the use of medical records in research. *Science*, **207**, 153–6.

Gordis, L., Gold, E., and Seltser, R. (1977). Privacy protection in epidemiologic and medical research: a challenge and a responsibility. *American Journal of Epidemiology*, **105**, 163–8.

Hayes, S. and Hayes, R. (1983). Third-party consent to medical procedures. *Medical Journal of Australia*, **2**, 90–2.

Holman, C. D. J. and Armstrong, B. K. (1984). Pigmentary traits, ethnic origin, benign naevi and family history as risk factors for cutaneous malignant melanoma. *Journal of the National Cancer Institute*, **72**, 257–66.

Jamrozik, K. (1984). Ethical considerations in clinical research. *Papua New Guinea Medical Journal*, **27**, 4–6.

Kricker, A., English, D. R., Randell, P. L., Heenan, P. J., Clay, C. D., Delaney, T. A., and Armstrong B. K. (1990). Skin cancer in Geraldton, Western Australia: a survey of incidence and prevalence. *Medical Journal of Australia*, **152**, 399–407.

Last, J. M. (1990). Guidelines on ethics for epidemiologists. *International Journal of Epidemiology*, **19**, 226–9.

Margetts, B. M., Beilin, L. J., Armstrong, B. K., and Vandongen, R. (1985). A randomized controlled trial of a vegetarian diet in the treatment of hypertension. *Clinical Experiments in Pharmacology and Physiology*, **12**, 263–6.

May, W. W. (1975). The composition and function of ethical committees. *Journal of Medical Ethics*, **1**, 23–9.

MRC (Medical Research Council) (1985). Responsibility in the use of personal medical information for research: principles and guide to practice. *British Medical Journal*, **290**, 1120-4.

Newman, S. C., Miller, A. B. and Howe, G. R. (1986). A study of the effect of weight and dietary fat on breast cancer survival time. *American Journal of Epidemiology*, **123**, 767-74.

NHMRC (National Health and Medical Research Council) (1985). *Report on ethics in epidemiological research*. Australian Government Publishing Service, Canberra.

NHMRC (National Health and Medical Research Council) (1988). *NHMRC statement on human experimentation and supplementary notes*. National Health and Medical Research Council, Canberra.

NHMRC (National Health and Medical Research Council) (1990). *Guidelines for the protection of privacy in the conduct of medical research*. National Health and Medical Research Council, Canberra.

Reynolds, P. D. (1979). *Ethical dilemmas and social science research*. Jossey-Bass, San Francisco.

Rose, G. (1989). Ethics and Public Policy. In *Assessment of inhalation hazards*, (ed. V. Mohr), pp. 349-56. Springer-Verlag, Berlin.

Rubehausen, O. M., and Brimm, O. G. Jr (1966). Privacy and behavioral research. *American Psychologist*, **21**, 423-44.

Savitz, D. A., Hamman, R. F., Grace, C., and Stroo, K. (1986). Respondents' attitudes regarding participation in an epidemiologic study. *American Journal of Epidemiology*, **123**, 362-6.

Schulte, P. A. (1985). The epidemiologic basis for the notification of subjects of cohort studies. *American Journal of Epidemiology*, **121**, 351-61.

Silverman, W. (1986). *Human experimentation*, p. 165. Oxford University Press, New York.

Soskolne, C. L. (1989). Epidemiology: Questions of science, ethics, law and morality. *American Journal of Epidemiology*, **129**, 1-18.

Steering Committee (1990). Proposed guidelines for ethical review procedures for epidemiological research and practice. Presented at the Conference on Development of International Ethical Guidelines for Epidemiological Research and Practice, held by the Council for International Organizations of Medical Sciences, Geneva, 7-9 November 1990.

USDHHS (US Department of Health and Human Services) (1981). Final regulations amending basic HHS policy for the protection of human research subjects. *Federal Register*, **46**, 8366-91.

Index